Baillière's
CLINICAL
GASTROENTEROLOGY
INTERNATIONAL PRACTICE AND RESEARCH

Editorial Board

M. J. P. Arthur (Great Britain)
Ian A. D. Bouchier (Great Britain)
David C. Carter (Great Britain)
W. Creutzfeldt (Germany)
John Dent (Australia)
Michael Gracey (Australia)
G. N. J. Tytgat (The Netherlands)

Baillière's
CLINICAL
GASTROENTEROLOGY
INTERNATIONAL PRACTICE AND RESEARCH

Volume 6/Number 3
September 1992

Portal Hypertension

R. SHIELDS Kt, DL, MD, DSc, FRCS, FACS, FCS(SA)
Guest Editor

Baillière Tindall
London Philadelphia Sydney Tokyo Toronto

This book is printed on acid-free paper.

Baillière Tindall 24–28 Oval Road
W.B. Saunders   London NW1 7DX, UK

The Curtis Center, Independence Square West
Philadelphia, PA 19106–3399, USA

55 Horner Avenue
Toronto, Ontario M8Z 4X6, Canada

Harcourt Brace Jovanovich Group (Australia) Pty Ltd
30–52 Smidmore Street, Marrickville, NSW 2204, Australia

Harcourt Brace Jovanovich Japan, Inc.
Ichibancho Central Building, 22–1
Ichibancho, Chiyoda-ku, Tokyo 102, Japan

ISSN 0950–3528

ISBN 0–7020–1624–1 (single copy)

© 1992 Baillière Tindall. All rights reserved. Authorization to make copies of items in this issue for internal or personal use, or for the personal or internal use of specific clients in the USA, may be given by Baillière Tindall on the condition, within the USA, that the copier pay the base fee of $05.00 per copy through the Copyright Clearance Center Inc., 27 Congress Street, Salem, MA 01970, USA, for copying beyond that permitted by Sections 107 or 108 of the US Copyright Law. This consent does not extend to other kinds of copying, such as copying for general distribution, for advertising or promotional purposes, for creating new collective works, for resale or for copying or distributing copies outside the USA. 0950–3528/92. $05.00.

Baillière's Clinical Gastroenterology is published four times each year by Baillière Tindall. Prices for Volume 6 (1992) are:

TERRITORY	ANNUAL SUBSCRIPTION	SINGLE ISSUE
Europe including UK	£65.00 post free	£27.50 post free
All other countries	Consult your local Harcourt Brace Jovanovich Office	

The editor of this publication is Seán Duggan, Baillière Tindall, 24–28 Oval Road, London NW1 7DX, UK.

Baillière's Clinical Gastroenterology was published from 1972 to 1986 as *Clinics in Gastroenterology*.

Typeset by Phoenix Photosetting, Chatham.
Printed and bound in Great Britain by Mackays of Chatham PLC, Chatham, Kent.

Contributors to this issue

HASAN ANSARI MD, Biometric Center for Therapeutic Studies, Pettenkofestrasse 2, 8000 Munich 2, Germany.

JAIME BOSCH MD, Professor of Medicine, University of Barcelona, Chief of Section, Liver Unit, Hospital Clinic i Provincial, Villarroel 170, Barcelona 08036, Spain.

ANDREW K. BURROUGHS MB, ChB(Hons), FRCP, Hepato-biliary and Liver Transplantation Unit, University Department of Medicine, Royal Free Hospital and School of Medicine, Pond Street, Hampstead, London NW3 2QG, UK.

FAUST FEU CABALLE MD, Post-Doctoral Research Associate, Hepatic Hemodynamics Laboratory, Liver Unit, Hospital Clinic i Provincial, Villarroel 170, Barcelona 08036, Spain.

DAVID C. CARTER MD, FRCS, Regius Professor of Clinical Surgery, University Department of Surgery, Royal Infirmary, Edinburgh EH3 9YW, UK.

O. JAMES GARDEN BSc, MBChB, MD, FRCS, Senior Lecturer in Surgery, Honorary Consultant Surgeon, University Department of Surgery, Royal Infirmary, Edinburgh EH3 9YW, UK.

PAOLO GENTILINI MD, Professor, Professor of Internal Medicine, Chief of Department of Internal Medicine and Liver Unit—Istituto di Clinica Medica Generale e Terapia Medica II, Università degli Studi di Firenze, Viale Morgagni 85, 50134 Florence, Italy.

YASUO IDEZUKI MD, FACS, Professor and Surgeon in Chief, 2nd Department of Surgery, University of Tokyo, Faculty of Medicine, 7–3–1 Hongo, Bunkyo-ku, Tokyo, Japan.

SHUNZABURO IWATSUKI MD, Falk Clinic 5-C, 3601 Fifth Avenue, Pittsburgh, Pennsylvania 15213, USA.

GERHARD KLEBER MD, Medical Department II, Klinikum Crosshadern, University of Munich, Marchioninish 15, 8000 Munich 70, Germany.

GIACOMO LAFFI MD, Associate Professor of Medicine, Istituto di Clinica Medica Generale e Terapia Medica II, Università degli Studi di Firenze, Viale Morgagni 85, 50134 Florence, Italy.

DEEPAK LAHOTI MD, DM, Pool Officer, Department of Gastroenterology, G. B. Pant Hospital and Maulana Azad Medical College, New Delhi 110002, India.

MERCEDES FERNÁNDEZ LOBATO PhD, Research Fellow, Hepatic Hemodynamics Laboratory, Liver Unit, Hospital Clinic i Provincial, Villarroel 170, Barcelona 08036, Spain.

ISABEL CIRERA LORENZO MD, Research Fellow, Hepatic Hemodynamics Laboratory, Liver Unit, Hospital Clinic i Provincial, Villarroel 170, Barcelona 08036, Spain.

ANGELO LUCA MD, Research Fellow, Hepatic Hemodynamics Laboratory, Liver Unit, Hospital Clinic i Provincial, Villarroel 170, Barcelona 08036, Spain.

P. AIDEN McCORMICK MB, BCR, MRCP, Lecturer in Medicine and Honorary Senior Registrar, University Department of Medicine, Royal Free Hospital School of Medicine, Pond Street, Hampstead, London NW3 2QG, UK.

JUAN CARLOS GARCÍA-PAGAN MD, Post-Doctoral Research Associate, Hepatic Hemodynamics Laboratory, Liver Unit, Hospital Clinic i Provincial, Villarroel 170, Barcelona 08036, Spain.

M. PILAR PIZCUETA PhD, Senior Research Associate, Hepatic Hemodynamics Laboratory, Liver Unit, Hospital Clinic i Provincial, Villarroel 170, 08036 Barcelona, Spain.

ROBERTO SANTAMBROGIO MD, Assistente, Università degli Studi di Milano, 1st Scienze Biomediche, Cl. Chir. Vi, Ospedale S. Paolo via A. di Rudinì 8, 20142 Milan, Italy.

SHIV K. SARIN MD, DM, Associate Professor, Department of Gastroenterology, G. B. Pant Hospital and Maulana Azad Medical College, New Delhi 110002, India.

TILMAN SAUERBRUCH Professor of Internal Medicine, Medical Department II, Klinikum Crossadern, University of Munich, Marchioninish 15, 8000 Munich 70, Germany.

ROBERT SHIELDS Kt, DL, MD, DSc, FRCS, FACS, FCS(SA), Head of Department, Department of Surgery, University of Liverpool, PO Box 147, Liverpool L69 3BX, UK.

GIANPAOLO SPINA MD, Professor Associate, Università degli Studi di Milano, 1st Scienze Biomediche Semeiotica Chirurgica, Ospedale S. Paolo, via A. di Rudinì 8, 20142 Milan, Italy.

THOMAS E. STARZL MD, PhD, Department of Surgery, University of Pittsburgh School of Medicine, Pittsburgh, Pennsylvania, USA.

DAVID R. TRIGER MA, BM, BCh, DPhil, FRCP, Professor and Postgraduate Medical Dean, University of Sheffield Medical School, Beech Hill Road, Sheffield, S10 2RX, UK.

KARIN WEISSENBORN PD, MD, Neurologische Klinik mit Klinischer Neurophysiologie, Medizinische Hocheschule Hannover, Konstanty-Gutschowstrasse 8, 3000 Hannover 61, Germany.

DAVID WESTABY MA, FRCP, Consultant Physician and Gastroenterologist, Charing Cross Hospital, Fulham Palace Road, London W6 8RF, UK.

Table of contents

Foreword/R. SHIELDS — ix

1 Hepatic, splanchnic and systemic haemodynamic abnormalities in portal hypertension — 425
J. BOSCH, M. P. PIZCUETA, M. FERNÁNDEZ, F. FEU, I. CIRERA, A. LUCA & J. C. GARCÍA-PAGÁN

2 Natural history and prognosis of variceal bleeding — 437
A. K. BURROUGHS & P. A. McCORMICK

3 Balloon tamponade and vasoactive drugs in the control of acute variceal haemorrhage — 451
O. J. GARDEN & D. C. CARTER

4 Emergency and elective endoscopic therapy for variceal haemorrhage — 465
D. WESTABY

5 Portal hypertensive gastropathy — 481
D. R. TRIGER

6 The role of portosystemic shunting in the management of portal hypertension — 497
G. P. SPINA & R. SANTAMBROGIO

7 Liver transplantation in the management of bleeding and oesophageal varices — 517
S. IWATSUKI & T. E. STARZL

8 Management of gastric varices — 527
S. K. SARIN & D. LAHOTI

9 Transection and devascularization procedures for bleeding oesophagogastric varices — 549
Y. IDEZUKI

10 Prophylaxis of first variceal bleeding — 563
G. KLEBER, H. ANSARI & T. SAUERBRUCH

11 Pathophysiology and treatment of ascites and the hepatorenal syndrome — 581
P. GENTILINI & G. LAFFI

12 Recent developments in the pathophysiology and treatment of hepatic encephalopathy — 609
K. WEISSENBORN

Index — 631

PREVIOUS ISSUES

October 1989
Liver and Pancreas Transplantation
W. CREUTZFELDT & R. PICHLMAYR

March 1990
Molecular Biology and its Impact on Gastroenterology
P. J. CICLITIRA

June 1990
Gastroenterological Aspects of AIDS
B. G. GAZZARD

September 1990
Virus Infections of the Gut and Liver
M. J. G. FARTHING

December 1990
Cancer of the Pancreas
J. P. NEOPTOLEMOS

March 1991
Endoscopy Update
D. L. CARR-LOCKE

June 1991
Practical Issues in Gastrointestinal Motor Disorders
J. DENT

September 1991
Gastrointestinal Emergencies: Part I
R. WILLIAMSON & J. N. THOMPSON

March 1992
Anorectal Disorders
M. HENRY

FORTHCOMING ISSUE

August 1992
Gastrointestinal Radiology
A. ADAM & D. J. ALLISON

November 1992
Diagnosis and Management of Biliary Stones
M. SACKMAN

Foreword

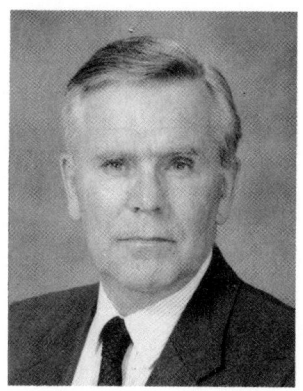

Portal hypertension represents one of the most challenging problems in modern gastroenterology. In the United Kingdom, almost half of the deaths due to gastrointestinal haemorrhage are caused by bleeding from gastro-oesophageal varices. The 6-week mortality of a first bleed from oesophageal varices is about 40%, of whom more than half die from the haemorrhage.

The reasons for this high mortality are not hard to find. Bleeding is often torrential and difficult to staunch. The patient may have been ravaged by the effect of the portal hypertension on other organs (for example the spleen) and the effect of the underlying disease (e.g. cirrhosis) on the functions of various organs, e.g. liver, brain, kidney. The assessment of the patient and the management of the clinical problem can therefore be exceedingly complex. Treatment involves both medical and surgical modalities. The large number of available treatments can make the choice of the most appropriate treatment for an individual patient difficult.

However, in the last few years, some relatively successful treatments have emerged, not only to control the acute variceal haemorrhage, but also to prevent recurrent bleeding subsequently. To treat the patient efficiently and effectively requires the mobilisation of the skills and expertise of medical and surgical teams.

The purpose of this monograph is to review current concepts of the pathophysiology of portal hypertension, the altered hepatic haemodynamics, and the complications of portal hypertension and bleeding oesophageal varices. Also reviewed are the contributions of the various treatment modalities to the successful management of the patient's condition. Their various roles are compared and contrasted to develop a management strategy for the care of these unfortunate patients.

R. SHIELDS

1

Hepatic, splanchnic and systemic haemodynamic abnormalities in portal hypertension

JAIME BOSCH
M. PILAR PIZCUETA
MERCEDES FERNÁNDEZ
FAUST FEU
ISABEL CIRERA
ANGELO LUCA
JOAN C. GARCÍA-PAGÁN

Portal hypertension is a clinical syndrome which is characterized by a pathological increase in portal venous pressure and by the formation of portosystemic collaterals that divert portal blood to the systemic circulation bypassing the liver (Bosch et al, 1989).

Although these two abnormalities are the circulatory hallmarks of the portal hypertension syndrome, many other haemodynamic disturbances are associated with portal hypertension. These include changes in the hepatic, splanchnic and systemic circulations, and are summarized in this chapter.

Not all patients with an increased portal venous pressure should be considered to have clinical portal hypertension. This is due to the fact that the complications of portal hypertension are only observed when the *portal pressure gradient* is increased above a threshold value of about 12 mmHg. This value therefore defines what is known as clinically significant portal hypertension (Bosch et al, 1989; Groszmann et al, 1990). The portal pressure gradient is the difference between portal pressure and the inferior vena cava pressure, and represents the hepatic perfusion pressure.

Haemodynamic factors influencing portal pressure

The portal pressure gradient is the result of the interrelationship of portal blood flow and the vascular resistance that opposes that flow. According to Ohm's law, this relationship is defined by the equation:

$$\Delta P = Q \times R \tag{1}$$

in which P is the portal pressure gradient, Q is blood flow within the entire portal venous system (including the portosystemic collaterals), and R is the vascular resistance of the portal venous system, which in turn represents the sum of the serial resistances of the portal vein and the hepatic vascular bed, and of the parallel resistance of the collaterals.

Therefore, an increased portal pressure gradient may be the result of increases in portal blood flow, of increases in vascular resistance, or of a combination of both.

For many years it was thought that portal hypertension was due to an increased resistance to portal blood flow, caused by a prehepatic, intrahepatic or posthepatic 'block' (backward theory of portal hypertension)

Table 1. Aetiology of portal hypertension.

Prehepatic:
    Portal vein thrombosis
    Splenic vein thrombosis
    External compression of portal vein

Intrahepatic
    Partial nodular transformation
    Nodular regenerative hyperplasia
    Congenital hepatic fibrosis
    Peliosis hepatis
    Polycystic disease
    Idiopathic portal hypertension
    Hypervitaminosis A
    Arsenic, copper sulphate and vinyl chloride monomer poisoning
    Schistosomiasis
    Sarcoidosis
    Tuberculosis
    Leprosy
    Primary biliary cirrhosis
    Sclerosing cholangitis
    Amyloidosis
    Mastocytosis
    Rendu–Osler disease
    Haematologic liver disease
    Acute fatty liver of pregnancy
    Fulminant and subfulminant acute viral hepatitis
    Chronic active hepatitis (autoimmune, viral)
    Hepatocellular carcinoma
    Cirrhosis (posthepatitic, haemochromatosis, Wilson's disease, cryptogenic)
    Alcoholic cirrhosis
    Alcoholic hepatitis
    Veno-occlusive disease

Posthepatic
    Budd–Chiari syndrome
    Congenital malformations and thrombosis of the inferior vena cava
    Constrictive pericarditis
    Tricuspid valve diseases

Miscellaneous
    Arteriovenous fistulae (splenic, aortomesenteric, aortoportal and hepatic artery–portal vein)

(Benoit et al, 1985; Bruix, 1990). This theory was supported by the finding that portal blood flow was frequently reduced in patients with cirrhosis.

This concept was challenged by studies using the radioactive microsphere technique in rats with portal hypertension due to partial portal vein ligation (PPVL) (Chojkier and Groszmann, 1981; Vorobioff et al, 1983). This technique allows the measurement of the portal venous inflow, which equals the sum of the portal blood flow and the collateral blood flow. These studies demonstrated that the portal venous inflow is markedly increased in portal hypertension, although most of it circulates through the collaterals (Vorobioff et al, 1983). These observations led to an opposite (forward flow) theory (Benoit et al, 1985; Bruix, 1990), which proposed that an increased portal venous inflow would play a key role in the pathophysiology of portal hypertension (Vorobioff et al, 1983). Subsequent studies in other models of portal hypertension (carbon tetrachloride-induced cirrhosis, chronic bile duct ligation and division) confirmed the presence of an increased portal venous inflow (Vorobioff et al, 1984; Pizcueta et al, 1989), which gave further support for this theory.

It is obvious, however, that in some cases, such as after PPVL, the factor that initiates portal hypertension is an increased resistance to portal blood flow. The relative role of an increased resistance and blood flow in the pathogenesis of portal hypertension has been clarified by studies showing that in the early phase following PPVL, portal resistance is markedly increased, while portal venous inflow is normal or low (Sikuler et al, 1985; Bruix, 1990), that removal of the ligature around the portal vein immediately normalized portal pressure in PPVL rats, although the portal inflow was still elevated (Sikuler and Groszmann, 1986), and that portocaval shunt rapidly brings portal pressure back to normal, despite further increasing the portal inflow (Kravetz et al, 1987a).

Thus, an increase in portal resistance does result in portal hypertension, but an increased portal venous inflow is not enough to cause portal hypertension. Increased portal blood inflow is an added factor contributing to the maintenance and, probably, the worsening of portal hypertension (Bosch et al, 1989).

CHANGES IN THE HEPATIC HAEMODYNAMICS AND THE PATHOPHYSIOLOGY OF PORTAL HYPERTENSION

Increased vascular resistance

Increased resistance to portal blood flow (at any site within the portal venous system) will result in portal hypertension. The more common causes of portal hypertension are diseases increasing the vascular resistance of the liver circulation (cirrhosis and other liver diseases) or within the portal vein (thrombosis, extrinsic compression) (Table 1).

In normal conditions, the principal site of resistance to portal blood flow is the hepatic microcirculation. However, this large vascular bed has a very low resistance, as indicated by the low perfusion pressure (<5 mmHg) required to maintain a normal portal blood flow. In addition, the liver circulation can accommodate large changes in portal blood flow with only minor changes in portal pressure (Bruix, 1990).

Factors influencing vascular resistance are interrelated by Poiseuille's law in the equation:

$$R = 8\mu L/\pi r^4 \tag{2}$$

in which μ is the coefficient of viscosity of the blood, L is the length of the vessel and r its radius. It is clear that the main factor influencing vascular resistance is the radius of the vessel(s). This can be influenced by passive changes (for example, dilatation in response to an increased pressure and blood flow, contraction in response to reduced blood volume) or actively, by factors acting on the vascular smooth muscle (neurogenic stimuli, humoral factors and pharmacological agents) (Bathal and Grossmann, 1985). Active changes in vascular resistance may occur at the liver microcirculation and at the prehepatic portocollateral system (Cummings et al, 1986; Valla et al, 1987; Navasa et al, 1989). The length of the vessels is another factor that may contribute significantly to the collateral resistance, since some collaterals are long and tortuous. Finally, blood viscosity changes (due to changes in haematocrit and plasma protein concentration) may also influence resistance.

Hepatic vascular resistance in cirrhosis

Increased hepatic vascular resistance in cirrhosis is thought to be located mainly at the hepatic sinusoids. This is supported by a number of pathological and micropuncture studies (Shibayama and Nakata, 1985). Presinusoidal and hepatic vein obstruction have also been suggested.

Increased hepatic vascular resistance of cirrhosis was thought to be a constant, mechanical consequence of the distortion of the liver vascular architecture caused by fibrosis, scarring and nodule formation (Bosch et al, 1989). However, there is increasing evidence that the hepatic vascular resistance is not constant in cirrhosis, but that there is an active component that can be modified by several stimuli (Bathal and Grossmann, 1985; Bosch, 1985). This may be related to the active contraction–relaxation of the myofibroblasts that are known to be present in the fibrous septa surrounding nodules and terminal venules (Bathal and Grossmann, 1985). Sustained contraction of these elements, as a result of neurogenic or humoral stimulation, may contribute to the increase of hepatic resistance to portal flow in cirrhosis. This has been suggested by studies in isolated perfused rat liver preparations (IPRLP) from cirrhotic animals (Bathal and Grossmann, 1985). The in vivo response of the hepatic resistance of cirrhotic animals or man to vasodilators is probably less pronounced (Navasa et al, 1988; García-Pagán et al, 1990). Nevertheless, these observations have offered new insights into the pathogenesis and pharmacological therapy of portal hypertension (Bosch, 1985).

CHANGES IN THE SPLANCHNIC HAEMODYNAMICS

Development of portosystemic collaterals

Increased portal pressure leads to the formation of portosystemic collaterals (Sikuler et al, 1985; Bruix, 1990). These develop by the opening, dilatation and hyperplasia of pre-existing vascular channels. Increased blood flow and active angiogenesis may also be involved in collateral formation.

Collateral formation is also a function of time. This is well illustrated by longitudinal studies in PPVL and chronic bile duct ligation (CBDL) rats (Bosch et al, 1983; Sikuler et al, 1985; García-Pagán et al, 1991a).

Maintenance of a patent collateral circulation requires that the vascular resistance in the collaterals be lower than in the obstructed portohepatic bed. The collaterals are able to respond to vasoactive stimuli, either endogenous or pharmacological. These vessels are probably hypersensitive to serotonin (Cummings et al, 1986), which markedly increases their vascular resistance, while this can be decreased by β-adrenergic stimulation (Mastai et al, 1987; Valla et al, 1987). Therefore, active changes of the collateral resistance may influence portal pressure. In addition, there is a possibility of influencing the formation and closure of the collaterals by means of pharmacological agents (Bosch et al, 1984b; Bosch, 1985; Kroeger and Groszmann, 1985; Cummings et al, 1986, 1988).

Splanchnic vasodilatation and increased portal venous inflow

As already mentioned, an increased portal venous inflow is characteristically observed in advanced stages of portal hypertension (Vorobioff et al, 1983, 1984). This plays a contributory role in maintaining and aggravating the portal hypertensive syndrome. Most attempts at the pharmacological treatment of portal hypertension have been aimed at correcting this factor (Bosch, 1985).

Increased portal venous inflow is the result of a marked arteriolar vasodilatation in splanchnic organs draining into the portal vein (Vorobioff et al, 1983; Pizcueta et al, 1989). The different mechanisms suggested as an explanation of the splanchnic vasodilatation associated with portal hypertension are summarized below.

Role of glucagon and other humoral factors

Cross-circulation studies between portal hypertensive and normal animals have demonstrated the development of splanchnic vasodilatation in the recipient, indicating that transferable humoral factors are implicated in the pathogenesis of the splanchnic hyperaemia (Benoit et al, 1984). Vasodilators of splanchnic origin, which undergo hepatic metabolism in normal conditions, may accumulate in the systemic circulation because of reduced hepatic uptake due to liver disease and/or portosystemic shunting (Benoit et al, 1984; Bosch et al, 1984a; Benoit and Granger, 1986). These include neuropeptides, prostacyclin, adenosine, bile acids, ammonia, endotoxin, and a variety of vasodilatory gastrointestinal hormones. However, available evidence is scarce for most of them. Studies inhibiting prostaglandin synthesis have shown a mild reduction in splanchnic blood flow in patients with cirrhosis (Bruix et al, 1985) and in portal hypertensive rats (Piqué et al, 1988), but this was not found in other studies (Blanchart et al, 1985). Other substances, including neuropeptides, secretin, cholecystokinin, pancreatic polypeptide and oestrogens, may induce splanchnic vasodilatation in pharmacological doses, but not in the range observed under physiological conditions (Benoit and Granger, 1986).

Probably, glucagon is the humoral vasodilator for which there is more evidence for a significant role promoting splanchnic hyperaemia in portal hypertension (Benoit et al, 1986; Kravetz et al, 1988; Pizcueta et al, 1990). A powerful splanchnic dilator, glucagon is markedly increased in cirrhosis and in experimental portal hypertensive models (Benoit et al, 1986; Kravetz et al, 1988; Silva et al, 1990). Studies increasing the circulating glucagon of normal rats to levels similar to those observed in portal hypertension have shown a significant increase in splanchnic blood flow. Conversely, in PPVL rats, the normalization of circulating glucagon by means of glucagon antibodies or by a somatostatin infusion partially reverses the increased splanchnic blood flow (Benoit et al, 1986; Kravetz et al, 1988). This response can be specifically blocked by preventing the fall in circulating glucagon by a concomitant glucagon infusion (Pizcueta et al, 1992). Hyperglucagonism has also been implicated in the splanchnic vasodilatation following surgical portocaval shunts (Kravetz et al, 1987a). It has been suggested that hyperglucagonism may account for approximately 30–40% of the splanchnic vasodilatation of chronic portal hypertension (Benoit et al, 1986). Glucagon may promote vasodilatation by two mechanisms: relaxing the vascular smooth muscle, and decreasing the sensitivity to endogenous vasoconstrictors, such as noradrenaline, angiotensin II and vasopressin (Richardson and Withrington, 1976; Pizcueta et al, 1990).

Role of endothelial-derived relaxing factor (EDRF)

The endogenous vasodilator nitric oxide, which has been identified as the EDRF, has also been suggested to contribute to the splanchnic vasodilatation associated with portal hypertension (Vallance and Moncada, 1991; Pizcueta et al, 1992). Studies using specific ERDF inhibitors have shown that this factor is implicated in the regulation of splanchnic and systemic haemodynamics in normal and portal hypertensive animals. Recent studies from our laboratory indicate that portal hypertensive rats are very sensitive to EDRF inhibition, which causes a normalization of splanchnic resistance and blood flow (Pizcueta et al, 1992). Thus, it is possible that an inadequate production of this powerful endogenous dilator contributes to the pathogenesis of the splanchnic vasodilatation observed in portal hypertension.

CHANGES IN THE SYSTEMIC HAEMODYNAMICS

Peripheral vasodilatation

Splanchnic vasodilatation in portal hypertension is characteristically associated with peripheral vasodilatation, with reduced arterial pressure and peripheral resistance (Bosch et al, 1980). It is likely that the pathogenesis of this circulatory abnormality shares common mechanisms with that of the splanchnic vasodilatation discussed above. Nitric oxide inhibitors rapidly correct arterial hypotension and reduced systemic resistance (Pizcueta et al, 1992). However, there is evidence indicating a different response of the splanchnic circulation compared to other peripherals beds. Specifically, some studies have indicated that hindquarter preparations of normal animals, that vasodilate when cross-perfused with hindquarters of portal hypertensive rats, are not vasodilated by glucagon (Korthuis et al, 1985).

Peripheral vasodilatation is thought to play a major role in the activation of neurohumoral systems leading to sodium retention, expansion of plasma volume and, finally, to the accumulation of ascites in patients with cirrhosis (Schrier et al, 1988). Vasodilatation and arterial hypotension would be even more severe if the sympathetic nervous system, the renin–angiotensin system, and plasma antidiuretic hormone (ADH) were not increased (Schrier et al, 1988). However, the response to endogenous vasoconstrictors is attenuated, so that the systemic effects of the activated neurohumoral systems are minimized (Kiel et al, 1985; Pizcueta et al, 1990). Nevertheless, studies in patients with cirrhosis and ascites have shown that, despite a low arterial pressure and systemic vascular resistance, there are vascular territories showing marked vasoconstriction, such as the femoral artery, the cubital artery and the kidneys (Fernández-Seara et al, 1989). Probably, most of the reduced peripheral resistance observed in these patients could be accounted for by the splanchnic vasodilatation. It has been suggested that if the splanchnic vasodilatation could be reversed, renal perfusion may be improved in patients with cirrhosis, ascites and hepatorenal syndrome (Bosch, 1990).

Expanded plasma volume and hyperkinetic circulation

Increased plasma volume is a ubiquitous finding in portal hypertension (Bosch et al, 1980; Kravetz et al, 1987b). It is thought that expansion of the plasma volume is due to transient renal sodium retention, which in turn is triggered by peripheral vasodilatation. The expanded plasma volume will thus represent a response directed to 'refill' the dilated arterial vascular tree (Schrier et al, 1988). Sequential studies have shown that this is a very early response: hypotension, sodium retention and expansion of the plasma volume occur prior to the increase in cardiac output which is observed in advanced portal hypertension (Albillos et al, 1990). It is likely that an expanded plasma volume plays a permissive role in the increase of the cardiac index.

In many experimental models and clinical situations, the expanded blood volume and hyperkinetic circulation allow a haemodynamic stabilization and no further sodium retention occurs (Bosch et al, 1980). However, when the disturbances are more pronounced and accompanied by increased transcapillary albumin escape, it is not possible to achieve haemodynamic compensation, and sodium retention continues, leading to the formation of ascites and oedema.

Expansion of the plasma volume has therefore a greater importance than it has traditionally been considered to have in the pathogenesis of circulatory disturbances in portal hypertension. This importance goes beyond changes in the systemic circulation. Studies in PPVL rats subjected to sodium restriction, and in patients with cirrhosis during the administration of spironolactone, show that this causes a significant decrease in plasma volume and cardiac index, as well as a reduction in portal pressure (Okumura et al, 1991; García-Pagán et al, 1991b).

These studies suggest that reduction of plasma volume with low sodium diet and spironolactone represents another possible treatment of portal hypertension, either alone or in combination with other drugs acting through different mechanisms. It has been shown that the administration of propranolol accentuates the fall in portal pressure caused by spironolactone (García-Pagán et al, 1991b). Also, administration of diuretics may be an important adjunct to therapy with nitrovasodilators, because a reduced blood volume may help to maintain and enhance the effects of these agents (Dupuis et al, 1990).

CHANGES IN THE GASTRIC AND PULMONARY CIRCULATION

Gastric microcirculatory changes

Portal hypertensive ('congestive') gastropathy is a recently recognized complication of portal hypertension which is characterized by diffuse gastric mucosal vascular ectasia (Quintero et al, 1987). At endoscopy, the lesions appear as multiple, small, cherry-red spots (severe gastropathy). In earlier stages the appearance is that of a 'mosaic' pattern or diffuse ('scarlatine') redness (Papazian et al, 1986). These lesions may also appear in the colon. Clinically, the disease may cause episodes of overt gastrointestinal haemorrhage (often only manifested by melaena and usually less severe than variceal bleeds) or manifest as chronic occult blood loss and microcytic anaemia requiring repeated blood transfusion and iron therapy (Quintero et al, 1987; D'Amico et al, 1990). Portal hypertensive gastropathy is the main cause of gastric bleeding in patients with cirrhosis.

Experimental and clinical studies have shown that gastric mucosal blood flow is markedly increased (Piqué et al, 1988; Pizcueta et al, 1989). The increased blood flow, combined with the increased outflow pressure caused by portal hypertension, may promote the dilatation of mucosal capillaries characteristic of this entity. The hyperaemia is partially corrected by propranolol administration (Piqué et al, 1990), which provides the rationale for the use of propranolol in treating patients with severe forms of the syndrome. Indeed, a recent randomized controlled study showed that propranolol therapy significantly reduced the incidence of recurrent bleeding and the transfusion requirements in patients who had bled from portal hypertensive gastropathy (Pérez-Ayuso et al, 1991).

The hepatopulmonary syndrome

It has been known for years that patients with advanced cirrhosis may have severe arterial hypoxaemia in the absence of intrinsic lung disease. Recent studies using the multiple inert gas dilution technique have shown that the hypoxaemia is not due to the presence of intrapulmonary shunts, but to marked ventilation–perfusion mismatching (Rodriguez-Roisin et al, 1987). This is caused by pulmonary vasodilatation, which is associated with an impaired hypoxic vasoconstriction of the pulmonary circulation. The syndrome is clearly functional, since there are no structural changes and the abnormalities have been shown to disappear following orthotopic liver transplantation (Agustí et al, 1990).

SUMMARY

Portal hypertension is characterized by a pathological increase in portal venous pressure that leads to the formation of portosystemic collaterals that divert portal blood to the systemic circulation, bypassing the liver.

Increased vascular resistance to portal blood flow is the initiating factor in portal hypertension. Increased resistance along the hepatic and porto-collateral circulation is in part modifiable by pharmacological agents. An additional factor is splanchnic vasodilatation with increased portal blood inflow, which contributes to the maintenance and aggravation of the portal hypertension.

Endogenous vasodilators are thought to be responsible for the splanchnic hyperaemia of portal hypertension. Vasodilatation is also prominent in the stomach and lungs, and plays an important role in the pathophysiology of portal hypertensive gastropathy and of the hepatopulmonary syndrome.

The systemic circulation is markedly hyperkinetic, with reduced arterial pressure and peripheral resistance and increased cardiac output. The plasma volume is expanded due to renal sodium retention. The expanded plasma volume enables the increase in cardiac output, and represents another mechanism contributing to the increase in portal pressure.

Acknowledgements

We are most grateful to Ms M. Angels Baringo for her expert technical assistance and to Ms Encarna Gutierrez and Mónica Masllorens for her secretarial help.

These studies have been supported by grants from the Fondo de Investigaciones Sanitarias (FIS 91/0374) and Ministerio de Educación y Ciencia.

REFERENCES

Albillos A, Colombato LA & Groszmann RJ (1990) Expansion of the sodium space in pre-hepatic portal hypertension: further support for the peripheral vasodilation hypothesis of sodium retention. *Hepatology* **12:** 854 (abstract).

Agustí AGN, Roca J, Bosch J & Rodriguez-Roisin R (1990) The lung in patients with cirrhosis. *Journal of Hepatology* **10:** 251–257.

Bathal PS & Grossmann HJ (1985) Reduction of the increased portal vascular resistance of the isolated perfused cirrhotic rat liver by vasodilators. *Journal of Hepatology* **1:** 325–337.

Benoit JN & Granger DN (1986) Splanchnic hemodynamics in chronic portal venous hypertension. *Seminars in Liver Disease* **6:** 287–298.

Benoit JN, Barrowman JA, Harper SL et al (1984) Role of humoral factors in the intestinal hyperemia associated with chronic portal hypertension. *American Journal of Physiology* **247:** G486–G493.

Benoit JN, Womack WA, Hernández L et al (1985) 'Forward' and 'backward' flow mechanisms of portal hypertension. Relative contributions in the rat model of portal vein stenosis. *Gastroenterology* **89:** 1092–1096.

Benoit JN, Zimmerman B, Premen AJ et al (1986) Role of glucagon in splanchnic hyperemia of chronic portal hypertension. *American Journal of Physiology* **251:** G674–G677.

Blanchart A, Hernando N, Fernández-Muñoz D et al (1985) Lack of effect of indomethacin on systemic and splanchnic hemodynamics in portal hypertensive rats. *Clinical Science* **68:** 605–607.

Bosch J (1985) Effect of pharmacological agents on portal hypertension: a hemodynamic appraisal. *Clinics in Gastroenterology* **14:** 169–183.

Bosch J (1990) Splanchnic vasodilation and renal vasoconstriction: a key to the hepatorenal syndrome? *Hepatology* **12:** 1445–1448.

Bosch J, Arroyo V, Betriu A et al (1980) Hepatic hemodynamics and the renin–angiotensin–aldosterone system in cirrhosis. *Gastroenterology* **78:** 92–99.

Bosch J, Enriquez R, Groszmann RJ et al (1983) Chronic bile duct ligation in the dog: hemodynamic characterization of a portal hypertensive model. *Hepatology* **3:** 1002–1007.

Bosch J, Gomis R, Kravetz D et al (1984a) Role of spontaneous portal-systemic shunting in hyperinsulinism of cirrhosis. *American Journal of Physiology* **247:** G206–G212.

Bosch J, Mastai R, Kravetz D et al (1984b) Effects of propranolol on azygos blood flow and on hepatic and systemic hemodynamics in cirrhosis. *Hepatology* **4:** 1200–1205.

Bosch J, Navasa M, García-Pagán JC et al (1989) Portal hypertension. *Medical Clinics of North America* **73:** 931–953.

Bruix J (1990) *Fisiopatología de la hipertensión portal. Estudio hemodinámico en ratas con hipertensión portal por ligadura parcial de la vena porta y en ratas con cirrosis hepática.* MD thesis, University of Barcelona.

Bruix J, Bosch J, Kravetz D et al (1985) Effects of prostaglandin inhibition on systemic and hepatic hemodynamics in patients with cirrhosis of the liver. *Gastroenterology* **88:** 430–435.

Chojkier M & Groszmann RJ (1981) Measurement of portal-systemic shunting in the rat by using labelled microspheres. *American Journal of Physiology* **240:** G371–G375.

Cummings SA, Groszmann RJ & Kaumann AJ (1986) Hypersensitivity of mesenteric veins to 5-hydroxytryptamine and ketanserin-induced reduction of portal pressure in portal hypertensive rats. *British Journal of Pharmacology* **89:** 501–513.

Cummings SA, Kaumann AJ & Groszmann RJ (1988) Comparison of the hemodynamic responses to ketanserin and prazosin in portal hypertensive rats. *Hepatology* **8:** 1112–1115.

D'Amico G, Montalbano L, Traina M et al (1990) Natural history of congestive gastropathy in cirrhosis. *Gastroenterology* **99:** 1558–1564.

Dupuis J, Lalonde G, Lemieux FR et al (1990) Tolerance to intravenous nitroglycerin in patients with congestive heart failure: role of increased intravascular volume, neurohumoral activation and lack of prevention with N-acetylcysteine. *Journal of the American College of Cardiologists* **16:** 923–931.

Fernández-Seara J, Prieto J, Quiroga J et al (1989) Systemic and regional hemodynamics in patients with liver cirrhosis and ascites with and without functional renal failure. *Gastroenterology* **97:** 1304–1312.

García-Pagán JC, Feu F, Ruiz del Arbol L et al (1990) Long-term haemodynamic effects of isosorbide-5-mononitrate in patients with cirrhosis and portal hypertension. *Journal of Hepatology* **11**: 189–195.

García-Pagán JC, Fernández M, Pizcueta P et al (1991a) Portal-systemic shunting influences haemodynamic abnormalities in bile duct ligated rats. *Journal of Hepatology* **13 (supplement 2)**: S30.

García-Pagán JV, Salmerón JM, Feu F et al (1991b) Spironolactone decreases portal pressure in patients with compensated cirrhosis. *Journal of Hepatology* **13 (supplement 2)**: S30.

Groszmann RJ, Bosch J, Grace ND et al (1990) Hemodynamic events in a prospective randomized trial of propranolol versus placebo in the prevention of a first variceal hemorrhage. *Gastroenterology* **99**: 1401–1407.

Kiel JW, Pitts V, Benoit J et al (1985) Reduced vascular sensitivity to norepinephrine in portal hypertensive rats. *American Journal of Physiology* **248**: G192–G195.

Korthuis RJ, Benoit JN, Kvietys PR et al (1985) Humoral factors may mediate increased rat hindquarter blood flow in portal hypertension. *American Journal of Physiology* **249**: H827–H833.

Kravetz D, Arderiu M, Bosch J et al (1987a) Hyperglucagonemia and hyperkinetic circulation after portocaval shunt in the rat. *American Journal of Physiology* **252**: G257–G261.

Kravetz D, Arderiu MT, Bosch J et al (1987b) Increased plasma volume in two models of portal hypertension in the rat: cirrhosis of the liver and partial portal vein ligation. *Revista Espanola de Fisiologia* **43**: 181–186.

Kravetz D, Bosch J, Arderiu MT et al (1988) Effects of somatostatin on splanchnic hemodynamics and plasma glucagon in portal hypertensive rats. *American Journal of Physiology* **254**: G322–G328.

Kroeger RJ & Groszmann RJ (1985) Increased portal venous resistance hinders portal pressure reduction during the administration of beta-adrenergic blocking agents in a portal hypertensive model. *Hepatology* **5**: 97–101.

Mastai R, Bosch J, Navasa M et al (1987) Effects of alpha-adrenergic stimulation and beta-adrenergic blockade on azygos blood flow and splanchnic haemodynamics in patients with cirrhosis. *Journal of Hepatology* **4**: 71–79.

Navasa M, Bosch J, Reichen J et al (1988) Effects of verapamil on hepatic and systemic hemodynamics and liver function in patients with cirrhosis and portal hypertension. *Hepatology* **8**: 850–854.

Navasa M, Chesta J, Bosch J & Rodés J (1989) Reduction of portal pressure by isosorbide 5-mononitrate in patients with cirrhosis. Effects on splanchnic and systemic hemodynamics and liver function. *Gastroenterology* **96**: 1110–1118.

Okumura H, Aramaki T, Katsuta Y et al (1991) Reduction in hepatic venous pressure gradient as a consequence of volume contraction due to chronic administration of spironolactone in patients with cirrhosis and no ascites. *American Journal of Gastroenterology* **86**: 47–52.

Papazian A, Braillon A, Dupas JL et al (1986) Portal hypertensive gastric mucosa: an endoscopic study. *Gut* **27**: 1199–1203.

Pérez-Ayuso RM, Piqué JM, Bosch J et al (1991) Propranolol in prevention of recurrent bleeding from severe portal hypertensive gastropathy in cirrhosis. *Lancet* **337**: 1431–1434.

Piqué JM, Leung FV, Kitahora T et al (1988) Gastric mucosal blood flow and acid secretion in portal hypertensive rats. *Gastroenterology* **95**: 727–733.

Piqué JM, Pizcueta MP, Pérez RM & Bosch J (1990) Effects of propranolol on gastric mucosal blood flow and acid secretion in portal hypertensive rats. *Hepatology* **12**: 476–480.

Pizcueta MP, De Lacy AM, Kravetz D et al (1989) Propranolol decreases portal pressure without changing portocollateral resistance in cirrhotic rats. *Hepatology* **10**: 953–957.

Pizcueta MP, Casamitjana R, Bosch J et al (1990) Decreased systemic vascular sensitivity to norepinephrine in portal hypertensive rats. Role of hyperglucagonism. *American Journal of Physiology* **258**: G191–G195.

Pizcueta MP, Piqué JM, Bosch J et al (1992) Effects of inhibiting nitric oxide biosynthesis on the systematic and splanchnic circulation of rats with portal hypertension. *British Journal of Pharmacology* (in press).

Pizcueta MP, García-Pagán JC, Fernández M et al (1991) Glucagon hinders the effects of somatostatin on portal hypertension: a study in rats with partial portal vein ligation. *Gastroenterology* **101**: 1710–1715.

Quintero E, Piqué JM, Bombi JA et al (1987) Gastric mucosal ectasia causing bleeding in cirrhosis. A distinct entity associated with hypergastrinemia and low serum levels of pepsinogen I. *Gastroenterology* **93:** 1054–1061.

Richardson PDI & Withrington PG (1976) The inhibition by glucagon of the vasoconstrictor actions of noradrenaline, angiotensin and vasopressin on the hepatic arterial vascular bed of the dog. *British Journal of Pharmacology* **57:** 93–102.

Rodriguez-Roisin R, Roca J, Agustí AGN et al (1987) Gas exchange and pulmonary vascular reactivity in patients with liver cirrhosis. *American Review of Respiratory Disease* **135:** 1085–1092.

Schrier RW, Arroyo V, Bernardi M et al (1988) Peripheral arterial vasodilation hypothesis: a proposal for the initiation of renal sodium and water retention in cirrhosis. *Hepatology* **8:** 1151–1157.

Shibayama Y & Nakata K (1985) Localization of increased hepatic vascular resistance in liver cirrhosis. *Hepatology* **5:** 643.

Sikuler E & Groszmann RJ (1986) Interaction of flow and resistance in maintenance of portal hypertension in a rat model. *American Journal of Physiology* **250:** G205–G212.

Sikuler E, Kravetz D & Groszmann RJ (1985) Evolution of portal hypertension and mechanisms involved in its maintenance in a rat model. *American Journal of Physiology* **248:** G618–G625.

Silva G, Navasa M, Bosch J et al (1990) Hemodynamic effects of glucagon in portal hypertension. *Hepatology* **11:** 668–673.

Valla D, Gaudin C, Geoffroy P et al (1987) Reversal of adrenaline-induced increase in azygos blood flow in patients with cirrhosis receiving propranolol. *Journal of Hepatology* **4:** 86–92.

Vallance P & Moncada S (1991) Hyperdynamic circulation in cirrhosis: a role for nitric oxide? *Lancet* **337:** 776–779.

Vorobioff J, Bredfeldt J & Groszmann RJ (1983) Hyperdynamic circulation in a portal hypertensive rat model: a primary factor for maintenance of chronic portal hypertension. *American Journal of Physiology* **244:** G52–G57.

Vorobioff J, Bredfeldt JE, Groszmann RJ (1984) Increased blood flow through the portal system in cirrhotic rats. *Gastroenterology* **87:** 1120–1126.

2

Natural history and prognosis of variceal bleeding

ANDREW K. BURROUGHS
P. AIDEN McCORMICK

Bleeding from oesophageal or gastric varices is a major complication of portal hypertension. Historically many of the first randomized clinical trials in the field of liver disease were concerned with the prevention of bleeding. In recent years there has been greater evaluation and understanding of the natural history of varices which has prompted studies of new prophylactic therapies against bleeding.

Information on the natural history of oesophageal varices comes from follow-up studies of patients with oesophageal varices, which include large numbers of patients in the control groups of the prophylactic and therapeutic trials for variceal bleeding. A number of important points emerge from these studies:

1. Oesophageal varices and congestive gastropathy develop in the majority (90%) of patients with alcoholic cirrhosis provided follow-up is long enough. It is likely that this is also true for other aetiologies of cirrhosis, but few data are available.
2. In most patients, oesophageal varices enlarge over time, although regression of varices in a minority of patients has also been observed.
3. The risk of a first variceal bleed is highest in the first 2 years after the identification of oesophageal varices. It is not clear if this is related to selection procedures for patients entering clinical studies or the natural evolution of varices and portal hypertension.
4. Mortality due to the first variceal bleed is very high (25–50%), and is dependent on the severity of liver disease.
5. Patients who have already had a variceal bleed have a high risk of recurrent bleeding—70% or more.

NATURAL HISTORY OF PORTAL HYPERTENSION IN CIRRHOTIC PATIENTS

Development of varices

Oesophageal varices develop and enlarge over time in patients with cirrhosis. Christensen et al (1981) studied the natural history of gastrointestinal bleeding in 532 cirrhotic patients included in a clinical trial evaluating the effect of prednisone. Regular follow-up continued for 12 years. Over this period the cumulative percentage of patients with varices increased from 12% to 90%. Calès et al (1990) prospectively followed 84 cirrhotic patients, 41 of whom had no varices and 43 of whom had small varices. Over a mean follow-up period of 16 months, 8 out of 41 (20%) developed new varices and of those with small varices 18 out of 43 (42%) enlarged. However, in chronic active liver disease treated with prednisolone the prevalence of oesophageal varices only increased from 8% to 13% over 5 years (Czaja et al, 1979). A similar development over time is seen with congestive gastropathy. In a large prospective study of 212 cirrhotic patients followed for a mean of 4 years the incidence of congestive gastropathy increased from 27% to 61% (D'Amico et al, 1990). The risk of bleeding from congestive gastropathy also increased over the period of study.

As well as enlarging over time, varices may also regress in a minority of patients (Baker et al, 1959; Dagradi, 1972; Calès et al, 1990; Muting et al, 1990). Baker et al studied 115 cirrhotic patients in whom varices were diagnosed prior to bleeding. Only 28 patients had repeated oesophagoscopies. The reason for this is not given but as both variceal bleeding and death were common in this study, patients who survived to have repeated oesophagoscopies probably represented a selected low-risk group. Nevertheless, varices disapperared in nine patients, decreased in extent in seven and remained unchanged in six. Regression of varices may be related to abstinence from alcohol. Dagradi found that variceal size decreased and cherry-red spots disappeared in 12 out of 15 patients with alcoholic cirrhosis who discontinued drinking, over a mean observation period of 3 years. Varices remained stable or enlarged and developed cherry-red spots in 17 alcoholic cirrhotics who continued drinking, over a similar period. More recently, Calès et al found that varices decreased in size in 7 out of 43 (16%) of patients with small varices followed for a mean of 16 months, although this was not clearly related to abstinence from alcohol. It may be that a decrease in variceal size is related to opening up of other collaterals, and in some patients varices may not develop, because of large spontaneous portosystemic shunts. These patients have chronic encephalopathy but do not bleed (Caturelli et al, 1991).

Experimentally, propranolol has been shown to ameliorate the development of portosystemic shunting in a chronic murine schistosomiasis model (Sarin et al, 1991), and similar results have been obtained in a rat cirrhotic model (D. Lebrec et al, personal communication). This opens up the possibility of altering the natural history of the development of varices in man.

Risk of first bleeding

The overall risk of bleeding from oesophageal varices has been evaluated many times. Baker et al (1959) reported that 33 out of 115 (29%) alcoholic cirrhotic patients with varices and no previous bleeding had a variceal haemorrhage over a mean follow-up period of 3.3 years, with a 48%

Table 1. Rebleeding and survival in the combined control and shunt refusal groups in the prophylactic shunt trials.

Trial	Year	No. of patients	Bleeding (%)	Survival (%)	Deaths due to variceal bleeding (%)	Follow-up period
Jackson et al	1968	75	19	72	43	5 years
Resnick et al	1969	45	27	58	26	8 years
Conn et al	1972	35	40	43	40	12 years
Conn et al	1972	24	29	46	45	6 years

mortality rate during the first variceal bleed. Most subsequent studies have confirmed these findings; for example, Christensen et al (1981) report a 50% mortality. In the prophylactic shunt trials the patients nearly all had alcoholic cirrhosis and the proportion bleeding in the non-surgical groups ranged from 19% to 40%, over follow-up periods of 5–12 years (Table 1). Over 70% of patients who bled did so during the first 2 years of follow-up. Mortality during the first bleeding episode was high, ranging from 42% to 71%. Between 28% and 57% of the patients died during these studies and about one-third of the total number of deaths was due to variceal bleeding.

The course of the control or placebo groups in the more recent prophylactic propranolol trials is summarized in Table 2. In common with the prophylactic shunt trials there was a high incidence of variceal haemorrhage during the first 2 years of follow-up (Table 2), but there were less patients with alcoholic cirrhosis. The incidence of bleeding appeared to be related to the severity of the underlying liver disease. Only 39% of patients were free of bleeding in the study by Pascal et al (1987), in which 46% of the patients had Pugh's grade C liver disease at entry to the trial. In contrast, in the other trials, which included patients with predominantly Pugh's class A and B disease, 68–78% of patients were free of bleeding after 2 years of follow-up. A similar trend is seen with regard to mortality (Table 2). Despite advances in the treatment of variceal bleeding, up to 40% of deaths in the control groups were related to bleeding. The risk of death due to the initial bleed, at 26% (Italian Multicenter Project for Propranolol in Prevention of Bleeding, 1989) and 29% (Idéo et al, 1988), is not much different from that reported by Baker et al (1959), allowing for the severity of liver disease.

Table 2. Variceal bleeding and survival in the control groups of the prophylactic propranolol and nadolol* trials in cirrhotic patients.

Trial	Year	No. of patients	Free of bleeding (%) 1 year	Free of bleeding (%) 2 years	Survival (%) 1 year	Survival (%) 2 years	Pugh's grade (%) (A/B/C)
Pascal et al	1987	112	73	39	67	51	17/37/46
Idéo* et al	1988*	49	81	70	84	78	78/22 (AB/C)
Lebrec* et al	1988*	47	80	—	80	—	62/38 (A/B)
IMPP†	1989	89	89	68	93	76	63/31/6
Conn	1991	51	78	78	80	76	47/47/6

† Italian Multicentre Project for Propranolol in the Prevention of Bleeding (1989).

However, the above data should be viewed with some caveats as the populations recruited into clinical trials may not be representative of all cirrhotics with varices (Burroughs et al, 1986). Firstly, asymptomatic patients with liver disease, who have varices diagnosed as part of their work-up, may be different from those with cirrhosis and complications, e.g. ascites. Secondly, knowledge that varices have been documented for many years without bleeding may mean that these patients have demonstrated that they will not bleed, and may have a different natural history. Indeed, most episodes of bleeding in the controlled trials occur within 2 years of the diagnostic endoscopy. Thirdly, the treatment received for bleeding may have influenced survival and in the controlled studies the acute treatment was not necessarily the same for all patients. In addition the degree of hepatic decompensation is not always documented, and this is well recognized to be the prime determinant of short-term survival following variceal bleeding. If many of these patients were in Child's grade C, or 'pre-terminal' patients, it might be expected that mortality would be high. For example, Baker et al (1959) record that 5 of the 16 deaths (32%) occurring after the first variceal haemorrhage in 33 patients were in terminally ill patients. Fourthly, the rate of deterioration of liver disease probably influences the risk of bleeding and the progression of varices (Cales et al, 1990). Abstention from alcohol may ameliorate liver function and the development of varices as suggested by Dagradi (1972).

Risk of recurrent bleeding

The incidence of bleeding is higher in trials of secondary prevention in which all patients had at least one previous episode of variceal bleeding than in the prophylactic trials. During long-term follow-up the majority of these patients will have further episodes of variceal haemorrhage (Tables 3 and 4). Inspection of Table 3 reveals, not surprisingly, that the risk appears to be related to the severity of the underlying liver disease. The highest incidences of rebleeding were recorded by Villeneuve et al (1986), 75% at 1 year, and Garden et al (1990), 70% at 1 year, both of whom included the largest number of patients with Pugh's grade C liver disease at entry (30% and 46% respectively). In contrast all the patients studied by Colombo et al (1989) had Pugh's grade A and B cirrhosis, and 51% bled from varices in the first year of follow-up. Similarly 96% of patients studied by Quieniet et al

Table 3. Rebleeding and survival in the control groups of the therapeutic shunt trials in cirrhotic patients with portal hypertension.

Trial	Year	No. of patients	Rebleeding (%)	Survival (%)	Follow-up period
Jackson et al	1971	77	65	36	5.5 years
Rueff et al	1976	49	71	47	3 years
Reynolds et al	1981	44	76 (1 yr) 90 (4 yr)	75	10 years
Resnick et al	1974	25	78	48	5 years

Table 4. Rebleeding and survival in the control groups of the propranolol trials for the prevention of variceal rebleeding in patients with cirrhosis.

Trial	Year	No. of patients	Rebleeding (%) 1 year	Rebleeding (%) 2 years	Survival (%) 1 year	Survival (%) 2 years	Pugh's grade (%) (A/B/C)
Lebrec et al	1984	36	58	68	84	57	Mostly A and B
Burroughs et al	1983	22	45	—	—	—	55/36/9
Villeneuve et al	1986	37	75	82	70	63	13/57/30
Quieniet et al	1987	48	48	—	80	—	46/48/6
Colombo et al	1989	30	51	60	68	—	47/53 (A/B)
Garden et al	1990	43	70	—	68	—	12/42/46

(1987) had Pugh's grade A and B liver disease and 48% bled in the first year of follow-up. Interestingly a percentage reduction of at least 12% in the hepatic venous pressure gradient in patients taking nadolol may indicate a greatly reduced risk of rebleeding (Sacerdoti et al, 1991).

PROGNOSIS OF ACUTE VARICEAL HAEMORRHAGE

Acute variceal bleeding is characterized by a high mortality and a high rate of early rebleeding (Burroughs et al, 1989). Mortality due to variceal bleeding is related to the degree of hepatic decompensation (Graham and Smith, 1981; Burroughs et al, 1989). The average mortality of the first haemorrhage is 50% in most studies, and is this high because of a high proportion of grade C patients. The average mortality for subsequent bleeding is about 25%, because the high-risk patients have mostly died following the first haemorrhage, but the mortality according to modified Child's classification remains the same: grade A, 5%, grade B, 25% or less; grade C, 50% or more.

In addition to the degree of liver dysfunction, renal dysfunction has been reported to be independently predictive of survival using serum creatinine (Garden et al, 1985; Christensen et al, 1989). The criteria used in Child–Pugh's classification (i.e. serum bilirubin, albumin, prothrombin time, ascites, hepatic encephalopathy) in a linear regression model have been found to be superior to other published scoring systems in predicting 30-day or 6-week mortality (Ohmann et al, 1990).

Amongst other prognostic factors for survival are a portohepatic gradient measured 2 weeks after haemorrhage (but it is unclear if this is independently predictive of the degree of liver cell dysfunction) (Vinel et al, 1986), early rebleeding or continued bleeding within 5 days (Cardin et al, 1990) in a study at the Royal Free Hospital, and active bleeding (oozing or spurting) at endoscopy in the Royal Free Hospital population (Cardin et al, 1990). However, the latter has not been confirmed by another group (Balanzo et al, 1991). We have also found that active bleeding at endoscopy, but not the presence of a white nipple sign, is independently associated with the risk of very early rebleeding (within 5 days), the other major factors being related to the severity of liver disease (Siringo et al, 1991). Ready et al (1991) have found that a higher hepatic venous pressure gradient (HVPG) was associated with continued bleeding or early rebleeding when measured on day 1 or 2 following admission for bleeding in 21 alcoholic cirrhotics. Patients whose HVPG was ≥ 16 mmHg on day 1 had more than a 50% chance of continued bleeding or rebleeding. In this study delerium tremens was also associated with early rebleeding. The severity of liver disease also affects the risk of very early rebleeding in response to somatostatin or placebo drug treatment (Burroughs et al, 1990).

The risk of both very early rebleeding and death decreases rapidly following admission (Burroughs et al, 1989). When expressed as a hazard function it can be seen that the risk of death becomes virtually constant about 6 weeks after bleeding (Graham and Smith, 1981; Burroughs et al, 1989)—this occurs earlier for patients with well-compensated cirrhosis (Burroughs et al, 1989). This has implications for the potential therapeutic impact of techniques to prevent rebleeding. Unless the measures are used, and are efficacious, within this high-risk interval they are unlikely to affect survival with respect to bleeding, given that all therapeutic measures, except liver transplantation, have no beneficial effect on liver function itself.

NATURAL HISTORY OF PORTAL HYPERTENSION IN PATIENTS WITHOUT CIRRHOSIS

Most patients with portal hypertension in the Western world have cirrhosis. A small minority will have other conditions such as extrahepatic portal venous obstruction, Budd–Chiari syndrome, nodular regenerative hyperplasia and so on. Non-cirrhotic portal hypertension or idiopathic portal hypertension is more commonly seen in India and Japan. Schistosomiasis is the most common cause of non-cirrhotic portal hypertension in the world. The major clinical difference between cirrhotic and non-cirrhotic portal hypertension is that good liver function is generally preserved in the latter conditions. As a result gastrointestinal bleeding and hypotension are better tolerated and thus there is a lower mortality. Quality of life between bleeding episodes also tends to be better than in cirrhosis.

Extrahepatic portal venous obstruction

This is the second most common cause of portal hypertension following cirrhosis in the Western countries. Prognosis depends on the underlying cause of the thrombosis and is worse in patients with underlying malignancies or serious haematological disorders. In some cases the venous obstruction is due to previous intra-abdominal sepsis or trauma but in most cases it is idiopathic. It has been suggested that a significant proportion of the 'idiopathic' adult cases may be due to the presence of a low-grade primary myeloproliferative disorder (Valla et al, 1988). As yet this has not been confirmed by others, and the mechanism of thrombosis is not clear. These putative myeloproliferative disorders do not seem to affect survival or bleeding (Cardin et al, 1992).

Extrahepatic portal venous obstruction most commonly presents in childhood but a significant proportion (about 40% in some series) present in adult life (Webb and Sherlock, 1979; Cardin et al, 1992). Most of the data relate to prognosis in the paediatric population, and are derived from series of cases treated for bleeding varices. As only a small proportion are diagnosed before variceal bleeding there is no information as regards risk of first bleeding. In addition there are no randomized trials using a control group, so that the real risk of rebleeding is difficult to assess. From our own data (Cardin et al, 1992), it seems to be less than for a group with well-compensated cirrhosis. However, from the paediatric information available, a number of points emerge (Aoyama and Myers, 1982; Boles and Birken, 1983; McPherson, 1984; Boles et al, 1986).

Firstly, bleeding is common as a clinical presentation with reported incidences ranging from 77% to 100%. Secondly, in comparison with cirrhosis, mortality during the initial bleed is very low. Aoyama and Myers (1982) studied 62 children with extrahepatic portal venous obstruction. None of their patients died as a result of the initial haemorrhage. Thirdly, long-term survival also appears to be good. McPherson (1984) reported a cumulative survival of 60% at 20 years in 20 children treated surgically. Aoyama and Myers (1982) reported 13% and Boles and Birken (1983) reported a 12% mortality respectively over long-term follow-up. Lastly, recurrent bleeding is frequent despite treatment. The probability of recurrent bleeding appears to depend on the interval from the previous bleed with an 80% probability if the patient has bled within the previous year and 13% if there has been no bleed for more than 10 years. The reason why the risk of rebleeding diminishes with time is not clear. There may be a change in variceal characteristics or in the collateral circulation affecting variceal blood flow, but this is speculative.

Less information is available with regard to prognosis in adult patients with extrahepatic portal venous obstruction. Kahn et al (1987) treated 39 adult and teenage patients with injection sclerotherapy. Mean follow-up was 4 years and there were no deaths during this period. Webb and Sherlock (1979) followed a mixed group of 97 children and adults. They reported that when the time of onset of portal venous thrombosis was known, the interval to first variceal haemorrhage was usually about 5 years, but could be delayed for as long as 10 years. Twenty-four of the 97 patients died (25%) and 60 survived for more than 10 years. Pande et al (1987) followed a cohort of 117 adults and children from India who had surgery for extrahepatic venous obstruction. Cumulative survival was 90% at 5 years and 75% at 10 years. Hepatic encephalopathy was not seen despite the fact that the majority of these patients had shunts, attesting to the importance of good liver function. However, ascites is sometimes seen in elderly adults following bleeding.

Idiopathic portal hypertension

This condition is particularly common in Japan and India. It is characterized by fibrotic obliteration of the intrahepatic portal vein radicals and most patients have marked splenomegaly. Liver function is well preserved in the majority of patients. As a consequence the prognosis appears to be better than that of cirrhosis with 91% of patients surviving for longer than 10 years in a large study from Japan (Okuda and Obata, 1991).

Schistosomiasis

Patients with schistosomiasis and portal hypertension have good liver function compared to those with cirrhosis (Rodriguez et al, 1955; Warren and Reboucas 1984). A patient who survived 33 episodes of upper gastrointestinal bleeding has been described (Garcia-Palmieri and Marcial-Rojas, 1959). Nevertheless bleeding varices is a frequent cause of death in this patient group. In a recent placebo-controlled trial using propranolol to prevent rebleeding, 20 out of 25 (80%) of the patients receiving placebo rebled within 1 year (Kiire, 1989). Over the same period, 5 of 25 patients in the control group died, four from bleeding varices and one from liver failure.

Nodular regenerative hyperplasia

Nodular regenerative hyperplasia of the liver is characterized by the presence of diffuse micronodular transformation of the hepatic parenchyma in the absence of fibrosis. A review of the literature revealed that 54% of reported cases had portal hypertension and that variceal haemorrhage had occurred in 19%. However, this is probably an overestimate as there were no cases of variceal haemorrhage among 64 patients with nodular regenerative hyperplasia identified at post mortem from a series of 2500 autopsies (Wanless, 1990). Similarly Colina et al (1989) identified 24 cases of nodular regenerative hyperplasia in a general hospital in Spain over 9 years. Nine patients had evidence of portal hypertension and three out of nine had upper gastrointestinal bleeding. Because liver function is well preserved, these patients tolerate variceal bleeding well. However, many have associated myeloproliferative disorders, collagen vascular diseases, or bone marrow transplants which may influence prognosis (Snover et al, 1989; Wanless et al, 1990).

PITFALLS IN ASSESSING PROGNOSIS

In evaluating prognosis the importance of the time when the initial observations are made relative to the start of the disease is frequently ignored. This fact can be crucial when comparing the results of clinical trials, particularly when those trials relate to an event with a high mortality such as variceal bleeding. Graham and Smith (1981) first suggested that the time interval between admission to hospital and the point used for the start of the survival analysis may be an important variable. We have confirmed these data in a cohort of 194 cirrhotic patients admitted with bleeding oesophageal varices but have also shown that changing the starting time for analysis significantly alters rebleeding rates (Burroughs et al, 1989). For rebleeding, if the starting point for the analysis is moved from 0 to 5 days the proportion free of rebleeding at 25 days changes from 75% to 41% ($p<0.0001$). For mortality, changing the starting point from 0 to 15 days changes the 1-year survival from 60% to 68% ($p<0.03$). Small changes in the starting time for analysis cause significant changes in outcome because the risk of mortality and rebleeding is very high immediately after a variceal haemorrhage and declines exponentially over the next 30 days or so. Delaying the start of the analysis selects out patients with better prognosis for both survival and risk of rebleeding because some poor-risk patients will already have rebled, or died, or both. Moreover the risk of dying following 6 weeks after admission for bleeding appears to be constant, suggesting that measures to prevent rebleeding which are used after this interval (e.g. surgery) or are only efficacious after this period of time (e.g. after obliteration of varices with chronic sclerotherapy) may not be able to influence mortality in a significant way.

In the setting of natural history and risk of first bleeding, there is a potential bias in the relationship between the time at which varices develop, the time of diagnosis and the time of recruitment into a clinical trial or clinical study. Thus, any relationship between entry in a clinical trial and the interval to first bleeding or death may be flawed because of inclusion of patients who were known to have varices for months or years before inclusion in a study. Such patients have already demonstrated that they are 'survivors' and not 'bleeders'. This may explain why the risk of first bleeding is not constant following the inclusion of patients in a clinical study or trial—70% of all bleeding occurs within 2 years of recruitment (Burroughs et al, 1986). The practical importance of this lies in trying to compare the results of different clinical trials evaluating the same treatments, as changes in the starting time for analysis can have such profound influences on outcomes. It is also important where two different treatments are being compared within the same trial. A good example is the trial by Rueff et al (1976) in which shunt surgery was compared with conservative medical treatment. In this trial shunt surgery was performed within 2 weeks of admission, but randomization for the medically treated group is stated to have been at least 2 weeks from admission. Thus, the medical group had an inherently less severe risk of dying or rebleeding. Interestingly this is the only shunt trial for secondary prevention which had a worse survival in the group randomized to surgery.

RISK FACTORS FOR FIRST BLEEDING

Identifying patients with varices who will bleed before they do so is clearly important in order to offer effective prophylactic therapy to those who need it and avoid it in those who do not, particularly if the therapy is invasive or has significant complications such as surgery and sclerotherapy. Indeed the latter two treatments should not be used as they have been shown to worsen survival (Pagliaro et al, 1989; Veterans Affairs Cooperative Variceal Sclerotherapy Group, 1991) despite reducing bleeding in most trials. Even in patients selected for high risk of first bleeding, prophylactic sclerotherapy confers no benefit (De Franchis et al, 1991). If a prophylactic therapy has few side-effects, such as β-blockers, selection of those likely to benefit may be less important in a general sense, but is still important when assessing individual cases for the risk of rebleeding versus likelihood of benefit from prophylactic therapy.

Risk factors for variceal bleeding have only been evaluated in cirrhotic patients. Their identification applies only to those cirrhotics with varices who have not bled. Most of those who have bled have similar characteristics, and as the risk of rebleeding is so high no clear-cut risk factors for rebleeding have been identified, except for the severity of liver disease, which influences very early rebleeding from varices (Burroughs et al, 1989; Cardin et al, 1990). In addition Sarcedoti et al (1991) suggest that in patients taking nadolol, a percentage reduction of HVPG of less than 12% is associated with rebleeding, when repeat hepatic venous pressure measurements are made at 1 month. These results need to be confirmed as they may represent crucial clinical information for individual patient management, but in addition it would be useful to know if a spontaneous reduction has the same significance.

Baker et al (1959) wrote, 'it is our impression that there is a correlation between the severity of liver impairment and the extent of varices, the frequency and severity of bleeding, and the mortality from haemorrhage.' This impression has proven to be correct, with recent studies confirming the relationships between varices at risk of bleeding, severity of liver disease, and death from bleeding.

Risk factors for first variceal bleeding include portal and/or intravariceal pressure, endoscopic appearances of varices, severity of liver disease and alcohol abuse. In patients with sinusoidal portal hypertension, such as alcoholic cirrhosis, the presence of varices indicates an HPVG of 12 mmHg or more (Viallet et al, 1975; Garcia-Tsao et al, 1985). Above this figure, there is no direct relationship between risk of bleeding and pressure, although HPVG tends to be higher in bleeders as well as in those cirrhotics with larger varices (Garcia-Tsao et al, 1985). Large varices have been associated with an increased risk of bleeding (Palmer and Brick, 1956; Lebrec, 1980), and it is believed that the tension on the variceal wall is the critical risk factor. This is related to the radius of the varix. This principle has been investigated in an artificial system, in which the increasing size of varix and the thinness of the wall resulted in rupture at lower intraluminal pressure (Polio and Groszmann, 1986). Thus, variceal wall tension is increased by variceal pressure, size of varix and decreased wall thickness. Very recently it has been shown that if the HVPG falls below 12 mmHg, no bleeding occurs (Groszmann et al, 1990) in a group of patients with varices that have not bled. This is the first time a haemodynamic index has correlated with the absence of bleeding.

Dagradi (1972) was the first to report the presence of cherry-red spots on varices, and found that they occurred and developed on large varices (5 mm diameter or more). Their presence indicated a higher risk of bleeding. In a retrospective study by the Japanese Research Society for Portal Hypertension (Beppu et al, 1981), the presence of red signs and blue varices were significant risk factors for bleeding—80% risk or more. These data were not reproduced by the Japanese themselves in a prophylactic trial (Inokuchi and

Co-operative Study Group of Portal Hypertension of Japan, 1990) or by the North Italian Endoscopic Club (NIEC) whose prospective study demonstrated a far lower risk of bleeding based on three independent risk factors: Child's class, size of varices and red weal markings (North Italian Endoscopic Club for the Study and Treatment of Oesophageal Varices, 1988). The range of risk for bleeding within a year ranges between 6% and 76%. Their model has been independently validated (Prada et al, 1990). A simplified NIEC index based on the presence or absence or red signs of varices, variceal size and Child class correlates well with the original index (De Franchis et al, 1990). Intravariceal pressure has been found to be an independent risk factor for first bleeding when evaluated with the NIEC index (Feu et al, 1990). HVPG has also been shown to be an independent risk factor (Merkel et al, 1991).

Fortunately, there is good interobserver correlation for the presence of varices, size (with direct measurement using the known span of a biopsy forceps) and presence of red signs at endoscopy (Calès et al, 1989). Other factors which have been reported as independent risk factors for bleeding are the presence of gastric varices (Kleber et al, 1991) and the velocity and direction of portal flow evaluated by echo doppler (Gaiani et al, 1991) but these have yet to be validated in independent groups.

All the factors mentioned above have been evaluated at single time points. There are very few studies on the evolution of these with time. However, data from the control groups of the old prophylactic shunt studies showed that persistence or development of ascites increased the risk of bleeding (Conn et al, 1972). The rate of deterioration of liver disease probably determines the risk of bleeding (Burroughs et al, 1989) and the earlier development of 'at-risk varices' (Calès et al, 1989). Alcohol abuse has been found to be more common in those who bleed than in those who do not, but it is not clear if these two groups are different in terms of their liver function. Dagradi (1972) suggested that abstinence from alcohol decreased the size of varices and the number of cherry-red spots and decreased risk of bleeding.

REFERENCES

Aoyama K & Myers NA (1982) Extra-hepatic portal hypertension: the significance of variceal haemorrhage. *Australian Paediatric Journal* **18:** 17–22.
Baker LA, Smith C & Lieberman G (1959) The natural history of esophageal varices. *American Journal of Medicine* **26:** 228–237.
Balanzo J, Villanueva C, Espinos J et al (1991) Predictive value of the endoscopic signs in variceal bleeding. *Journal of Hepatology* **13 (supplement 2):** S93 (abstract).
Beppu K, Inokuchi K, Koyanagi N et al (1981) Prediction of variceal haemorrhage by oesophageal endoscopy. *Gastrointestinal Endoscopy* **27:** 213–218.
Boles ET & Birken G (1983) Extrahepatic portal hypertension in children: long term evaluation. *Chirurgie Pediatrique* **24:** 23–28.
Boles ET, Wise WE & Birken G (1986) Extrahepatic portal hypertension in children: long-term evaluation. *American Journal of Surgery* **151:** 734–739.
Burroughs AK, Jenkins WJ, Sherlock S et al (1983) Controlled trial of propranolol for the prevention of recurrent variceal hemorrhage in patients with cirrhosis. *New England Journal of Medicine* **309:** 1539–1542.

Burroughs AK, D'Heygere F & McIntyre N (1986) Pitfalls in studies of prophylactic therapy for variceal bleeding in cirrhotics. *Hepatology* **6:** 1407–1413.

Burroughs AK, Mezzanotte G, Phillips A et al (1989) Cirrhotics with variceal hemorrhage: the importance of the time interval between admission and the start of the analysis for survival and rebleeding rates. *Hepatology* **9:** 801–807.

Burroughs AK, McCormick PA, Hughes MD et al (1990) Randomized double-blind placebo controlled trial of somatostatin for variceal bleeding. *Gastroenterology* **99:** 1388–1395.

Calès P, Buscail L, Bretagne JF et al (1989) Concordance inter-obserateurs intercentres des signes endoscopiques gastro-oesophagiens au cours de la cirrhose. *Gastroenterologie Clinique et Biologique* **13:** 967–973.

Calès P, Desmorat H, Vinel JP et al (1990) Incidence of large oesophageal varices in patients with cirrhosis: application to prophylaxis of first bleeding. *Gut* **31:** 1298–1302.

Cardin F, Gori G, McCormick PA & Burroughs AK (1990) A predictive model for very early rebleeding from varices. *Gut* **31:** A1204 (abstract).

Cardin F, Graffeo M, McCormick PA et al (1992) Adult 'idiopathic' extra hepatic venous thrombosis: importance of putative 'latent' myeloproliferative disorders and a comparison with cases of a known aetiology. *Digestive Diseases and Sciences* (in press).

Caturelli E, Sperandeo G, Squillante MM & Andriulli A (1991) Spontaneous porto-systemic shunts preventing esophageal varices formation: an echo-doppler study. *Hepatology* **14:** 237A (abstract).

Christensen E, Faverholdt L, Schlicthing P et al (1981) Aspects of the natural history of gastrointestinal bleeding in cirrhosis and the effect of prednisolone. *Gastroenterology* **81:** 944–952.

Christensen E, Krintel JJ, Hansen M, Krogh S et al (1989) Prognosis after the first episode of gastrointestinal bleeding or coma in cirrhosis. *Scandinavian Journal of Gastroenterology* **24:** 999–1006.

Colina F, Alberti N, Solis JHA & Martinez-Tello FJ (1989) Diffuse nodular regenerative hyperplasia of the liver (DNRH). A clinicopathologic study of 24 cases. *Liver* **9:** 253–265.

Colombo M, De Franchis R, Tommasini M et al (1989) β-blockade prevents recurrent gastrointestinal bleeding in well-compensated patients with alcoholic cirrhosis: a multicenter randomized controlled trial. *Hepatology* **9:** 433–438.

Conn HO, Lindenmuth WW, May CJ et al (1972) Prophylactic portacaval anastomosis. A tale of two studies. *Medicine* **51:** 27–40.

Conn HO, Grace ND, Bosch J et al (1991) Propranolol in the prevention of the first hemorrhage from esophagogastric varices: A multicenter, randomized clinical trial. *Hepatology* **13:** 902–912.

Czaja AJ, Wolf AM & Summerskill WH (1979) Development and early prognosis of esophageal varices in severe chronic active liver disease (CALD) treated with prednisolone. *Gastroenterology* **77:** 629–633.

Dagradi A (1972) The natural history of oesophageal varices in patients with alcoholic liver disease. *American Journal of Gastroenterology* **57:** 520–540.

D'Amico G, Montalbano L, Traina M et al (1990) Natural history of congestive gastropathy in cirrhosis. *Gastroenterology* **99:** 1558–1564.

De Franchis R, Arcidiacono P, Nolte A et al (1990) Development of a simplified prognostic index to predict the first oesophageal bleed in cirrhotics. *Journal of Hepatology* **11 (supplement 2):** S18 (abstract).

De Franchis R, Primigiani M, Arcidiacono PG et al (1991) Prophylactic sclerotherapy in high risk cirrhotics selected by endoscopic criteria. *Gastroenterology* **101:** 1087–1093.

Feu F, Bordes JM, Garcia-Pagan JC et al (1990) Endoscopic measurement of variceal pressure in patients with cirrhosis. Correlation with the NIEC index (NI) and with the risk of variceal haemorrhage. *Journal of Hepatology* **11 (supplement 2):** S22 (abstract).

Gaiani S, Bolondi L, Li Bassi S et al (1991) Prevalence of spontaneous hepatofugal portal flow in liver cirrhosis. *Gastroenterology* **100:** 160–167.

Garcia-Palmieri MR & Marcial-Rojas RA (1959) Portal hypertension due to schistosomiasis Mansoni. *American Journal of Medicine* **27:** 811–816.

Garcia-Tsao G, Groszmann RJ, Fisher RL et al (1985) Portal pressure presence of gastroesophageal varices and variceal bleeding. *Hepatology* **5:** 419–424.

Garden OJ, Motyl H, Gilmour WH et al (1985) Prediction of outcome following acute variceal haemorrhage. *British Journal of Surgery* **72:** 91–95.

Garden OJ, Mills PR, Birnie GG et al (1990) Propranolol in the prevention of recurrent variceal hemorrhage in cirrhotic patients. A controlled trial. *Gastroenterology* **98:** 185–190.

Graham DY & Smith JL (1981) The course of patients after variceal hemorrhage. *Gastroenterology* **80:** 800–809.

Groszmann RJ, Bosch J, Grace ND et al (1990) Hemodynamic events in a prospective randomized trial of propranolol versus placebo in the prevention of a first variceal hemorrhage. *Gastroenterology* **99:** 1401–1407.

Idéo G, Bellati G, Fesce E & Grimoldi D (1988) Nadolol can prevent the first gastrointestinal bleeding in cirrhotics; a prospective, randomized study. *Hepatology* **8:** 6–9.

Inokuchi K & Co-operative Study Group of Portal Hypertension of Japan (1990) Improved survival after prophylactic portal non-decompression surgery for oesophageal varices: a randomized clinical trial. *Hepatology* **12:** 1–6.

Italian Multicenter Project for Propranolol in Prevention of Bleeding (1989) Propranolol prevents first gastrointestinal bleed in non-ascitic cirrhotic patients. Final report of a multicenter randomized trial. *Journal of Hepatology* **9:** 75–83.

Jackson FC, Perrin EB, Smith AG et al (1968) A clinical investigation of the portacaval shunt. II. Survival analysis of the prophylactic operation. *American Journal of Surgery* **115:** 22–42.

Jackson FC, Perrin EB, Felix R & Smith AG (1971) A clinical investigation of the portacaval shunt: V. Survival analysis of the therapeutic operation. *Annals of Surgery* **174:** 672–700.

Kahn D, Terblanche J, Kitano S & Bornman P (1987) Injection sclerotherapy in adult patients with extrahepatic portal venous obstruction. *British Journal of Surgery* **74:** 600–602.

Kiire CF (1989) Controlled trial of propranolol to prevent recurrent variceal bleeding in patients with non-cirrhotic portal fibrosis. *British Medical Journal* **298:** 1363–1365.

Kleber G, Sauerbruch T, Ansari H & Paumgartner G (1991) Prediction of variceal hemorrhage in cirrhosis: a prospective follow-up study. *Gastroenterology* **100:** 1332–1337.

Lebrec D (1980) Portal hypertension size of esophageal varices, and risk of gastrointestinal bleeding in alcoholic cirrhosis. *Gastroenterology* **79:** 1139–1144.

Lebrec D, Poynard T, Bernuau J et al (1984) A randomized controlled study of propranolol for prevention of recurrent gastrointestinal bleeding in patients with cirrhosis; a final report. *Hepatology* **4:** 355–358.

Lebrec D, Poynard T, Capron JP et al (1988) Nadolol for prophylaxis of gastrointestinal bleeding in patients with cirrhosis. A randomized trial. *Journal of Hepatology* **7:** 118–125.

McPherson AIS (1984) Portal hypertension in children: an experience of 33 cases. *Scottish Medical Journal* **29:** 6–14.

Merkel C, Bolognesi M, Bellon S et al (1991) Hepatic vein catheterization in the prognostic evaluation of cirrhotics with esophageal varices. *Journal of Hepatology* **13 (supplement 2):** S53 (abstract).

Muting D, Kalk JF, Fischer R & Wiewel D (1990) Spontaneous regression of oesophageal varices after long-term conservative treatment. Retrospective study in 20 patients with alcoholic liver cirrhosis, posthepatic cirrhosis and haemochromatosis with cirrhosis. *Journal of Hepatology* **10:** 158–162.

North Italian Endoscopic Club for the Study and Treatment of Oesophageal Varices (1988) Prediction of the first variceal haemorrhage in patients with cirrhosis of the liver and oesophageal varices: a prospective multicentre study. *New England Journal of Medicine* **319:** 983–989.

Ohmann C, Stoltzing H, Wins L et al (1990) Prognostic scores in oesophageal or gastric variceal bleeding. *Scandinavian Journal of Gastroenterology* **25:** 501–512.

Okuda K & Obata H (1991) Idiopathic portal hypertension (hepatoportal sclerosis). In Okuda K & Benhamou JP (eds) *Portal Hypertension: Clinical and Physiological Aspects*, pp 271–287. Tokyo: Springer-Verlag.

Pagliaro L, Burroughs AK, Sorensen TIA et al (1989) Therapeutic controversies and randomised controlled trials (RCT's): prevention of bleeding and re-bleeding in cirrhosis. *Gastroenterology International* **2:** 71–84.

Palmer ED & Brick IB (1956) Correlation between severity of esophageal varices in portal cirrhosis and their propensity toward hemorrhage. *Gastroenterology* **30:** 85–90.

Pande GK, Reddy VM, Kar P et al (1987) Operations for portal hypertension due to extrahepatic obstruction: results and 10 year follow up. *British Medical Journal* **295:** 1115–1117.

Pascal JP, Calès P & Multicentre Study Group (1987) Propranolol in the prevention of first upper gastrointestinal tract haemorrhage in patients with cirrhosis of the liver and oesophageal varices. *New England Journal of Medicine* **317:** 856–861.

Polio J & Groszmann RJ (1986) Hemodynamic factors involved in the development and rupture of oesophageal varices: a physiological approach to treatment. *Seminars in Liver Disease* **6:** 318–331.

Prada A, Bortoli A, Minoli G et al (1990) The prediction of esophageal variceal bleeding: NIEC's score validation by an independent group. *Gastroenterology* **98:** A108 (abstract).

Quieniet AM, Czernichow P, Lerebours E et al (1987) Etude controlee du propranolol dans la prevention des recidives hemorragiques chez les patients cirrhotiques. *Gastroenterologie Clinique et Biologique* **11:** 41–47.

Ready JB, Robertson AD, Goffs JS & Rector WG (1991) Assessment of risk of bleeding from esophageal varices by continuous monitoring or portal pressure. *Gastroenterology* **100:** 1403–1410.

Resnick RH, Chalmers TC, Ishihara AM et al (1969) A controlled study of the prophylactic portacaval shunt. A final report. *Annals of Internal Medicine* **70:** 675–688.

Resnick RH, Iber FL, Ishihara AM et al (1974) A controlled study of the therapeutic portacaval shunt. *Gastroenterology* **67:** 843–857.

Reynolds TB, Donovan AJ, Mikkelsen WP et al (1981) Results of a 12-year randomized trial of portacaval shunt in patients with alcoholic liver disease and bleeding varices. *Gastroenterology* **80:** 1005–1011.

Rodriguez HF, Garcia-Palmieri MR, Rivera JV & Rodriguez-Molina R (1955) A comparative study of portal and bilharzial cirrhosis. *Gastroenterology* **29:** 235–246.

Rueff B, Prandi D, Degos F et al (1976) A controlled study of therapeutic portacaval shunt in alcoholic cirrhosis. *Lancet* **1:** 655–659.

Sarcedoti D, Merkel C & Gratta A (1991) Importance of the 1 month effect of nadolol on portal pressure in predicting failure of prevention of rebleeding in cirrhosis. *Journal of Hepatology* **12:** 124–125 (letter).

Sarin SK, Groszmann RJ, Mosca PG et al (1991) Propranolol ameliorates the development of portal-systemic shunting in a chronic murine schistosomiasis model of portal hypertension. *Journal of Clinical Investigation* **87:** 1032–1036.

Siringo S, McCormick PA, Mistry P et al (1991) Prognostic significance of the white nipple sign in variceal bleeding. *Gastrointestinal Endoscopy* **37:** 51–55.

Snover DC, Weisdorf S, Bloomer J et al (1989) Nodular regenerative hyperplasia of the liver following bone marrow transplantation. *Hepatology* **9:** 443–448.

Valla D, Cadadevall N, Huisse MG et al (1988) Etiology of portal vein thrombosis in adults: a prospective evaluation of primary myeloproliferative disorders. *Gastroenterology* **94:** 1063–1069.

Veterans Affairs Cooperative Variceal Sclerotherapy Group (1991) Prophylactic sclerotherapy for esophageal varices in men with alcoholic liver disease. *New England Journal of Medicine* **324:** 1779–1784.

Viallet A, Marleau D, Huet M et al (1975) Haemodynamic evaluation of patients with intrahepatic portal hypertension. *Gastroenterology* **69:** 1297–1300.

Villeneuve JP, Pomier-Layrargues G, Infante-Rivard C et al (1986) Propranolol for the prevention of recurrent variceal haemorrhage: a controlled trial. *Hepatology* **6:** 1239–1243.

Vinel JP, Cassingeul J, Levade M et al (1986) Assessment of short term prognosis after variceal bleeding in patients with alcoholic cirrhosis by early measurement of porto-hepatic gradient. *Hepatology* **6:** 116–117.

Wanless IR (1990) Micronodular transformation (nodular regenerative hyperplasia) of the liver: a report of 64 cases among 2,500 autopsies and a new classification of benign hepatocellular nodules. *Hepatology* **11:** 787–797.

Wanless IR, Peterson P, Das A et al (1990) Hepatic vascular disease and portal hypertension in polycythemia vera and agnogenic myeloid metaplasia: a clinicopathological study of 145 patients examined at autopsy. *Hepatology* **12:** 1166–1174.

Warren KS & Reboucas G (1964) Blood ammonia during bleeding from esophageal varices in patients with hepatosplenic schistosomiasis. *New England Journal of Medicine* **271:** 921–926.

Webb LJ & Sherlock S (1979) The aetiology, presentation and natural history of extra-hepatic portal venous obstruction. *Quarterly Journal of Medicine* **48:** 627–639.

3

Balloon tamponade and vasoactive drugs in the control of acute variceal haemorrhage

O. JAMES GARDEN
DAVID C. CARTER

The acute management of bleeding oesophageal varices continues to prove controversial. Despite changing trends in treatment, morbidity and mortality remain high. The range of therapeutic options has increased steadily and includes the use of drugs, such as vasopressin and somatostatin, to lower portal pressure, oesophageal tamponade, both per-oesophageal and trans-hepatic injection sclerotherapy, oesophageal transection with or without a devascularization procedure and selective and non-selective portocaval shunting. Each of these options may have a place in management but there is still considerable debate over their role in controlling acute variceal haemorrhage. Endoscopic and surgical means of arresting haemorrhage are discussed elsewhere and this chapter will focus on balloon tamponade and pharmacological control of bleeding.

OESOPHAGEAL TAMPONADE

Historical background

Although Westphal had shown in 1930 that compression of a bleeding oesophageal varix with an oesophageal sound was a simple method of arresting haemorrhage, it was Rowntree et al (1947) who suggested that an inflatable balloon could be used to compress the tributaries of the coronary veins as they communicate with the varices. Sengstaken and Blakemore (1950) described the use of a three-lumen oesophagogastric tube which compressed both the fundal and oesophageal veins and provided a third channel for aspiration of the stomach. With the more widespread use of balloon tamponade to control variceal haemorrhage, it became apparent that aspiration of blood and pharyngeal secretions by the patient gave rise to frequent and significant respiratory complications. Linton and Ellis (1956) described the use of a tube with only a gastric balloon and a distal aspirating lumen. The balloon, unlike the gastric balloon of the Sengstaken–Blakemore tube, could be inflated to a volume of 600 ml. This tube could be used to determine whether bleeding originated above or below the gastric cardia but it soon became apparent that it was also an effective means of controlling haemorrhage from gastric or oesophageal varices. Nachlas (1956) modified the system by adding an extra channel to aspirate the oesophagus and nasopharynx (Linton–Nachlas tube). There remained, however, a vogue for using a tube providing both oesophageal and gastric balloons and Boyce (1962) attached a standard nasogastric tube to the Sengstaken–Blakemore tube to provide aspiration above the upper end of the oesophageal balloon, thereby minimizing the risk of aspiration pneumonia. Edlich et al (1968) developed a four-lumen oesophagogastric tube at the University of Minnesota, the upper and lower balloons being inflated through two separate channels whilst the remaining lumen incorporated within the tube allowed aspiration of the stomach contents and the oesophagus above the oesophageal balloon.

Despite the introduction of this four-lumen Minnesota tube, the use of tamponade for primary control of haemorrhage in patients with bleeding oesophageal varices has remained controversial. Difficulties in insertion of the tube, the need for constant medical and nursing supervision, and the potential for complications, has resulted in a reluctance to use this method to control acute variceal haemorrhage in some centres.

Technique of balloon tamponade

The indications for tamponade to control bleeding from varices are not standardized but the technique has been the primary means of arresting variceal haemorrhage in our own experience (Garden et al, 1983). Endoscopy is performed as part of the initial assessment of each patient following initial resuscitation. When variceal haemorrhage is demonstrated at endoscopy and deemed to be so severe that it is unlikely to cease spontaneously, tamponade is instituted using the Minnesota four-lumen modification of the Sengstaken–Blakemore tube. If such proven variceal haemorrhage is minimal and thought likely to cease without intervention, tamponade is not instituted until it is clear that bleeding is continuing as evidenced by further overt haematemesis or occult haemorrhage as reflected in a rising pulse rate and/or falling blood pressure. It has rarely been necessary to institute oesophageal tamponade before adequate resuscitation and endoscopy but on occasion this has proved to be a life-saving manoeuvre in patients known to have cirrhosis or portal hypertension.

The tube must be inserted by medical staff trained in its use. The balloons of the Minnesota tube are first checked carefully for leaks and channels tested for patency. Although our initial practice was to pass the tube through the mouth, in recent years the nasogastric route has been preferred. Ideally the stomach should first be emptied by means of a nasogastric tube to reduce the possibility of vomiting and aspiration but, in practice, skilled insertion in the co-operative patient carries a small risk of these complications. Once the tube has been passed, the gastric balloon is inflated with

100 ml water and 20 ml sodium and meglumine iodamide (Uromiro 340, Merck Ltd). The oesophageal balloon is inflated with air to a pressure of 40 mmHg as measured by an aneroid barometer. The position of the tube is confirmed by abdominal radiography immediately after insertion. Continuous drainage of the gastric and pharyngeal channels of the Minnesota tube is supplemented by hourly syringe aspiration to detect continued bleeding and to prevent inhalation of pharyngeal secretions. The tube position is maintained simply by taping the tube to the side of the nose or to a spatula at the side of the mouth. Sedatives and analgesics are avoided whenever possible. Nursing patients in an intensive care unit does not guarantee the absence of complications but the patient must be supervised constantly by trained nursing staff. In our experience endotracheal intubation is rarely required before passage of the tube. Antacids and lactulose can be delivered through the tube into the stomach to minimize the risk of gastric and duodenal erosions and encephalopathy.

The Minnesota tube is kept in position with both balloons inflated for 24 h. The oesophageal balloon is then deflated and the tube left in place for an additional 12 h. If bleeding does not recur, the tube is then removed and destroyed to prevent reuse. If bleeding recurs while the tube is still in place, the balloons are reinflated for a further 24 h. When the condition of the patient permits, injection sclerotherapy can be undertaken.

Results of balloon tamponade

Over a 7-year period in our own unit (Haddock et al, 1989), 138 patients with portal hypertension presented on 223 occasions with endoscopically proven acute variceal haemorrhage. Haemorrhage ceased spontaneously on 92 occasions (41%) but on 126 occasions (57%) passage of the Minnesota tube was required with successful control of haemorrhage in 98% of cases. On only five occasions was intubation refused by the patient (2%). Haemorrhage recurred during these 223 admissions on 47 occasions (21%); on 11 occasions a second rebleed occurred and on two occasions a third. Tamponade was required during all of these rebleeds and arrest of haemorrhage was achieved in 87% of the episodes. Thus the overall rate of control in the total of 186 episodes of haemorrhage requiring tamponade was 94%.

Our own results are similar to those of other studies which have shown that variceal haemorrhage will be controlled by tamponade in 85–92% of patients (Boyce, 1962; Pitcher, 1967; Mitchell et al, 1981; Sarin and Nundy, 1984; Panes et al, 1988). It might be expected that bleeding is less likely to be controlled by tamponade in patients with severely impaired liver function. Panes et al (1988) recently reported control in 92% of patients, only 20% of whom were Child's grade C patients. Our own control rate of 94% was achieved in a predominantly poor-risk group of patients, 63% of whom were in modified Child's grade C (Tables 1 and 2). However, patients in whom haemorrhage was not controlled by tamponade in our experience had, with few exceptions, a poor prognostic score with advanced liver disease and severe coagulopathy (Garden et al, 1985).

Table 1. Control of haemorrhage by tamponade and relationship to modified Child's grade.

	Modified Child's grade		
	A	B	C
Initial bleeds	4	42	80
No. of patients in whom initial bleed controlled	4 (100%)	42 (100%)	77 (96%)
Rebleeds	2	17	41
No. of patients in whom rebleed controlled	2 (100%)	16 (94%)	34 (83%)

After Haddock et al (1989).

Table 2. Complications of oesophageal tamponade.

	Modified Child's grade		
	A	B	C
Aspiration → chest infection (no sclerotherapy)			4 (3)
Aspiration → chest infection (post-sclerotherapy)		4 (1)	5 (3)
Oesophageal tear on intubation			2 (2)
Pulled up tube	1	2	5 (1)
Cardiac arrest		1	3 (1)
Unexplained death			1 (1)
Total	1	7 (1)	20 (11)

Figures in parentheses denote deaths related to use of Minnesota tube.
After Haddock et al (1989).

Complications of tamponade

There is much controversy regarding the true incidence of serious complications associated with tamponade (Conn, 1958; Read et al, 1960; Conn and Simpson, 1967; Pitcher, 1967; Conn, 1971; Bauer et al, 1974; Chojkier and Conn, 1980; Panes et al, 1988). Conn and Simpson (1967) proposed that oesophageal tamponade should be used only as a last resort because of the high complication rate observed in their centre. They suggested that prophylactic tracheostomy or endotracheal intubation prior to insertion of the tube should be seriously considered in an attempt to prevent these complications. The favourable results of our own management policy suggest that endotracheal intubation may complicate unnecessarily the medical and nursing care of these patients.

Conn and Simpson (1967) found that 14 out of 40 patients (35%) admitted with acute variceal haemorrhage and treated by oesophageal tamponade suffered major complications; death was attributed to the use of the tube in nine patients (22%). Pitcher (1967) has shown that the incidence of complications can be minimized by strict nursing and medical care. The mortality rate attributed to tamponade in our series of patients was 6.4% with an overall complication rate per bleed of 15% (Haddock et al, 1989). It is unfortunate that in the centre most critical of the use of oesophageal tamponade, the identified deficiencies of management were not rectified and there was little change in subsequent morbidity and mortality rates over 10 years later (Chojkier and Conn, 1980).

We have shown previously that three factors, namely prothrombin ratio, serum creatinine and the presence of encephalopathy, were found to have independent significance in the prediction of outcome following acute variceal haemorrhage (Garden et al, 1985). The regression equation derived using these factors accurately predicted outcome in 90% of cases and patients with prognostic scores of 0.66 or greater would be expected to survive admission. It is interesting to note that in our own experience of managing variceal haemorrhage by tamponade (Haddock et al, 1989), only four of the tube-related deaths occurred in patients with a prognostic score of >0.66. Thus it could be argued that factors other than tamponade contributed significantly to the deaths of those patients with poor prognostic scores, although the possibility cannot be ignored that the two patients who suffered oesophageal tears on intubation might otherwise have survived.

Aspiration of secretions is the most common complication of tamponade and is reported in 10–20% of cases (Conn and Simpson, 1967; Chojkier and Conn; 1980; Barsoum et al, 1982; Sarin and Nundy, 1984). Our policy has been to avoid sedation of patients when passing the tube in the hope of reducing the risk of aspiration pneumonia although intubation in restless patients may be hazardous. The incidence of pneumonia per intubation (7%) in our own series may reflect unfairly on oesophageal tamponade given that most of these patients proceeded to sclerotherapy, conducted in some cases under general anaesthesia (McKee et al, 1991). The use of a four-lumen tube undoubtedly minimizes the risk of aspiration and respiratory complications (Pitcher, 1967) but the importance of constant expert nursing supervision and care cannot be overemphasized.

Rupture of the oesophagus can occur if the gastric balloon is inflated in the oesophagus (Chojkier and Conn, 1980) or if the tube is withdrawn precipitously with the balloons inflated (Garden et al, 1983). Perforation and tearing of the oesophagus may also occur during passage of the tube (Conn and Simpson, 1967). Excessive traction should be avoided and traction using pulleys and weights has been replaced in most centres by simple taping of the tube to the nose or cheek. Removal of the tube by patients is, in our own experience, infrequent; limited inflation of the gastric balloon may account for the fact that only one of our eight patients who pulled out their tube sustained oesophageal rupture.

In a prospective controlled randomized study comparing a programme of endoscopic sclerotherapy with tamponade alone in acute variceal haemorrhage, Paquet and Feussner (1985) reported an initial control rate of 73% for tamponade as opposed to 95% for sclerotherapy. This difference was not statistically significant although, not surprisingly, definitive control of haemorrhage at 30 days was significantly better in the sclerotherapy group. While it may be desirable to attempt emergency sclerotherapy of bleeding varices, injection is undoubtedly easier when haemorrhage has ceased, and may not be practical in the face of torrential bleeding. Furthermore many centres do not have the necessary expertise to provide an emergency sclerotherapy service. Tamponade may therefore offer a useful means of arresting haemorrhage until definitive sclerotherapy can be instituted.

VASOPRESSIN AND ITS ANALOGUES

The posterior pituitary hormone, vasopressin (also known as antidiuretic hormone) is a short-lived peptide with vasoconstrictive properties when introduced into the circulation. It was first used to treat presumed variceal haemorrhage in 1957, when bleeding in two patients was arrested (Kehne et al, 1956). Vasopressin is thought to cause splanchnic arteriolar constriction, resulting in reduced portal inflow and a consequent fall in portal venous pressure (Texter et al, 1964; Freedman et al, 1978). Catheterization studies in dog and man have confirmed that vasopressin reduces portal pressure by 23–32% (Sirinek et al, 1977; Bosch et al, 1981; Groszmann et al, 1982; Mols et al, 1984) when wedged hepatic venous pressure gradient is used as an index. However, wedged hepatic venous pressure gradient does not fall in all patients, giving rise to the suggestion that vasopressin is only of use in patients who have reversed flow in the portal system and established oesophageal collaterals (Kallio and Lempinen, 1983). Azygos blood flow, as measured by thermodilution, is decreased by 25% by vasopressin (Bosch et al, 1985), again suggesting that portal pressure is diminished.

Much of our understanding of the portal haemodynamic effects of vasopressin has been derived from studies involving animal models of portal hypertension or stable patients with cirrhosis. There is some evidence that the effects of vasopressin may be less marked after bleeding has occurred. For example, rats with portal hypertension subjected to bleeding required much larger doses of vasopressin (ten-fold) to produce the decrease in portal flow and pressure seen when vasopressin was given during a controlled stable state (Kravetz et al, 1987). On the other hand, Ready et al (1991) have recently demonstrated that intravenous infusion of relatively small doses of vasopressin (0.2 units/min) significantly decreased wedged hepatic venous pressure, transhepatic venous pressure gradient (wedged minus free hepatic venous pressure) and heart rate in patients with alcoholic liver disease during bleeding from oesophageal varices. Tachyphylaxis did not occur over the 26-h study, doubling the infusion rate did not produce further decreases in the parameters studied, and there was no evidence of a 'rebound' effect when the infusion was stopped.

Despite the widespread clinical use of vasopressin in patients with variceal haemorrhage for some 35 years, there have been few randomized controlled trials to evaluate its efficacy. In essence, despite varied methods and routes of administration (intravenous versus intra-arterial; bolus, constant infusion, multiple dose schedules), vasopressin has proved no better than placebo (Fogel et al, 1982), conventional medical management (Conn et al, 1975) or balloon tamponade (Corrila et al, 1984) in terms of need for surgery, transfusion requirement or mortality. In comparison with other pharmacological agents also, vasopressin has failed to produce impressive results. For example, Freeman et al (1982) found that vasopressin controlled bleeding in only 9% of cases whereas a control rate of 70% was achieved with terlipressin, while Kravetz et al (1984) reported that while vasopressin and somatostatin gave comparable control rates (58% versus 53% respectively), somatostatin had a much lower complication rate.

A major problem attending the use of vasopressin has been its propensity to cause cardiac complications. Coronary vasoconstriction, reduced cardiac output, myocardial ischaemia and infarction, and fatal arrhythmias are all well-recognized complications. Vasodilators such as nitroprusside and nitroglycerin have been used in an attempt to minimize these adverse cardiocirculatory effects while maintaining or even enhancing the effect of vasopressin on portal flow and pressure. In a controlled study from Taiwan involving 39 patients with bleeding varices, vasopressin infusion alone was compared to vasopressin with sublingual nitroglycerin (0.6 mg every 6 h). No differences in bleeding control or survival rates were observed but 32% of patients treated with vasopressin alone had to stop treatment compared to 10% in the group receiving combination treatment (Tsai et al, 1986). In a study from London, Gimson et al (1986) compared vasopressin alone with the combination of vasopressin and intravenous nitroglycerin (40–400 μg/min). Bleeding was controlled significantly more often in the combination therapy group (68% versus 44%) and complications necessitating cessation of therapy were less frequent (3% versus 21%); no differences in survival rates were observed.

Thus, considerable controversy still surrounds the use of vasopressin in variceal bleeding. It has been our view that the evidence in its favour was unconvincing and that the danger of adverse cardiocirculatory side-effects was sufficiently real to preclude its use. Attempts have been made to retain the portal haemodynamic effects of vasopressin and reduce undesirable side-effects by giving its synthetic triglycyl-lysine derivative, terlipressin (Glypressin). This agent has less antidiuretic hormone activity and does not increase plasminogen activator concentrations (Douglas et al, 1979); it is in effect an expensive slow-release form of vasopressin and a bolus intravenous injection of 1–2 mg is given every 6 h. As mentioned earlier, terlipressin controlled bleeding much more effectively than vasopressin and reduced transfusion requirements in controlled trials (Freeman et al, 1982, 1989) although systemic haemodynamic complications have still been observed. As might be anticipated, the combination of terlipressin and nitroglycerin has also been evaluated (Lin et al, 1990) and encouraging preliminary results underline the need for further study to define the value of this approach. As pointed out by MacDougall et al (1991), the combination of a bolus injection of terlipressin and the skin patch administration of nitroglycerin would provide an appealing method of controlling variceal bleeding during the transfer of patients to specialist centres.

SOMATOSTATIN

Somatostatin is a 14-amino-acid peptide which in most studies has been shown to reduce splanchnic blood flow in animals and man. However, it must be stressed that some studies have failed to demonstrate any significant effect on portal tributary blood flow (Sonnenberg et al, 1981; Merkel et al, 1985) or intravariceal pressure (Kleber et al, 1988). Varying doses, varying forms of somatostatin and the presence or absence of general anaesthesia have given rise to some confusion, as has the use of different indices of portal venous pressure and flow. Studies using the synthetic analogue SMS 201-995 in conscious rats with portal hypertension have shown that this long-acting preparation (half-life 1–2 h as opposed to 2–3 min for naturally occurring somatostatin) significantly decreased portal venous tributary flow by 18–27% depending on whether the portal hypertension was non-cirrhotic or cirrhotic (Cerini et al, 1988). The analogue decreased cardiac output by approximately 20% while increasing mean arterial pressure and systemic vascular resistance. It was concluded that SMS 201-995 reduces portal pressure principally by reducing portal tributary flow and that this is achieved through a direct vasoconstrictive effect or by an indirect effect mediated by reduced release of vasoactive hormone(s). In our own study of haemodynamically stable cirrhotic patients, SMS 201-995 reduced cardiac index while increasing systemic vascular resistance and producing a fall in wedged hepatic venous pressure and transhepatic venous gradient (Pringle et al, 1988).

Uncontrolled studies in patients with variceal bleeding have shown benefit in two studies (Thulin et al, 1979; Limberg and Kommerell, 1980) but no benefit in one (Raptis and Zoupas, 1979). Early controlled comparison showed that in one small study, all somatostatin-treated patients stopped bleeding without complications as opposed to only one-third of vasopressin-treated patients (Jenkins et al, 1985). In a larger study mentioned earlier, the two agents proved equally effective (53% versus 58% control rate) but somatostatin appeared safer in that one-quarter of vasopressin-treated patients had to have therapy withdrawn (Kravetz et al, 1984).

In more recent placebo-controlled studies, one multicentre trial (Valenzuela et al, 1989) failed to show significant benefit in that in the 30-h study period 65% of patients given somatostatin stopped bleeding as opposed to 83% of those given placebo. Despite the somewhat surprising 'success' of placebo, transfusion requirements and mortality rates were similar in the two groups. In a trial from the Royal Free Hospital, London, somatostatin proved significantly more effective than placebo in controlling bleeding (64% versus 41%), and when rebleeding occurred it did so earlier in the placebo group (Burroughs et al, 1990). Somatostatin significantly reduced blood and plasma transfusion requirements and halved the need for balloon tamponade. Although it was concluded that somatostatin was safe and more effective at controlling bleeding than placebo, 30-day mortality was not affected. As pointed out by Resnick (1990), the Royal Free trial continued with the same concentration of intravenous infusion (250 μg/h) for 5 days, suggesting that a longer period of drug administration may be necessary to avoid rebleeding.

In our own prospective controlled comparison of SMS 201-995 and balloon tamponade in patients with endoscopically proven acute variceal bleeding, there was no significant difference in time to control bleeding, transfusion requirement or number of patients requiring cross-over to the other treatment arm (R. F. McKee et al, unpublished data). However, all patients randomized to receive SMS 201-995 survived to leave hospital as opposed to 15 of the 20 allocated to balloon tamponade ($p = 0.047$).

OTHER DRUGS AND ACUTE VARICEAL BLEEDING

Propranolol is a non-selective β-adrenergic blocking drug which reduces cardiac output and heart rate, and produces a fall in portal venous blood flow. Acute administration decreases wedged hepatic venous pressure by a variable extent in man and the effect can be maintained by continued oral administration (Hillon et al, 1982; Mills et al, 1984; Westaby et al, 1984; Groszmann et al, 1990). Animal experiments also indicate that portal venous flow is reduced by 30% by propranolol (Calès et al, 1985; Kroeger and Groszmann, 1985) and a similar decrease in azygos flow has been reported in man (Bosch et al, 1984; Calès et al, 1984). The reductions in portal venous pressure and flow by propranolol are not solely the result of diminished cardiac output in that cardioselective β-blockers such as atenolol cause lesser falls in portal venous pressure, the magnitudes of which are directly proportional to the reduction in cardiac output (Mills et al, 1984). It appears that splanchnic vasoconstriction resulting from blockade of $β_2$-adrenergic receptors in the splanchnic bed is also implicated.

Propranolol has been shown in most controlled studies to reduce the risk of rebleeding in portal hypertension (Lebrec et al, 1984; Garden et al, 1990; Hayes et al, 1990) although some trials have shown no benefit (Burroughs et al, 1983). Despite its potential value in prevention of bleeding and its acute effects on portal venous pressure and flow, propranolol is not recommended for use as a vasoactive agent in the control of acute variceal bleeding.

Other vasoactive drugs, such as the α-adrenergic blocker prazosin, also reduce portal pressure (Mills et al, 1984) but, like propranolol, they are not used in the control of acute variceal haemorrhage.

Agents which affect the lower oesophageal sphincter such as pentagastrin and metoclopramide may also prove to have a beneficial effect on portal venous pressure (Miskowiak et al, 1981; Hosking et al, 1988), but as yet they have no established place in patient management.

SUMMARY

Successful pharmacological arrest of haemorrhage might avoid the risk of aspiration associated with tamponade and early studies have suggested that the vasoactive agent somatostatin may be as effective and perhaps safer than tamponade in controlling variceal haemorrhage. In our view, vasopressin has not established a role in management but we retain an open mind regarding the potential use of terlipressin in combination with nitroglycerin. It is unlikely that any of these agents can improve significantly our ability to control variceal haemorrhage when compared to balloon tamponade but they may reduce the incidence of pulmonary complications and thereby reduce subsequent mortality.

Tamponade has proved successful in controlling acute haemorrhage from oesophageal varices in our hands. Late complications continue to give cause for concern but until effective safe alternatives to tamponade are developed, we continue to advocate its use for emergency control of acute variceal haemorrhage. Our own studies have shown that the high mortality seen in this patient population may reflect the severity of the underlying liver disease rather than failure of a management policy employing oesophageal tamponade for the initial control of acute variceal haemorrhage.

REFERENCES

Barsoum MS, Bolous FI, El-Rooby AA et al (1982) Tamponade and injection sclerotherapy in the management of bleeding oesophageal varices. *British Journal of Surgery* **69:** 76–78.

Bauer JJ, Kreel I & Kark AE (1974) The use of the Sengstaken–Blakemore tube for immediate control of bleeding esophageal varices. *Annals of Surgery* **179:** 273–277.

Bosch J, Kravetz D & Rodes J (1981) Effects of somatostatin on hepatic and systemic haemodynamics in patients with cirrhosis of the liver: comparison with vasopressin. *Gastroenterology* **80:** 518–525.

Bosch J, Mastai R, Kravetz D et al (1984) Effects of propranolol on azygos venous blood flow and hepatic and system haemodynamics in cirrhosis. *Hepatology* **4:** 1200–1205.

Bosch J, Mastai R, Kravetz D et al (1985) Measurement of azygos blood flow in the evaluation of portal hypertension in patients with cirrhosis. *Journal of Hepatology* **1:** 125–129.

Boyce HW (1962) Modification of the Sengstaken–Blakemore balloon tube. *New England Journal of Medicine* **267:** 195–196.

Burroughs AK, Jenkins WJ, Sherlock S et al (1983) Controlled trial of propranolol for the prevention of recurrent variceal haemorrhage in patients with cirrhosis. *New England Journal of Medicine* **309:** 1539–1542.

Burroughs AK, McCormick PA, Hughes MD et al (1990) Randomized, double-blind, placebo-controlled trial of somatostatin for variceal bleeding. *Gastroenterology* **99:** 1388–1395.

Calès P, Braillon A, Jiron MI & Lebrec D (1984) Superior portosystemic collateral circulation estimated by azygos blood flow in patients with cirrhosis. *Journal of Hepatology* **1:** 37–46.

Calès P, Braillon A, Girod C & Lebrec D (1985) Effects of propranolol on splanchnic circulation in portal hypertensive rats. *Gastroenterology* **88:** 857 (letter).

Cerini R, Lee SS, Hadengue A et al (1988) Circulatory effects of somatostatin analogue in two conscious rat models of portal hypertension. *Gastroenterology* **94:** 703–708.

Chojkier M & Conn HO (1980) Esophageal tamponade in the treatment of bleeding varices: a decadal progress report. *Digestive Diseases and Sciences* **25:** 267–272.

Conn HO (1958) Hazards attending use of esophageal tamponade. *New England Journal of Medicine* **259:** 701–707.

Conn HO (1971) Sengstaken–Blakemore tube revisited. *Gastroenterology* **62:** 398–400.

Conn HO & Simpson JA (1967) Excessive mortality associated with balloon tamponade of bleeding varices: a critical reappraisal. *Journal of the American Medical Association* **202:** 587–591.

Conn HO, Ramsey GR, Storer EH et al (1975) Intra-arterial vasopressin in the treatment of upper gastrointestinal haemorrhage: a prospective controlled clinical trial. *Gastroenterology* **68:** 211–221.

Corrila JP, Alves MM, Alexandrino P & Silveira J (1984) Controlled trial of vasopressin and balloon tamponade in bleeding oesophageal varices. *Hepatology* **4:** 885–888.

Douglas JG, Forest JAH, Prowse CV et al (1979) Effects of lysine, vasopressin and glypressin on the fibrinolytic system in cirrhosis. *Gut* **20:** 565–567.

Edlich RF, Lande AJ, Goodale RL & Wangensteen OH (1968) Prevention of aspiration pneumonia by continuous esophageal aspiration during esophagogastric tamponade and gastric cooling. *Surgery* **64:** 405–408.

Fogel MR, Knauer M, Ljudevit L et al (1982) Continuous intravenous vasopressin in active upper gastrointestinal bleeding—a placebo controlled trial. *Annals of Internal Medicine* **96:** 565–569.

Freedman AR, Kerr JC, Swan KG et al (1978) Primate mesenteric blood flow. Effect of vasopressin and its route of delivery. *Gastroenterology* **74:** 875–878.

Freeman JG, Cobden I, Lishman AH & Record CO (1982) Controlled trial of terlipressin (glypressin) versus vasopressin in the early treatment of oesophageal varices. *Lancet* **ii:** 66–68.

Freeman J, Cobden I & Record C (1989) Placebo controlled trial of glypressin in the management of acute variceal bleeding. *Journal of Clinical Gastroenterology* **11:** 58–60.

Garden OJ, Osborne DH, Blamey SL & Carter DC (1983) The management of acute variceal haemorrhage. *Australian and New Zealand Journal of Surgery* **53:** 197–202.

Garden OJ, Motyl H, Gilmour WH et al (1985) Prediction of outcome following acute variceal haemorrhage. *British Journal of Surgery* **72:** 91–95.

Garden OJ, Mills PR, Birnie GG et al (1990) Propranolol in the prevention of recurrent variceal hemorrhage in cirrhotic patients. A controlled trial. *Gastroenterology* **98:** 185–190.

Gimson AES, Westaby D, Hegarty J et al (1986) A randomised trial of vasopressin and vasopressin plus nitroglycerin in the control of acute variceal haemorrhage. *Hepatology* **6:** 410–413.

Groszmann RJ, Kravetz D, Bosch J et al (1982) Nitroglycerin improves the haemodynamic response to vasopressin in portal hypertension. *Hepatology* **2:** 757–762.

Groszmann RJ, Bosch J, Grace ND et al (1990) Hemodynamic events in a prospective randomized trial of propranolol versus placebo in the prevention of a first variceal haemorrhage. *Gastroenterology* **99:** 1401–1407.

Haddock G, Garden OJ, McKee RF et al (1989) Esophageal tamponade in the management of acute variceal hemorrhage. *Digestive Diseases and Sciences* **34:** 913–918.

Hayes PC, Davis JM, Lewis JA & Bouchier IAD (1990) Meta-analysis of value of propranolol in prevention of variceal haemorrhage. *Lancet* **336:** 153–156.

Hillon P, Lebrec D, Munoz C et al (1982) Comparison of the effects of a cardioselective and non-cardioselective β-blocker on portal hypertension in patients with cirrhosis. *Hepatology* **2:** 528–531.

Hosking SW, Doss W, el-Zeiny H et al (1988) Pharmacological constriction of the lower oesophageal sphincter: a simple method of arresting variceal haemorrhage. *Gut* **29:** 1098–1102.

Jenkins SA, Baxter JN, Corbett WA et al (1985) A prospective randomised controlled clinical trial comparing somatostatin and vasopressin in controlling acute variceal haemorrhage. *British Medical Journal* **290:** 275–278.

Kallio H & Lempinen M (1983) Effect of vasopressin on portal venous pressure. *Acta Chirurgica Scandinavica* **149:** 49–52.

Kehne JH, Hughes FA & Compertz ML (1956) Use of surgical pituitrin in control of oesophageal varix bleeding: experimental study and report of two cases. *Surgery* **39:** 917–925.

Kleber G, Sauerbruch T, Fischer G & Paumgartner G (1988) Somatostatin does not reduce oesophageal variceal pressure in liver cirrhotics. *Gut* **29:** 153–156.

Kravetz D, Bosch J, Teres J et al (1984) Comparison of intravenous somatostatin and vasopressin infusions in treatment of acute variceal haemorrhage. *Hepatology* **4:** 442–446.

Kravetz D, Cummings SA & Groszmann RJ (1987) Hyposensitivity to vasopressin in a hemorrhaged-transfused rat model of portal hypertension. *Gastroenterology* **93:** 170–175.

Kroeger RJ & Groszmann RJ (1985) Increased portal venous resistance during the administration of β-adrenergic blocking agents in a portal hypertensive model. *Hepatology* **5:** 97–101.

Lebrec D, Poynard T, Bernuau J et al (1984) A randomised controlled study of propranolol for prevention of recurrent gastrointestinal bleeding in patients with cirrhosis: a final report. *Hepatology* **4:** 355–358.

Limberg B & Kommerell B (1980) Somatostatin and bleeding esophageal varices: peer review anyone? *Gastroenterology* **78:** 658–659.

Lin HC, Tsai YT, Lee FY et al (1990) Systemic and portal haemodynamic changes following triglycyllysine vasopressin plus nitroglycerin administration in patients with hepatitis B-related cirrhosis. *Journal of Hepatology* **10:** 370–374.

Linton RR & Ellis DS (1956) Emergency and definitive treatment of bleeding esophageal varices. *Journal of the American Medical Association* **160:** 1017–1023.

MacDougall BRD, Westaby D & Blendis LA (1991) Portal hypertension—25 years of progress. *Gut* **32 (supplement)** S18–S24.

McKee RF, Garden OJ & Carter DC (1991) Injection sclerotherapy for bleeding varices: risk factors and complications. *British Journal of Surgery* **78:** 1098–1101.

Merkel C, Gatta A, Zuin R et al (1985) Effect of somatostatin on splanchnic haemodynamics in patients with liver cirrhosis and portal hypertension. *Digestion* **32:** 92–98.

Mills PR, Rae AP, Farah DA et al (1984) Comparison of three adrenoreceptor blocking agents in patients with cirrhosis and portal hypertension. *Gut* **25:** 73–78.

Miskowiak J, Burcharth F & Jensen LI (1981) Effect of lower oesophageal sphincter on oesophageal varices: a portographic study. *Scandinavian Journal of Gastroenterology* **16:** 957–960.

Mitchell K, Silk DBA & Williams R (1981) Prospective comparison of two Sengstaken tubes in the management of patients with variceal haemorrhage. *Gut* **21:** 570–573.

Mols P, Hallemans R, Van Kuyk M et al (1984) Haemodynamic effects of vasopressin, alone and in combination with nitroprusside in patients with liver cirrhosis and portal hypertension. *Annals of Surgery* **199:** 176–181.

Nachlas MM (1956) Experience of the triple-lumen single balloon tube in massive upper gastrointestinal haemorrhage. *Gastroenterology* **30:** 913–928.

Novis BH, Duys P, Barbezat GO et al (1976) Fibreoptic endoscopy and the use of the Sengstaken tube in acute gastrointestinal haemorrhage in patients with portal hypertension and varices. *Gut* **17:** 258–263.

Panes J, Teres J, Bosch J & Rodes J (1988) Efficacy of balloon tamponade in treatment of bleeding gastric and esophageal varices: results in 151 consecutive episodes. *Digestive Diseases and Sciences* **33:** 454–459.

Paquet K-J & Feussner H (1985) Endoscopic sclerosis and balloon tamponade in acute hemorrhage from esophagogastric varices: prospective controlled randomised trial. *Hepatology* **5:** 580–583.

Pitcher JL (1967) Safety and effectiveness of the modified Sengstaken–Blakemore tube: a prospective study. *Gastroenterology* **61:** 291–298.

Pringle SD, McKee RF, Garden OJ et al (1988) The effect of a long-acting somatostatin analogue on portal and systemic haemodynamics in cirrhosis. *Alimentary Pharmacology and Therapeutics* **2:** 451–459.

Pugh RNH, Murray-Lyon IM, Dawson JL et al (1973) Transection of the oesophagus for bleeding oesophageal varices. *British Journal of Surgery* **60:** 646–649.

Raptis S & Zoupas C (1979) Somatostatin not helpful in bleeding oesophageal varices. *New Zealand Journal of Medicine* **300:** 736.

Read AE, Dawson AM, Kerr DNA & Turner MD (1960) Bleeding oesophageal varices treated by oesophageal compression tube. *British Medical Journal* **1:** 227–231.

Ready JB, Robertson AD & Rector WG Jr (1991) Effects of vasopressin on portal pressure during hemorrhage from esophageal varices. *Gastroenterology* **100:** 1411–1416.

Resnick RH (1990) Somatostatin for variceal bleeding. *Gastroenterology* **99:** 1524–1526.

Rowntree LG, Zimmerman EF, Todd MH & Ajac J (1947) Intra-esophageal venous tamponade: its use in a case of variceal hemorrhage from the esophagus. *Journal of the American Medical Association* **13:** 630–631.

Sarin SK & Nundy S (1984) Balloon tamponade in the management of bleeding oesophageal varices. *Annals of the Royal College of Surgeons of England* **66:** 30–32.

Sengstaken RW & Blakemore AH (1950) Balloon tamponade for the control of hemorrhage from esophageal varices. *Annals of Surgery* **131:** 781–789.

Sirinek KR, Thomford NR & Pace WG (1977) Adverse cardio-dynamic effects of vasopressin not avoided by selective intra-arterial administration. *Surgery* **81:** 723–728.

Sonnenberg GE, Keller V, Perruchoud A et al (1981) Effect of somatostatin on splanchnic haemodynamics in patients with cirrhosis and normal subjects. *Gastroenterology* **80:** 526–532.

Texter CE, Chou CC, Merrill SL et al (1964) Direct effect of vasoactive agents on sequential

resistances of the mesenteric and portal circulation. *Journal of Laboratory and Clinical Medicine* **64:** 624–633.
Thulin L, Tyden G, Samnegard H et al (1979) Treatment of bleeding oesophageal varices with somatostatin. *Acta Chirurgica Scandinavica* **145:** 395–397.
Tsai YT, Lay CS, Lai KW et al (1986) Controlled trial of vasopressin alone in the treatment of bleeding oesophageal varices. *Hepatology* **6:** 406–409.
Valenzuela JE, Schubert T, Fogel MR et al (1989) A multicenter randomized double-blind trial of somatostatin in management of acute hemorrhage from esophageal varices. *Hepatology* **10:** 958–961.
Westaby D, Bihari DJ, Gimson AE et al (1984) Selective and non-selective beta-receptor blockade in the reduction of portal pressure in patients with cirrhosis and portal hypertension. *Gut* **25:** 121–124.
Westphal K (1930) Uber Eine Kompression Behandlung Der Blutungen Aus Esophagus Varizen. *Deutsche Medizinische Wochenschrift* **56:** 1135.

4

Emergency and elective endoscopic therapy for variceal haemorrhage

D. WESTABY

A little more than 50 years have passed since the first case report of the transoesophageal injection of a sclerosing agent into oesophageal varices to prevent rebleeding (Crafoord and Frenckner, 1939). The next 30 years saw fewer than 20 further reports which originated from a small group of enthusiasts who considered injection sclerotherapy superior to the major alternative of portosystemic shunt surgery (Westaby and Williams, 1983). The last two decades have seen a remarkable expansion of reports relating to injection sclerotherapy, culminating in a number of important controlled trials to assess the efficacy of the technique.

Up until the last five years the injection of sclerosing agents was the only local endoscopic therapy in widespread use. However, two new local treatments have been introduced, firstly the direct intravariceal injection of tissue adhesives and secondly the placement of prestressed rubber bands to ligate the variceal cords. The initial reports of these techniques have been encouraging and there is some evidence to suggest that in the future the endoscopic therapy used will be selected on an individual basis governed by the clinical setting and the observed variceal anatomy.

TECHNIQUES OF LOCAL ENDOSCOPIC THERAPY

Injection sclerotherapy

The earliest experience with injection sclerotherapy, by necessity, used the rigid oesophagoscope under general anaesthesia. However, it was the introduction of fibreoptic endoscopes in the early 1970s which led to a massive increase in the availability of the technique. Many of those experienced with the use of the rigid oesophagoscope maintained that this offered enhanced control of a varix bleeding point and enabled more accurate injection of the sclerosant. However, the only control trial to compare the rigid and flexible techniques, carried out by a group who were extremely experienced in both disciplines, failed to show any benefit for the rigid instrument (Bornman et al, 1988).

Two very different approaches to the injection of sclerosant have been developed. In the USA and the UK, most workers inject the sclerosant directly into the varix lumen, with the aim of luminal obliteration. Groups in Austria and Germany developed an alternative concept in which multiple small injections of sclerosant were placed immediately adjacent to the varix, with the aim of initiating local fibrogenesis which would then provide a protective covering over an intact varix. However, the differences between these two techniques may be more theoretical than real as local vessel thrombosis and extensive scarring are a uniform response to the diffuse action of sclerosing agents, whichever site they are injected at (Helpap and Bollweg, 1981; Evans et al, 1982). In experienced hands the results of these two techniques appear to be very similar, although the only controlled trial reported suggests an advantage for the intravariceal approach (Sarin et al, 1986b). A combination of the two techniques has been described (Soehendra et al, 1983) and has been widely adopted. Attempts to improve the efficacy of injection sclerotherapy have included the use of an outer oesophageal sheath, which was designed to offer some of the control associated with the rigid endoscope with the ease of manipulation found with the flexible instrument (Williams and Dawson, 1979). A controlled trial comparing sclerotherapy with or without this outer oesophageal sheath did confirm some benefits for the former, particularly with respect to early obliteration of varices (Westaby et al, 1983). However, this and a more recent encouraging report describing an alternative technique utilizing an outer oesophageal sheath (Kitano et al, 1987) have not led to widespread adoption.

There is now a sizeable list of compounds that have been used as sclerosing agents and their efficacy has been evaluated both in vivo and in vitro (Jensen et al, 1986; Kitano et al, 1988; Sarin et al, 1988; Balanzo et al, 1989). This type of study is notoriously difficult to interpret, but it is reasonable to summarize that a number of sclerosing agents (Table 1) when used in experienced hands have a similar efficacy and safety profile.

Table 1. Sclerosing agents.

Ethanolamine oleate
Polidocanol
Sodium tetradecyl sulphate
Sodium morrhuate
Alcohol (50% or 100%)
Thrombin

The extent to which therapy should extend orally above the gastro-oesophageal junction has largely remained an empirical decision. Primarily, this is influenced by the size and length of the variceal cords. However, recent studies of the normal venous anatomy of the lower oesophagus and that observed in portal hypertension have provided some objective information as to the optimal sites of injection (Vianna et al, 1987). These studies have confirmed a number of different pathways by which portal venous blood might reach the lower oesophageal vessels. Of particular importance are large perforating veins communicating between the intrinsic and para-oesophageal vessels (Figure 1). These perforating vessels have been confirmed in vivo by doppler ultrasound with evidence of bidirectional flow

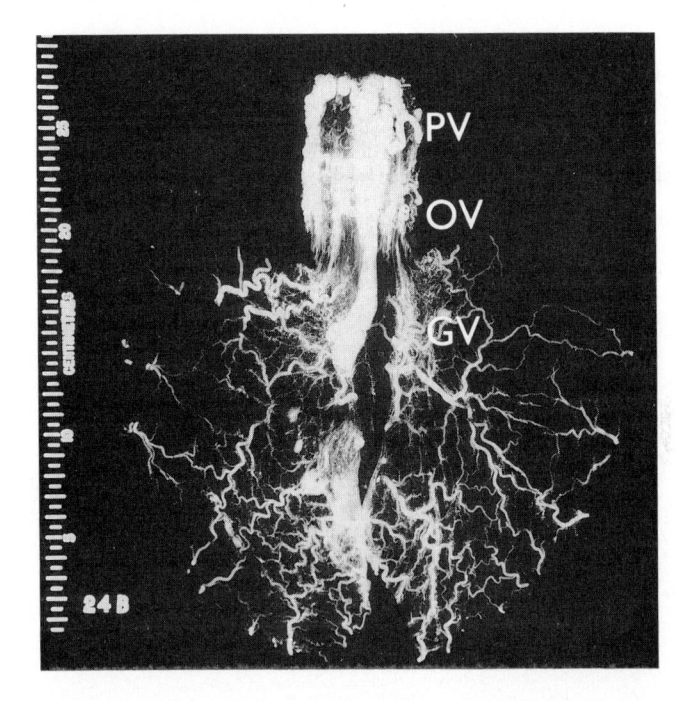

Figure 1. A radiograph taken of a post mortem preparation demonstrating the venous system of the gastro-oesophageal junction from a patient with portal hypertension. The portal vein has been infused with a barium-gelatin mixture. GV, gastric varix; OV, oesophageal varices; PV, perforating veins.

(MacCormack et al, 1983). It is reasonable to assume that, in portal hypertension, retrograde flow through these perforating vessels might maintain the patency of the intrinsic oesophageal varices. Therefore, any local endoscopic therapy should plan to obliterate not only the intrinsic vessels crossing the gastro-oesophageal junction but also the perforating vessels in the zone 3–5 cm proximal in the oesophagus.

The endoscopic injection of tissue adhesive

The tissue adhesives in n-butyl-2-cyanoacrylate (histoacryl) and isobutyl-2-cyanoacrylate (bucrylate) have both been used for the treatment of oesophageal and gastric fundal varices (Ramond et al, 1986; Soehendra et al, 1986). These agents solidify almost instantaneously when brought into contact with blood (Yamamoto and Suzuki, 1989). The aim of the technique is to produce rapid obliteration of the varix lumen. As a consequence, accurate intravariceal injection is a prerequisite for this to be achieved. The technique of injection requires care in providing a clean and dry needle to minimize the risk of premature adhesive hardening. The risk of the adhesive occluding the endoscope channels may be reduced by applying silicone oil to the tip of the instrument. The mixing of the tissue adhesive with the contrast agent lipiodol has been used to reduce the risk of premature hardening and also to allow radiological monitoring of the injections (Soehendra et al, 1986, 1987).

Endoscopic banding ligation of varices

Endoscopic ligation of varices is carried out using a device that attaches to the end of a conventional forward-viewing gastroscope. The technique is

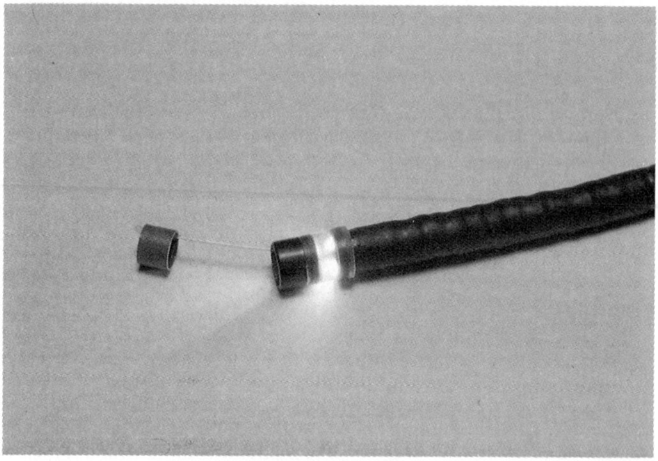

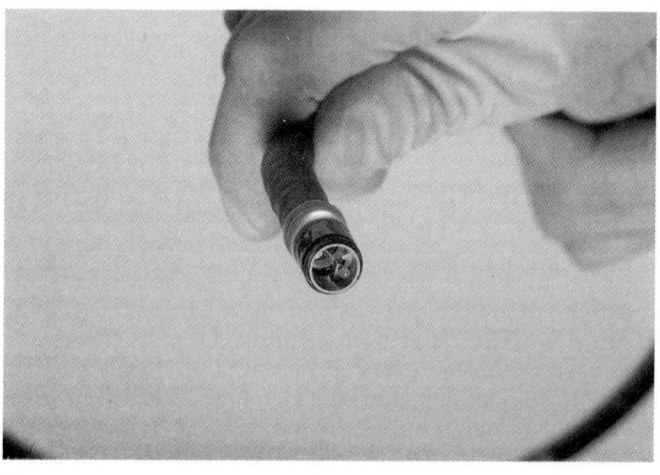

(a)

(b)

Figure 2. The equipment used for banding ligation. A short cylinder is attached to the tip of the endoscope. Placed within this is an inner cylinder, the prestressed rubber band at its distal end. A nylon thread passed through the biopsy channel and attached to the inner cylinder facilitates band release.

based upon the same concept as that used for banding ligation of internal haemorrhoids. The banding device consists of two cylinders, the outer one being in a fixed position attached to the endoscope tip; the inner cylinder has a prestressed rubber band positioned at its distal end and is free to move within the outer cylinder (Figure 2). The endoscope and attached banding device are brought into close apposition to a varix cord which is then drawn into the device by using continuous suction. When the inner banding cylinder is filled with the varix this is retracted within the outer cylinder by a trip wire running through the biopsy channel of the endoscope. This manoeuvre serves to roll the prestressed band over the entrapped varix, leaving a strangulated length of vessel (Figure 3). Placement of the bands

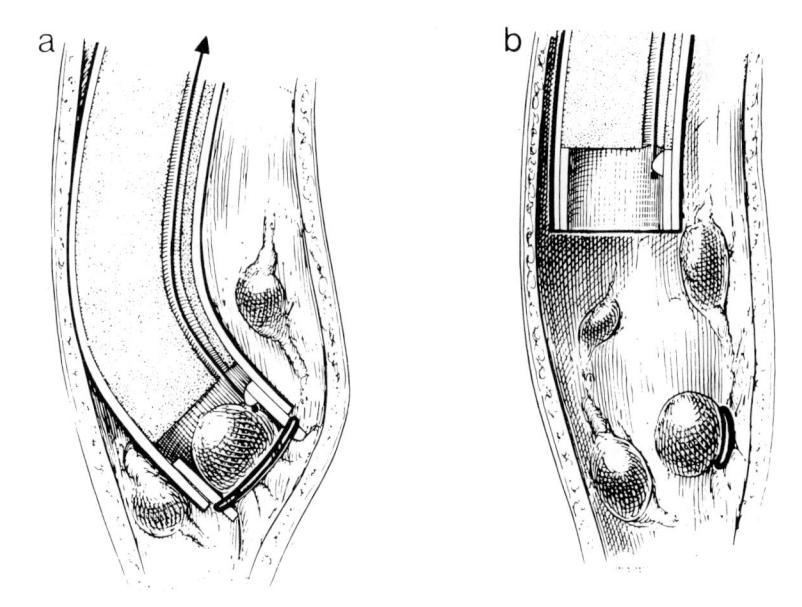

Figure 3. A diagrammatic representation of the banding technique. The varix is aspirated into the inner cylinder and the band released, leaving a 'polyp-like' strangulated varix.

starts caudally at the gastro-oesophageal junction and extends about 5 cm orally (see above). A median of 6–8 bands are placed on the first session. The repeated intubation that is required for this technique is facilitated by the initial insertion of an oesophageal sheath. The strangulated sections of varix slough off within 5–7 days, leaving a small discrete ulcer. The depth of ligated tissue provides a considerable safety margin to avoid full-thickness oesophageal wall necrosis; however, this risk may arise in children under the age of 5 in whom banding ligation should be avoided. The technique is also unsuitable for fundal gastric varices, the size of which exceeds the capacity of the banding cylinder. This would result in partial vessel ligation and a high risk of precipitating further bleeding.

Schedules of repeated endoscopic therapy

The aim of long-term local endoscopic therapy is to obliterate the oesophageal varices to prevent recurrent bleeding. The optimal time interval between sessions of therapy has been the subject of a number of studies. In the early uncontrolled reports of injection sclerotherapy it was common to use an arbitrary three-week interval between sessions, but this led to very protracted periods to achieve variceal obliteration and theoretically exposed the patient to an increased risk of rebleeding. The reluctance to use shorter intervals reflected a concern that the complication rate might be increased, particularly oesophageal mucosal damage, stricture formation and full-thickness oesophageal wall necrosis. Two controlled trials have compared injection sclerotherapy carried out at three- and one-week intervals (Westaby et al, 1984; Sarin et al, 1986a). Both confirmed more rapid obliteration of varices using the shorter interval without any increased risk of complication. In one of the studies (Westaby et al, 1984) there was no difference in the frequency of rebleeding, but in the second there was a significant benefit associated with the shorter interval (Sarin et al, 1986a). A more recent study has assessed a shorter, three-day interval between sessions, but encountered an increased risk of mucosal damage without reducing the risk of early rebleeding (Akriviadis et al, 1989). Based on these investigations a one-week interval between sessions of injection sclerotherapy may be considered the optimal schedule. Similar timing has been adopted both for the injection of tissue adhesives and banding ligation, although this has not been assessed in any objective way.

The initial concept of long-term injection sclerotherapy envisaged a surveillance programme to follow the initial period of variceal obliteration. The aim of the surveillance programme was to detect recurrence of varices before they could be a source of further bleeding. The schedule for follow-up endoscopy has varied between centres, but has been based upon the observation that the majority of rebleeding episodes occur within the first 6–12 months after the initial obliteration of varices (Westaby and Williams, 1984). The efficacy of long-term surveillance programmes has never been fully established and is currently a subject of considerable controversy (see below).

COMPLICATIONS OF LOCAL ENDOSCOPIC THERAPY

Not surprisingly, the majority of the information concerning complications refers to the use of injection sclerotherapy. The most frequently observed complication is oesophageal mucosal damage. Ulceration at the site of previous injection is a very common finding, the frequency being dependent upon the timing of subsequent follow-up endoscopy (Westaby et al, 1984), reflecting the fact that most lesions heal spontaneously over a short period of time. Many workers would consider that ulceration observed at follow-up endoscopy is an integral part of injection sclerotherapy and should only be considered a complication when symptoms such as pain and particularly bleeding occur. In a study aimed specifically at identifying mucosal ulceration as a site of recurrent bleeding this was observed in almost 20% of patients (Polson et al, 1989). Oesophageal stricture formation was a frequent observation in the early reports of injection sclerotherapy, with an incidence of up to 15% of cases (Terblanche et al, 1979; MacDougall et al, 1982). This might, in part, reflect the use of the rigid oesophagoscope in the early reports (Kahn et al, 1989). In more recent reports this complication has been observed in less than 5% of cases and is seldom a cause of protracted symptoms, being easily managed by oesophageal dilatation.

Perforation of the oesophagus has been reported in up to 5% of cases undergoing sclerotherapy, but has been much less frequently observed since the replacement of the rigid oesophagoscope by fibreoptic instruments (Kahn et al, 1989). Perforation may occur as a result of direct trauma or more frequently by full-thickness oesophageal wall necrosis in response to the excessive injection of sclerosant. The former presents soon after the procedure, whereas the latter may produce insidious symptoms over a few days before the development of free perforation. Management is usually by conservative means, including pleural and mediastinal drainage, antibiotics, and parenteral nutrition. The overall mortality of oesophageal perforation is in excess of 50%, rising to almost 100% if surgical intervention is required.

Considerable attention has been directed towards the investigation of oesophageal motility following long-term injection sclerotherapy. The results of these studies have been conflicting. Abnormalities of the lower oesophageal sphincter have been documented with increased periods of acid reflux (Reilly et al, 1984; Snady and Korsten, 1986). Other studies have shown no abnormalities of oesophageal motility whatsoever (Sauerbruch et al, 1986; Siemens et al, 1989). Reflux-related symptoms are seldom a protracted problem in the post-sclerotherapy period and as such this militates against the importance of any documented motility disturbance.

The complications associated with tissue adhesive injection have not been extensively documented but appear to be similar to those experienced with the injection of sclerosing agents (Ramond et al, 1986; Soehendra et al, 1986). There is a report of two patients developing cerebrovascular accidents following bucrylate injection which was attributed to the dissemination of the tissue adhesive into the cerebral arterial system (See et al, 1986).

Reported complications associated with banding ligation have been encouragingly few (Stiegmann et al, 1990). One of the major aims of the technique was to minimize the local mucosal damage association with the injection of sclerosing agents. Discrete ulceration at the site of banding is the norm, but unlike the effect of sclerosing agents the extent is limited by the intrinsic design of the banding device. Thus, to date, there are no recorded cases of full-thickness oesophageal wall necrosis and perforation. Recurrent bleeding from the banding-related ulcer has been observed in approximately 10% of cases (Stiegmann et al, 1990).

RESULTS OF LOCAL ENDOSCOPIC TECHNIQUES FOR THE MANAGEMENT OF ACTIVE VARICEAL BLEEDING

Injection sclerotherapy

Two large, uncontrolled series were the first reports to strongly support the use of sclerotherapy for an episode of variceal bleeding (Johnston and Rodgers, 1973; Terblanche et al, 1981). Control of bleeding for the period of admission was achieved in 93% and 92% of cases respectively. In the majority of the cases reported, variceal haemorrhage had been initially controlled by balloon tamponade, prior to carrying out sclerotherapy. Subsequently, a number of controlled trials have been carried out in which injection sclerotherapy has been compared to conservative measures such as balloon tamponade or vasoconstrictor therapy, either as a single therapy or in combination (Barsoum et al, 1982; Paquet and Feussner, 1985; Soderlund and Ihre, 1985; Larson et al, 1986; Moreto et al, 1988). In four of these five trials (Barsoum et al, 1982; Paquet and Feussner, 1985; Soderlund and Ihre, 1985; Moreto et al, 1988) control of bleeding was improved by sclerotherapy, but in none was a survival benefit observed, although a trend was evident. From these trials comparing injection sclerotherapy with conservative measures it is important to recognize that the former provides the ability not only to control active haemorrhage but also to prevent early rebleeding. Thus, when comparisons are extended over the full period of admission there is a bias towards injection sclerotherapy as compared to balloon tamponade or vasoconstrictor therapy, which are only effective for their period of application.

An important question that remained unanswered was the optimum timing of injection sclerotherapy with respect to the active bleeding episode. The options are immediate treatment, with the associated risks of complication and technical difficulties, or initial delay in order to allow vasoconstrictor drugs or balloon tamponade to provide temporary haemostasis. Preliminary data came from a report in which patients with active variceal bleeding were treated by immediate injection sclerotherapy and compared with a historical control group (Prindiville and Trudeau, 1986). Immediate sclerotherapy was able to control active bleeding in 89% of cases by the end of 48 hours, as compared to 64% in the historical control group ($p = 0.05$). In a subsequent randomized controlled trial, immediate sclerotherapy was compared to initial treatment with a regimen of vasopressin and nitroglycerine, the control of bleeding being assessed over the first 12 hours after randomization (Westaby et al, 1989). Both groups were then entered into a regimen of long-term injection sclerotherapy. Immediate sclerotherapy achieved control of bleeding in 88% of cases, compared to 65% of those treated by the vasoconstrictor therapy ($p = 0.05$). The frequency of rebleeding during the period of admission was the same for both groups (31%), reflecting the use of long-term sclerotherapy in each arm of the trial. There were significantly fewer patients in the immediate sclerotherapy group with blood transfusion requirements exceeding eight units. Admission mortality was not different for the two groups (27% versus 39% respectively, $p = 0.20$).

A number of studies have compared injection sclerotherapy with surgical measures for the management of variceal bleeding. Criteria for inclusion in these trials, however, has usually extended to patients with recent bleeding as well as those with active ongoing haemorrhage. Only one trial has compared injection sclerotherapy to the portocaval shunt and this was restricted to patients with decompensated liver disease (Cello et al, 1987). Whilst early rebleeding was significantly less in the shunt group, survival was unchanged. There were early cost benefits for injection sclerotherapy but these were subsequently diminished by a high rate of long-term recurrent bleeding in this group (75%). A further three trials have compared sclerotherapy with oesophageal transection and devascularization procedures (Huizinga et al, 1985; Teres et al, 1987; Burroughs et al, 1989b). In two of these trials (Huizinga et al, 1985; Burroughs et al, 1989b) oesophageal transection significantly reduced the risk of early rebleeding as compared to sclerotherapy, whilst in the third (Teres et al, 1987) this was similar. There was no survival benefit observed for either treatment.

The endoscopic injection of tissue adhesive

There has been no controlled comparison of this technique with other measures for the management of active variceal haemorrhage. In a small number of uncontrolled series, initial control of bleeding was obtained in approximately 90% of cases, although the subsequent rate of rebleeding was not dissimilar from that observed with injection sclerotherapy (Ramond et al, 1986; Soehendra et al, 1987). An important distinction from the other local endoscopic techniques is the successful application of tissue adhesive injection for fundal variceal bleeding.

Endoscopic banding ligation

There are no completed controlled trials comparing endoscopic banding ligation with other techniques. In an uncontrolled study, control of active variceal bleeding was obtained in 18 (86%) of 21 patients so treated (Stiegmann et al, 1990). In a second study, 10 patients who were considered failures of injection sclerotherapy were treated by banding ligation and control of active haemorrhage was achieved in 9 of these (Saeed et al, 1990).

Table 2. Interim results of an ongoing trial (King's College Hospital) comparing banding ligation and injection sclerosis for active variceal bleeding.

	Sclerotherapy $n=20$	Banding $n=18$
Child-Pugh grade A	4	2
B	8	7
C	8	9
Control of bleeding (12 h)	18 (90%)	15 (85%)
30-day rebleed	10 (50%)	8 (44%)
30-day mortality	7 (35%)	8 (44%)

There are two ongoing controlled comparisons of banding ligation with injection sclerotherapy, the preliminary results of which suggest similar efficacy for the two techniques (Stiegmann et al, 1991; Gimson and Westaby, unpublished data; Table 2).

THE LONG-TERM EFFICACY OF LOCAL ENDOSCOPIC THERAPY

Injection sclerotherapy

The use of repeated courses of injection sclerotherapy to prevent recurrent haemorrhage has been extensively investigated in a number of controlled trials (Barsoum et al, 1982; Terblanche et al, 1983; Copenhagen Oesophageal Varices Sclerotherapy Project, 1984; Korula et al, 1984; Paquet and Feussner, 1985; Soderlund and Ihre, 1985; Westaby et al, 1985; Burroughs et al, 1989a). Taken on an individual basis, all trials have shown a reduction in the total number of bleeding episodes, as compared to the control group. However, it must be stressed that the median rate of rebleeding in the sclerotherapy-treated patients was in excess of 50%, underlining one of the major limitations of this therapy. The effect of long-term sclerotherapy upon survival has been a topic of considerable controversy, with only three of the controlled trials showing clear significant benefit (Barsoum et al, 1982; Paquet and Feussner, 1985; Westaby et al, 1985). In an attempt to clarify the data from these divergent trials, the statistical tool of meta-analysis has been utilized (L'Abbe et al, 1987). This analysis involves the calculation and then pooling of the relative risk of both bleeding and death between the sclerotherapy and control groups. The pooled relative risk and its 95% confidence intervals then give an estimate of the overall efficacy of the treatment as extrapolated from the trials under review. The analysis is only valid if there is a degree of homogeneity between the different trials that are incorporated. Two such analyses have been carried out (Infante-Rivarde et al, 1989; Pagliari et al, 1989). Both have confirmed a significant benefit for long-term injection sclerotherapy for rebleeding and survival and in each case this approximated to a 50% reduction. While this provides important support for the use of long-term injection sclerotherapy, controversy still exists as to the interpretation of the available data. This revolves around the treatment that was offered to the patients in the control arms of the different trials when they presented with rebleeding. The majority of the studies incorporated into a protocol the use of conservative measures such as vasoconstrictor drugs or balloon tamponade as initial treatment for rebleeding. However, in two of the trials a single session of injection sclerotherapy was carried out when rebleeding occurred (Terblanche et al, 1983; Burroughs et al, 1986). These latter two trials were notable for their failure to show any trend towards improved survival. It has therefore been suggested that the survival benefits accrued from long-term injection sclerotherapy might only reflect the failure to use acute sclerotherapy for episodes of active rebleeding in the control group.

A number of controlled studies have compared long-term injection sclerotherapy to alternative measures. In four of these trials the comparison has been with shunt surgery; in three to the distal splenorenal shunt (Rikkers et al, 1987; Teres et al, 1987; Henderson et al, 1990) and in the fourth to the portocaval shunt (Cello et al, 1987). As might be anticipated, there were significantly fewer rebleeding episodes in those undergoing shunt surgery as compared to sclerotherapy. However, in one of the studies (Henderson et al, 1990) there was a clear survival benefit observed in the injection sclerotherapy group. The authors of this trial emphasize the frequent use of rescue shunt surgery in patients who are considered failures of injection sclerotherapy (almost 30% of the sclerotherapy group). In the remaining three trials (Cello et al, 1987; Rikkers et al, 1987; Teres et al, 1987) survival for the two treatment groups was almost identical.

With the introduction of non-selective β-adrenergic blockade as long-term therapy to prevent rebleeding, injection sclerotherapy represented the most established treatment against which this could be compared. From three reported comparisons (Fleig et al, 1987; Alexandrino et al, 1988; Westaby et al, 1990) only one (Alexandrino et al, 1988) confirmed a benefit for sclerotherapy with respect to rebleeding and none have shown any survival benefit for either treatment.

Injection of tissue adhesive

The long-term use of tissue adhesive injection has not been assessed in a controlled way. In an uncontrolled series of 49 patients, bucrylate was used in repeated sessions to prevent rebleeding (Ramond et al, 1986). Recurrent haemorrhage occurred in 42% of the patients within the first 12 months with an overall one-year survival of 53%. Such a rebleeding rate is not dissimilar from that which would be anticipated using long-term injection sclerotherapy.

Endoscopic banding ligation

No controlled studies of endoscopic banding ligation have been reported in their entirety, although such studies are ongoing (see below). In a large consecutive series of 100 patients treated by banding ligation 88 were entered into a long-term programme (Stiegmann et al, 1990). Varices were successfully obliterated in 60 (68%) of these 88 patients with a median of five

Table 3. Interim results of an ongoing trial (King's College Hospital) comparing banding ligation and injection sclerosis for long-term control of variceal bleeding.

	Banding $n = 48$	Sclerotherapy $n = 40$	p value
Child-Pugh score	8.8	8.1	N.S.
Sessions to obliteration	3.4	5.1	<0.01
Patients rebleeding	15 (32%)	21 (53%)	<0.10

sessions (range 1–12). Episodes of rebleeding were experienced in 41 (45%) of the 88 patients with a total of 72 episodes. Only 9 of the original 100 patients were considered failures of treatment and were managed by alternative methods. Results of an ongoing comparison of banding ligation to injection sclerotherapy (Gimson and Westaby, unpublished data) suggests benefits for the former with respect to earlier obliteration of varices and fewer rebleeding episodes (see Table 3).

LOCAL ENDOSCOPIC TECHNIQUES COMBINED WITH OTHER MEASURES

The high rebleeding rate observed with all the endoscopic techniques, particularly injection sclerotherapy, has led to a number of studies assessing the use of additional measures. One such approach has been based on the observation that many early rebleeding episodes are precipitated by sclerotherapy-induced mucosal damage. Whilst H_2-receptor antagonists have been employed in this setting there is no objective evidence to support their use. However, a large control trial of the mucosal protectant sucralfate has confirmed benefit for the reduction of early rebleeding, particularly in patients with well-compensated cirrhosis (Polson et al, 1989). A small percentage of sclerotherapy-induced ulcers, particularly straddling the gastro-oesophageal junction, may become chronic and a cause of repeated bleeding and/or pain. A recent publication has shown that omeprazole is highly effective at achieving healing of these ulcers, although relapse was observed in a number of cases when the drug was discontinued (Gimson et al, 1990).

A number of controlled trials have been carried out to assess whether the combination of oral propranolol and long-term injection sclerotherapy enhanced the efficacy of each. The results of these relatively small trials have been conflicting and provide little support for the widespread adoption of this combination (Westaby et al, 1986; Jensen and Krarup, 1989; O'Connor et al, 1989). A single report, to date only in abstract form, has shown considerable benefit for the combination of the somatostatin analogue octreotide (given in the long term subcutaneously) and injection sclerotherapy (Jenkin et al, 1991). These results require confirmation.

THE CURRENT STATUS OF LOCAL ENDOSCOPIC THERAPY FOR VARICEAL BLEEDING

The use of local endoscopic techniques, particularly injection sclerotherapy, has been well proven for an episode of variceal haemorrhage. The diagnostic endoscopy, as an integral part of any management regime, provides the optimum time to intervene with sclerotherapy. This can then provide haemostasis in patients who continue to bleed actively, but also to prevent early rebleeding in those in whom bleeding may have stopped spontaneously. The value of the newer techniques for active variceal bleeding has not been fully established. The injection of tissue adhesives appears to be highly effective at arresting bleeding but further evidence is required with respect to their safety profile. Tissue adhesive injection remains the only endoscopic technique that may be recommended for the management of fundal variceal bleeding. Banding ligation appears to be a safe alternative treatment but is no more effective than injection sclerotherapy for the arrest of active bleeding. Further evaluation is required to assess whether this technique has value in any particular subgroup of patients. Whichever endoscopic technique is employed it is of paramount importance that a definition for failure of treatment is established. Most workers would justify a second intervention with endoscopy therapy, particularly if there had been technical difficulties on the first attempt. However, if haemostasis is not obtained with the second intervention then there should be no delay in arranging alternative measures, which would usually involve one of the surgical techniques.

Following initial control of bleeding with an endoscopic technique there is almost a logical progression for this to be used as a long-term measure. There is now considerable evidence that long-term injection sclerotherapy is of proven benefit for both rebleeding and perhaps survival, but there are increasing doubts concerning the need for the intensive regimens that have been utilized for the last 15 years. The value of variceal obliteration as an end-point and the need for subsequent surveillance endoscopy are areas that require investigation. It is in the area of long-term therapy that the new technique of banding ligation may have an important role as there is already some evidence of more rapid obliteration of varices and fewer rebleeding episodes. If this is confirmed, it may be envisaged that in the future active bleeding may be controlled by the injection of a sclerosant, then to be followed by a short course of banding ligation to achieve partial or complete obliteration of the varices. As in the case of active variceal bleeding it is extremely important to establish the definition for failed treatment so that other measures can be employed at the most optimal time. In the setting of long-term therapy it is usually the occurrence of a life-threatening rebleed or multiple small rebleeds that dictate a move to alternative measures.

One of the encouraging trends over the last decade has been the justifiable move to local endoscopic techniques being the initial treatment of choice for active variceal bleeding and to prevent recurrence. However, there is no doubt that a higher proportion of such patients are subsequently undergoing surgical intervention. Whilst such changes are open to a number of interpretations, the most likely explanation is an increasing awareness of the strengths and weaknesses of the treatments available, and patients are being managed by means of a treatment protocol rather than a single measure in isolation.

REFERENCES

Akriviadis E, Korula J, Gupta S et al (1989) Frequent endoscopic variceal sclerotherapy increases risk of complications: a prospective randomised controlled study of two treatment schedules. *Digestive Diseases and Sciences* **34**: 1068–1074.

Alexandrino PJ, Alves MM & Pinto-Correia J (1988) Propranolol or endoscopic sclerotherapy in the prevention of recurrence of variceal bleeding. A prospective, randomised controlled trial. *Journal of Hepatology* **7:** 175–185.

Balanzo J, Sainz S, Espinos J et al (1989) Efficacy of ethanolamaine and polidocanol in the eradication of oesophageal varices: a prospective randomised trial. *Endoscopy* **21:** 251–253.

Barsoum MS, Boulous FI, El-Robby A et al (1982) Tamponade and injection sclerotherapy in the management of bleeding oesophageal varices. *British Journal of Surgery* **69:** 76–78.

Bornman PC, Kahn D, Terblanche J et al (1988) Rigid versus fibreoptic endoscopic injection sclerotherapy: a prospective randomized controlled trial in patients with bleeding oesophageal varices. *Annals of Surgery* **208:** 175–178.

Burroughs A, d'Heygere F & McIntyre N (1986) Pitfalls in studies of prophylactic therapy for variceal bleeding in cirrhotics. *Hepatology* **6:** 1407–1413.

Burroughs AK, McCormick PA, Siringo S et al (1989a) Prospective randomized trial of long-term sclerotherapy for variceal rebleeding using the same protocol to treat rebleeding in all patients (abstract). *Journal of Hepatology* **9:** S12.

Burroughs A, Hamilton G, Phillips A et al (1989b) A comparison of sclerotherapy with staple transection of the esophagus for the emergency control of bleeding from oesophageal varices. *New England Journal of Medicine* **321:** 857–862.

Cello JP, Grendell JH, Crass RA et al (1987) Endoscopic sclerotherapy versus portacaval shunt in patients with severe cirrhosis and acute variceal haemorrhage: long-term follow-up. *New England Journal of Medicine* **316:** 11–15.

Copenhagen Oesophageal Varices Sclerotherapy Project (1984) Sclerotherapy after first variceal hemorrhage in cirrhosis. A randomized multicenter trial. *New England Journal of Medicine* **311:** 1594–1600.

Crafoord C & Frenckner P (1959) New surgical treatment of varicose veins of the oesophagus. *Acta Otolaryngologica (Stockholm)* **27:** 422–429.

Evans D, Jones D, Cleary D et al (1982) Oesophageal varices treated by sclerotherapy: a histopathological study. *Gut* **23:** 615–620.

Fleig WE, Stange EF, Hunecke R et al (1987) Prevention of recurrent bleeding in cirrhotics with recent variceal haemorrhage: prospective, randomised comparison of propranolol and sclerotherapy. *Hepatology* **7:** 355–361.

Gimson A, Polson R, Westaby D et al (1990) Omeprazole in the management of intractable oesophageal ulceration following injection sclerotherapy. *Gastroenterology* **99:** 1829–1831.

Helpap B & Bollweg L (1981) Morphological changes in the terminal oesophagus with varices, following sclerosis of the wall. *Endoscopy* **13:** 229–233.

Henderson J, Kutner M, Millikan W et al (1990) Endoscopic variceal sclerosis compared with distal spleno-renal shunt to prevent recurrent variceal bleeding in cirrhosis. *Annals of Internal Medicine* **112:** 262–269.

Huizinga W, Angorn P & Baker L (1985) Oesophageal transection versus injection sclerotherapy in the management of bleeding oesophageal varices in patients at high risk. *Surgery, Gynaecology and Obstetrics* **160:** 539–546.

Infante-Rivard C, Esnaola S & Villeneuve J-P (1989) Role of endoscopic variceal sclerotherapy in the long-term management of variceal bleeding: a meta-analysis. *Gastroenterology* **96:** 1087–1092.

Jenkins SA, Ellenbogen S, Baxter JN et al (1991) Sandostatin in the long-term management of portal hypertension—a preliminary prospective randomised controlled clinical trial. *Gut* **32:** A838.

Jensen L & Krarup N (1989) Propranolol in prevention of recurrent bleeding from oesophageal varices during the course of endoscopic sclerotherapy. *Scandinavian Journal of Gastroenterology* **24:** 339–345.

Jensen D, Machicado G & Silpa M (1986) Oesophageal varix haemorrhage and sclerotherapy—animal studies. *Endoscopy* **18:** 18–22.

Johnston GW & Rodgers HW (1973) A review of 15 years experience in the use of sclerotherapy in the control of acute haemorrhage from oesophageal varices. *British Journal of Surgery* **60:** 797–800.

Kahn D, Jones B, Bornman PC et al (1989) Incidence and management of complications after injection sclerotherapy: a 10-year prospective evaluation. *Surgery* **105:** 160–165.

Kitano S, Koyanagi N, Iso Y et al (1987) Prevention of recurrence of oesophageal varices after endoscopic injection sclerotherapy with ethanolamine oleate. *Hepatology* **7**: 810–815.
Kitano S, Iso Y, Yamaga H et al (1988) Trial of sclerosing agents in patients with oesophageal varices. *British Journal of Surgery* **75**: 751–753.
Korula J, Balart LA, Radvan G et al (1984) A prospective, randomized controlled trial of chronic oesophageal variceal sclerotherapy. *Hepatology* **5**: 584–589.
L'Abbe K, Detsky A & O'Rouke K (1987) Meta-analysis in clinical research. *Annals of Internal Medicine* **107**: 224–233.
Larson A, Cohen H, Zweiban B et al (1986) Acute oesophageal variceal sclerotherapy: results of a prospective randomized controlled trial. *Journal of the American Medical Association* **255**: 497–500.
MacCormack T, Smith P, Rose J et al (1983) Perforating veins and blood flow in oesophageal varices. *Lancet* **2**: 442–444.
MacDougall BRD, Westaby D, Theodossi A et al (1982) Increased long-term survival in variceal haemorrhage using injection sclerotherapy. *Lancet* **1**: 124–127.
Moreto M, Zaballa M, Bernal A et al (1988) A randomized trial of tamponade or sclerotherapy as immediate treatment for bleeding oesophageal varices. *Surgery, Gynaecology and Obstetrics* **167**: 331–334.
O'Connor K, Lehman G, Yune H et al (1989) Comparison of three non-surgical treatments for bleeding oesophageal varices. *Gastroenterology* **96**: 899–906.
Pagliari L, Burroughs AK, Sorensen TA et al (1989) Therapeutic controversies and randomised controlled trials: prevention of bleeding and rebleeding in cirrhosis. *Gastroenterology International* **2**: 71–84.
Paquet KJ & Feussner H (1985) Endoscopic sclerosis and oesophageal balloon tamponade in acute haemorrhage from oesophagogastric varices: a prospective controlled randomized trial. *Hepatology* **5**: 580–583.
Polson RJ, Westaby D, Gimson AES et al (1989) Sucralfate for the prevention of early rebleeding following injection sclerotherapy for oesophageal varices. *Hepatology* **10**: 279–283.
Prindiville T & Trudeau W (1986) A comparison of immediate versus delayed endoscopic injection sclerosis of bleeding oesophageal varices. *Gastrointestinal Endoscopy* **32**: 385–388.
Ramond MJ (1986) Endoscopic obliteration of oesophagogastric varices with bucrylate. *Gastroentérologie Clinique et Biologique* **10**: 575–583.
Ramond MJ, Valla D, Gotlib JP et al (1986) Obturation endoscopique des varices oesogastriques par le Bucrylate. *Gastroentérologie Clinique et Biologique* **10**: 575–579.
Reilly J, Schade R & Van Thiel D (1984) Esophageal function after injection sclerotherapy: pathogenesis of esophageal stricture. *American Journal of Surgery* **147**: 85–88.
Rikkers LF, Burnett DA, Volentine GD et al (1987) Shunt surgery versus endoscopic sclerotherapy for long-term treatment of variceal bleeding: early results of a randomized trial. *Annals of Surgery* **206**: 261–271.
Saeed Z, Michaletz P, Winchester C et al (1990) Endoscopic variceal ligation in patients who have failed sclerotherapy. *Gastrointestinal Endoscopy* **36**: 572–574.
Sarin SK, Sachdev G, Nanda R et al (1986a) Comparison of the two time schedules for endoscopic sclerotherapy: a prospective randomised controlled study. *Gut* **27**: 710–713.
Sarin S, Nanda R, Sachdev G et al (1986b) Intravariceal versus paravariceal sclerotherapy: a prospective controlled randomised trial. *Gut* **28**: 657–662.
Sarin S, Mishra S, Sachdev G et al (1988) Ethanolamine oleate versus absolute alcohol as a variceal sclerosant: a prospective randomized controlled trial. *American Journal of Gastroenterology* **8**: 526–530.
Sauerbruch T, Wirschung R, Holl J et al (1986) Effects of repeated injection sclerotherapy on acid gastroesophageal reflux. *Gastrointestinal Endoscopy* **32**: 81–83.
See A, Florent C, Lamy P et al (1986) Accidents vasculaires cérébraux après obturation endoscopique des varices oesophagiennes par l'Isobutyl-2 Cyanoacrylate chez deux malades. *Gastroentérologie Clinique et Biologique* **10**: 604–607.
Siemens F, Paquet K, Koussouris P et al (1989) Long-term injection sclerotherapy of bleeding oesophageal varices. A prospective analysis of results by endoscopy, menometry and 24 hours pH monitoring. *Surgical Endoscopy* **3**: 137–141.
Snady H & Horsten M (1986) Esophageal acid-clearance and motility after endoscopic sclerotherapy of esophageal varices. *American Journal of Gastroenterology* **81**: 419–422.

Soderlund C & Ihre T (1985) Endoscopic sclerotherapy versus conservative management of bleeding oesophageal varices. A 5-year prospective controlled trial of emergency and long-term treatment. *Acta Chirurgica Scandinavica* **151:** 449–456.

Soehendra N, de Heer K, Kempeneers I et al (1983) Sclerotherapy of oesophageal varices: acute arrest of gastrointestinal haemorrhage or long-term therapy? *Endoscopy* **15:** 136–140.

Soehendra N, Ham V, Grimm H et al (1986) Endoscopic obliteration of large oesophagogastric varices with bucrylate. *Endoscopy* **18:** 25–25.

Soehandra N, Grimm H, Nam VC et al (1987) N-glutyl-2-cyanoacrylate: a supplement to endoscopic sclerotherapy. *Endoscopy* **19:** 221–223.

Stiegmann GV, Goff JS, Michaletz P et al (1990) Endoscopic variceal ligation versus sclerotherapy for bleeding oesophageal varices: early results of a prospective randomized trial. *Gastrointestinal Endoscopy* **36:** 188 (abstract).

Terblanche J, Northover J, Bamman P et al (1979) A prospective controlled trial of sclerotherapy in the long-term management of patients after esophageal variceal bleeding. *Surgery, Gynecology and Obstetrics* **148:** 323–333.

Terblanche J, Yakoob H, Bornman P et al (1981) Acute bleeding varices: a five-year prospective evaluation of tamponade and sclerotherapy. *Annals of Surgery* **194:** 521–530.

Terblanche J, Bornman PC, Kahn D et al (1983) The failure of long-term injection sclerotherapy after variceal bleeding to improve survival. *Lancet* **2:** 1328–1332.

Teres J, Baroni R, Bordas J et al (1987) Randomized trial of portacaval shunt, stapling transection and endoscopic sclerotherapy in uncontrolled variceal bleeding. *Journal of Hepatology* **4:** 159–167.

Vianna A, Hoyes P, Moscosco G et al (1987) Normal venous circulation of the gastroesophageal junction: a route to understanding varices. *Gastroenterology* **93:** 876–881.

Westaby D & Williams R (1983) History and development of sclerotherapy. *Gastrointestinal Endoscopy* **29:** 303–307.

Westaby D & Williams R (1984) Follow-up study after sclerotherapy. *Scandinavian Journal of Gastroenterology* **19:** 71–75.

Westaby D, MacDougall BRD, Melia WM et al (1983) A prospective randomized study of two sclerotherapy techniques for oesophageal varices. *Hepatology* **3:** 681–684.

Westaby D, Melia WM, MacDougall BR et al (1984) Injection sclerotherapy for oesophageal varices: a prospective randomized trial of different treatment schedules. *Gut* **25:** 129–132.

Westaby D, MacDougall BRD & Williams R (1985) Improved survival following injection sclerotherapy for oesophageal varices: final analysis of a controlled trial. *Hepatology* **5:** 627–631.

Westaby D, Melia W, Hegarty J et al (1986) Use of propranolol to reduce the rebleeding rate during injection sclerotherapy prior to variceal obliteration. *Hepatology* **6:** 673–675.

Westaby D, Hayes P, Gimson A et al (1989) Controlled clinical trial of injection sclerotherapy for active variceal bleeding. *Hepatology* **9:** 274–277.

Westaby D, Polson RJ, Gimson AES et al (1990) A controlled trial of oral propranolol compared with injection sclerotherapy for the long-term management of variceal bleeding. *Hepatology* **11:** 353–359.

Williams KGD & Dawson JL (1979) Fibreoptic injection of oesophageal varices. *British Medical Journal* **2:** 766–767.

Yamamoto M & Suzuki H (1989) Endoscopic sclerotherapy with Histoacryl. *Digestive Endoscopy* **6:** 851–857.

5

Portal hypertensive gastropathy

DAVID R. TRIGER

Gastric mucosal abnormalities have long been recognized in association with portal hypertension. At the turn of the century Osler (1898) considered one of the causes of chronic gastritis to be 'conditions of the portal circulation causing chronic engorgement of the mucous membrane as in cirrhosis'. Two years later, in a review of 60 cases of fatal gastrointestinal bleeding due to cirrhosis, Preble (1900) observed that 'not all cirrhotics who bleed have varices as a source of haemorrhage, simultaneous rupture of many capillaries may cause bleeding in some'.

Despite these observations attention throughout this century has largely been focused on oesophageal varices as the major source of upper gastrointestinal bleeding in cirrhosis and this has been reflected by the enormous literature relating to portocaval shunt surgery and to variceal sclerotherapy. During the 1960s and 1970s a number of reports of gastritis in cirrhotics appeared (McCray et al, 1969; Dagradi et al, 1970; Khodadoost and Glass, 1972; Thomas et al, 1979), but since most patients had alcoholic liver disease this lesion was generally attributed to the effects of alcohol. Two advances during the last 20 years have done much to reawaken interest in the gastric mucosa in cirrhosis. First, the widespread availability of fibreoptic endoscopy has meant that both the site and cause of gastrointestinal haemorrhage can be defined with greater accuracy than previously. Second, the advent of endoscopic sclerotherapy has given us a tool which enables us to obliterate oesophageal varices without altering the vascular haemodynamics of the portal circulation. In the past when patients with portal hypertension and patent large oesophageal varices have presented with upper gastrointestinal tract bleeding it has been customary to ascribe such haemorrhage to the varices even if they were not actively seen to be bleeding at the time. Experience in recent years has resulted in an increasing recognition of gastric bleeding in patients with portal hypertension, particularly when the varices have been obliterated by sclerotherapy. This chapter will consider the gastric abnormalities associated with portal hypertension and review the current state of knowledge concerning this condition.

DEFINITION

The literature includes many terms which are both inaccurate and misleading. Early descriptions have included the terms 'gastritis', 'gastric erosions', 'gastric mucosal hyperaemia', 'haemorrhagic gastritis' and 'gastric mucosal ectasia'. The term 'gastritis' implies that there is inflammation of the stomach but recent studies have shown that this is not a prominent histological feature. As will be discussed later in greater detail, venous dilatation of the mucosal vessels is the most obvious abnormality and because of this we (McCormack et al, 1985) coined the term 'congestive gastropathy'. Others have preferred the descriptive term 'portal vasculopathy' (Sarfeh and Tarnawski, 1987). More recently the term 'portal hypertensive gastropathy' has found favour and since this makes no assumption about the pathogenesis it will be used in this chapter.

There is at present no generally agreed definition of portal hypertensive gastropathy. Suspicion of the condition should be raised by the macroscopic appearances seen on endoscopy and this may be confirmed by the presence of appropriate histological changes when other disorders have been excluded. For practical purposes I have chosen to define portal hypertensive gastropathy as 'a condition in which there are macroscopic changes of the gastric mucosa associated with mucosal and submucosal vascular ectasia and dilatation without significant histological changes of inflammation'. The details of the definition will be discussed below.

MACROSCOPIC APPEARANCES

The abnormal macroscopic appearances in this condition may be classified as either mild or severe.

Mild gastropathy

A fine speckling or 'scarlatina' appearance and superficial reddening are commonly seen in the gastric mucosa but these are non-specific findings which may occur in the absence of liver disease or portal hypertension. A much more characteristic observation is a mosaic or 'snakeskin' appearance in which areas of raised pink oedematous mucosa are separated by a fine white reticular pattern resembling the skin of a snake. This appearance is thought to be due to oedema and congestion highlighting the normal areae gastricae pattern of the gastric mucosa (Mackintosh and Keel, 1977). A French study (Papazian et al, 1986) has reported the snakeskin appearance in 94 out of 100 patients with cirrhosis and seven out of eight with non-cirrhotic portal hypertension, compared with 1 out of 300 control subjects and 0 out of 100 alcoholics without liver disease. A similar prevalence has been reported in another study from France (Calès et al, 1990) but a recent survey from Italy (D'Amico et al, 1990) found that only 110 out of 212 cirrhotics had macroscopic abnormalities of the gastric mucosa, suggesting that it is by no means an invariable finding in chronic liver disease.

Severe gastropathy

Cherry-red spots arising in islands of gastric mucosa are a characteristic sign of severe gastropathy. These are identical in appearance to the cherry-red spots which, when overlying oesophageal varices, are known to be associated with a high risk of haemorrhage. Similarly, their presence on the gastric mucosa is also associated with a high risk of bleeding. Isolated red spots are less frequently associated with haemorrhage but in more severe cases they progress to form confluent areas of diffuse bleeding, generally termed haemorrhagic gastritis. Although gastropathy may occur throughout the stomach the mucosal abnormalities tend to be more prominent in the fundus. It is important to recognize this regional variation since this part of the stomach can easily be overlooked on endoscopy unless the instrument is specifically everted. In a small group of patients the mucosal abnormalities appear to be confined to the antrum (Van Vliet et al, 1978; Quintero et al, 1985). This has been termed 'antral mucosal hyperaemia': in many cases, however, the abnormality is not confined to the antrum and the condition is probably merely a variant of portal hypertensive gastropathy.

HISTOLOGICAL APPEARANCES

Although the reddened macroscopic appearance of the gastric mucosa suggests the probability of inflammation, neutrophil infiltration of the superficial layers of the stomach is conspicuously absent. Dilatation of the mucosal and submucosal vessels together with capillary and venous ectasia are the most striking histological changes (McCormack et al, 1985). Unfortunately these abnormalities are not always detectable on biopsy since the samples that can be taken using ordinary endoscopic forceps are usually too small and superficial to permit assessment of the vessels. Adequate material can be obtained if a snare biopsy technique is used (Saperas et al, 1989) but this is not recommended for routine clinical practice. Ultrastructural studies have confirmed dilatation of the mucosal capillaries and have also shown capillary fenestrations to be widened as well as increased in number (Haung, 1989).

From a histological point of view the distinction between mild and severe gastropathy appears to be quantitative. Quintero et al (1987), using morphometric analysis, have found a gradation in gastric mucosal capillary cross-sectional area from control subjects without portal hypertension ($353 \pm 20\ \mu m^2$) through cirrhotics without gastric lesions ($541 \pm 61\ \mu m^2$) to cirrhotics with gastric lesions ($1371 \pm 320\ \mu m^2$). Routine light microscopy studies without such objective measurements, however, are not able to distinguish readily between the grades of gastropathy. Iwao et al (1990) have confirmed the Spanish workers' morphometric studies and in addition have shown that the gastric red spots are characterized on electronmicroscopy by extravasation of red cells through the defective portions of the endothelium as well as being present within the interepithelial spaces.

The morphology of the gastric circulation has been studied by Hashizume et al (1983). This was carried out by excising the stomach at either surgery or autopsy and injecting the vessels with silicone rubber. Using this technique the authors were able to demonstrate that precapillaries, capillaries, and mucosal and submucosal vessels were all dilated and in addition the arterioles were much straighter in cirrhotics than in non-cirrhotics. They also observed the presence of a number of arteriovenous anastomoses ranging from 15 to 50 μm in diameter.

CLINICAL FEATURES

Mild portal hypertensive gastropathy is asymptomatic and should be considered as an incidental finding on routine gastroscopy in patients with portal hypertension. It is never responsible for symptoms of abdominal pain or dyspepsia and when macroscopic abnormalities are observed in patients with such complaints alternative explanations should be sought. Severe gastropathy is similarly painless but as mentioned earlier is associated with a high risk of bleeding. McCormack et al (1985) reported that it was responsible in 9 out of 114 patients with portal hypertension presenting for the first time with gastrointestinal bleeding, but this proportion rose to 30% in those suffering further bleeds after endoscopic sclerotherapy, while others (McCray et al, 1969; Dagradi et al, 1970; Khodadoost and Glass, 1972; Waldram et al, 1974; Thomas et al, 1979), have reported that gastric mucosal lesions account for 10–60% of all bleeds. These figures probably overestimate the contribution of portal hypertensive gastropathy as the studies were performed before the recognition of the entity and they undoubtedly included other conditions such as *Helicobacter* infection. Nevertheless there is general agreement that severe portal hypertensive gastropathy is a significant cause of acute bleeding, but its role in chronic anaemia is less certain. D'Amico et al (1990) studied 212 cirrhotic patients prospectively and reported that both anaemia and overt bleeding were significantly more common in patients with severe gastropathy compared with those with mild or absent gastropathy. This study included a substantial proportion of patients without portal hypertension—thus making interpretation difficult. In contrast neither Calès et al (1989) nor Granai et al (1991b) were able to show any correlation between the presence of mild or severe gastropathy and the haemoglobin level.

Other than the presence of portal hypertension there appear to be no discernible clinical features which determine the presence of either mild or severe gastropathy. Although the condition is more frequently found in cirrhotics with oesophageal varices there is no clear association between the two pathologies (Papazian et al, 1986; Quintero et al, 1987; Calès et al, 1990). Sacchetti et al (1988) reported that the prevalence of gastric erosions increases with deterioration in hepatic function, being found in 21% with Child A, 26% with Child B and 48% with Child C cirrhotics, but such an association was not confirmed by another Italian study (D'Amico et al, 1990) and it is not clear whether this increase, if real, is a consequence of the severity of liver damage or the duration of the portal hypertension. Portal hypertensive gastropathy occurs with similar frequency in both alcoholic and non-alcoholic cirrhosis and it is also found in non-cirrhotic portal hypertension (McCormack et al, 1985). It appears to be uncommon in young people in India where portal hypertension is largely due to non-cirrhotic causes (S. K. Sarin, personal communication) but formal studies have yet to be carried out. The prevalence of gastropathy is also related to sclerotherapy, being found more commonly in patients who have undergone the procedure compared with those who have not (D'Amico et al, 1990) and it is also more frequently found in those who have had more prolonged courses of such treatment (McCormack et al, 1985). However, acute gastric mucosal changes may be induced by sclerotherapy and this will be discussed later. There is no evidence to suggest that portal hypertensive gastropathy is related to age, gender or administration of any drugs.

DIFFERENTIAL DIAGNOSIS

As mentioned earlier, the definition of portal hypertensive gastropathy should ideally be based upon both macroscopic and histological appearances, but this is often not possible. Many endoscopists, when faced with an actively bleeding lesion in the stomach of a patient with portal hypertension and coagulation disturbances, are reluctant to biopsy the mucosa and, even if a histological sample is obtained, it may prove too small to permit a confident diagnosis. In practice, the diagnosis is often made by the exclusion of other conditions (Table 1).

Table 1. Differential diagnosis of portal hypertensive gastropathy.

Helicobacter pylori gastritis
Alcoholic gastritis
Gastric ulcers/erosions
Drug-associated gastric lesions
Bile gastritis
Water melon stomach
Gastric angiodysplasia
Disseminated intravascular coagulopathy

Helicobacter pylori

H. pylori is such a common feature in gastric mucosal biopsies that its presence must be considered in any patient with macroscopic abnormalities in the stomach. In our experience the presence of *H. pylori* in patients with portal hypertension is almost invariably associated with a histological inflammatory cell infiltrate (Laing et al, 1990) in addition to which the organism is usually detectable by specific histochemical or other techniques. Although the studies are small, evidence to date does not suggest any correlation between portal hypertensive gastropathy and the presence of this organism (Pretolani et al, 1988; Foster et al, 1989).

Alcoholic gastritis

Since alcohol is the most common aetiological cause of cirrhosis in the Western world, it is particularly important to distinguish alcoholic gastritis from portal hypertensive gastropathy as both lesions may be macroscopically similar and both may be haemorrhagic. Subepithelial haemorrhages are a characteristic histological lesion in the alcoholic stomach (Laine et al, 1989) and this is readily distinguishable from gastropathy.

Gastric ulcers/erosions

The earlier literature on gastric lesions in portal hypertension (Lam, 1976) suggesting that erosions were particularly common in cirrhosis was probably based on a confusion between portal hypertensive gastropathy and erosive gastritis. Whether or not true gastric ulcers are more common in portal hypertension is uncertain; it is probable, however, that they are more frequently complicated by haemorrhage due to a bleeding diathesis which often accompanies cirrhosis and portal hypertension.

Drugs

Rats in whom portal hypertension has been induced by portal vein ligation are unduly susceptible to aspirin-induced gastric mucosal damage (Sarfeh et al, 1988). The histological lesions produced in this model differ considerably from portal hypertensive gastropathy in man and its relevance to the clinical situation is uncertain. Our own clinical observations do not suggest an association between portal hypertensive gastropathy and drug ingestion (McCormack et al, 1985) but to date no formal case control studies have been conducted to exclude this possibility.

Bile gastritis

As with aspirin, the gastric mucosa in portal vein-ligated animals is unduly susceptible to the irritant effect of bile (Sarfeh et al, 1984). On the other hand, taurocholate does not produce significant gastric lesions in animals with carbon tetrachloride-induced cirrhosis and portal hypertension (Angerson et al, 1992), suggesting that either the method or the time course for producing the haemodynamic disturbance in the portal venous system may be important. Bile reflux is not usually a significant problem in patients with portal hypertension, and there is no clinical evidence to suggest that it plays a significant role in portal hypertensive gastropathy.

Water melon stomach/gastric angiodysplasia

Water melon stomach is the name given to a condition in which erythematous lesions resembling 'water melon stripes' are found in the gastric antrum. Histologically they are characterized by dilated capillaries and tortuous submucosal venous channels, and larger series usually include several patients with cirrhosis (Jabbari et al, 1984; Gostout et al, 1989). It is not clear whether this is synonymous with antral vascular ectasia referred to earlier and its relation to gastric angiodysplasia is similarly uncertain. These localized lesions, however, are usually amenable to diathermy (Gostout et al, 1989) or laser treatment (Petrini and Johnston, 1989) whereas portal hypertensive gastropathy is usually too diffuse to allow such therapy.

Variceal sclerotherapy

As discussed earlier, there is considerable evidence to suggest that portal hypertensive gastropathy is seen more frequently in patients who have undergone endoscopic sclerotherapy and its frequency appears to increase with time as more sclerotherapy is performed. It is important to distinguish between transient changes occurring as a consequence of the procedure of variceal injection and longer term abnormalities. McCormack et al (1985) observed that injection of oesophageal varices led to the early appearance of fundal gastropathy in a number of patients, but also resulted in its disappearance in an equal number. This may have been due to obliteration of the veins producing local haemodynamic disturbances which might either acutely raise or lower local venous pressure depending upon the direction of the superficial venous blood flow. Such changes, however, are usually transient and reverse when venous collaterals develop over a period of a few days or weeks.

Disseminated intravascular coagulopathy

A generalized coagulopathy associated with diffuse gastrointestinal bleeding, endotoxaemia and renal failure is well recognized in terminal hepatic failure (Clemente et al, 1977). Haemorrhagic gastropathy is common but on clinical grounds such patients should be readily distinguishable from those with portal hypertensive gastropathy.

PATHOGENESIS

Experimental animal studies

Attempts to produce an experimental animal model have largely concentrated on portal vein ligation in the rat. Although this procedure undoubtedly produces both portal hypertension and gastric mucosal changes, the relevance to human portal hypertensive gastropathy is questionable for a number of reasons. The haemodynamic changes affecting the portal venous circulation are known to be unstable following portal vein ligation and vary according to the time following the procedure (Groszmann and Colombato, 1988). Furthermore, the histological changes in the rat model of acute portal hypertension show striking submucosal oedema rather than vascular ectasia (Tarnawski et al, 1988). The topical application of bile acid (Sarfeh et al, 1984) and alcohol (Sarfeh et al, 1983) produces deep ulceration and necrosis which is histologically unlike the lesion seen in portal hypertensive gastropathy in man. Finally, there is no evidence that spontaneous haemorrhage from the gastric mucosa has been observed in any rat subjected to portal vein ligation alone. There are at present very few studies in which portal hypertension has been induced by experimental cirrhosis (Manabe et al, 1978; Angerson et al, 1992): it is clear that more data are required.

Human studies

Portal haemodynamics

Portal hypertension is unquestionably a key requirement for the condition. Not only are the histological and some of the macroscopic changes unique to portal hypertension but they are reliably and effectively reversed by portosystemic decompression shunt surgery (Sarfeh et al, 1982). Once portal hypertension is present, however, the degree of elevation of portal pressure does not appear to be important since there is no direct correlation between wedge hepatic vein pressure and the presence or absence of gastropathy (McCormack et al, 1985).

The association of portal hypertension and venous mucosal and submucosal dilatation led to the notion that the gastric mucosal abnormalities occurred as a consequence of venous congestion, thus giving rise to the term 'congestive gastropathy' (McCormack et al, 1985). This, however, is unlikely to be the complete explanation since (1) it fails to take into account the arteriolar changes that have been reported by Hashizume et al (1983), as described earlier in the chapter, and (2) one would as a consequence predict a direct association between venous pressure and vascular dilatation.

Recently attention has been directed to the gastric mucosal blood flow in this condition. Measurement of mucosal blood flow in man is technically difficult and there is at present no consensus on the accuracy and reliability of the currently available methods. Several workers have used a hydrogen gas clearance technique in which the subject breathes hydrogen which is absorbed into the circulation and then diffuses across the gastric mucosa at a rate proportional to the mucosal blood flow. This technique is difficult to reproduce but two Japanese groups have claimed that mucosal blood flow in both the body and antrum of the stomach is reduced in cirrhosis, particularly in patients with gastric mucosal redness (Adachi et al, 1989; Nishiwaki et al, 1990). Using laser doppler velocimetry, however, Chung et al (1988) have reported increased fundal mucosal blood flow in cirrhotics while Eleftheriadis et al (1990) have found significant reduction in the body of the stomach with a corresponding increase in the antrum. We have used a radio-isotope technique in which we measured the gastric clearance of [^{99m}Tc]pertechnetate injected intravenously and found gastric mucosal blood flow to be reduced in cirrhotics compared with controls, although we failed to observe any further alteration in the presence of gastropathy (Walsh et al, 1988). This technique, however, gives only a global measurement of blood flow and fails to distinguish between mucosal and submucosal flow. More studies are required to establish satisfactory techniques for measuring mucosal blood flow in humans not only in order to estimate total blood flow but also to distinguish reliably between mucosal and submucosal flow. Results to date on experimental animals have not been useful since most are based on the portal vein-ligated rat model. In this, Geraghty et al (1988) have shown that this is clearly an unstable model for measuring gastric blood flow since different results are obtained according to the time of study following venous ligation.

Since portal hypertension appears to result in changes in both venous and arteriolar vessels, it is tempting to speculate that the factors critical to the production of gastropathy may relate to inappropriate balance between the two. Such a hypothesis, however, is unlikely to be amenable to testing in man in the foreseeable future although it could be usefully explored in a suitable animal model when appropriate techniques have been developed.

Gastric mucosal function

Metabolic function is impaired in a number of ways in portal hypertension. Patients with cirrhosis and portal hypertension have normal basal acid output but significantly reduced maximal acid output in response to pentagastrin; the acid secretion does not appear to be further influenced by the presence of portal hypertensive gastropathy (Granai et al, 1991a).

Quintero et al (1987) have reported hypergastrinaemia and low levels of pepsinogen I in cirrhotics bleeding from antral vascular ectasia compared with both non-bleeding cirrhotics and non-cirrhotic controls. The same group has also shown that although many of these patients had achlorhydria there appeared to be no correlation between the circulating hormone levels and the lack of acid production (Perez-Ayuso et al, 1989). Gastric mucosal potential difference has been shown to be low in cirrhosis and to be even further reduced in patients with severe gastropathy (Pienkowski et al, 1989). Abnormalities in gastric prostaglandin E_2 (PGE_2) metabolism have also been recorded but with conflicting results, a Spanish group reporting increased levels in antral vascular ectasia (Saperas et al, 1990) while reduced levels have been found in a Japanese study of patients with alcoholic cirrhosis (Arakawa et al, 1987). Further work is needed to establish whether these differences are due to methodology or patient selection.

Additional information is available from experimental animals undergoing portal vein ligation, but the relevance of these studies to the human situation has already been discussed. Impaired response to pentagastrin stimulation (Pique et al, 1988), reduced mucosal potential difference (Sarfeh et al, 1983) and gastric mucosal hypoxia (Sarfeh et al, 1989) with reduction in secretion of gastric mucus (Kameyama et al, 1989) have all been reported.

It is not difficult to imagine how the impairment of gastric mucosal function might result in perturbation of the gastric defence mechanism to such a degree that pathological changes leading to rupture of the surface might occur—particularly in the presence of the vascular changes already described. It remains to be determined, however, whether the metabolic disturbances are a primary phenomenon or merely occur as a consequence of the vascular and possibly other hitherto undefined disturbances.

TREATMENT

As indicated earlier, mild hypertensive gastropathy requires no treatment and the natural progression from mild to severe changes occurs so infrequently and unpredictably that there is no justification for prophylactic therapy (Triger and Hosking, 1989).

Patients with severe haemorrhagic gastropathy require active therapeutic intervention since if left untreated bleeding may be prolonged and considerable (Triger, 1989). Decompression shunt surgery has been shown to be highly effective in abolishing the bleeding in this condition (Sarfeh et al, 1982; Babb and Mitchell, 1988), but treatment with propranolol is to be preferred. Two open studies have shown this drug to be effective in controlling haemorrhage from the gastric mucosa in portal hypertension. Quintero et al (1985) reported successful control in five out of six patients bleeding from antral mucosal hyperaemia while our own group (Hosking et al, 1987) found that by titrating the dose of propranolol it was possible to arrest haemorrhage in 14 consecutive patients—the dose required ranging from 80 to 320 mg/day. A multicentre placebo-controlled study from Spain has also produced strong evidence in favour of the efficacy of propranolol (Perez-Ayuso et al, 1991). Fifty-four patients with anaemia and endoscopic evidence of multiple gastric red spots were randomized to receive either propranolol (26) or placebo (28). Those receiving propranolol were given the drug in increasing dosage until the resting heart rate fell by 25% or below 55 beats/min—the dose required ranging from 40 to 320 mg daily. Both

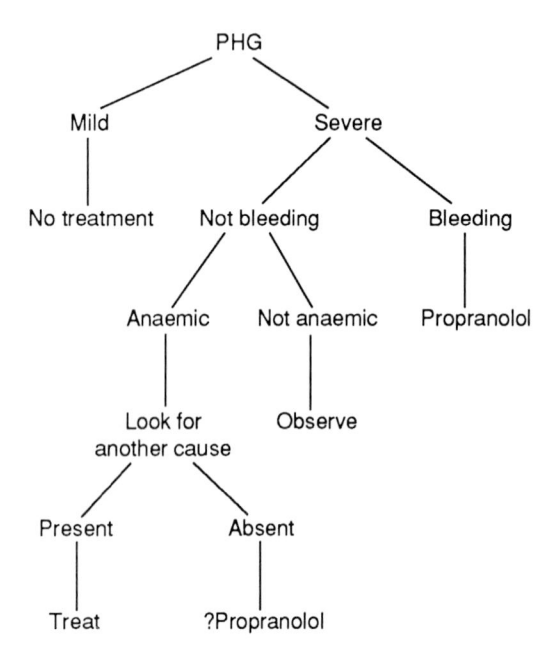

Figure 1. Treatment of portal hypertensive gastropathy.

groups were followed for a mean of over 18 months and actuarial analysis showed that at 12 months a significantly higher proportion of controls had rebled from portal hypertensive gastropathy compared with propranolol-treated subjects (62% versus 35%, $p<0.05$).

Although this study is convincing in terms of demonstrating the efficacy of propranolol it is disappointing to note how many patients had rebled while taking β-blocker (30 months follow-up showed that 48% had rebled from gastropathy). This contrasts with our own experience where we have found that once bleeding has been arrested propranolol remains effective over long periods of time (Triger, 1989). While this difference may be due to problems of long-term patient compliance, a further explanation may relate to the selection criteria for entry in the trial. The Spanish study included all patients with multiple gastric red spots irrespective of whether they were seen to be bleeding. While cherry-red spots usually indicate a high risk of gastrointestinal haemorrhage their presence does not exclude the possibility of bleeding lesions lower down the gastrointestinal tract which may not readily respond to β-blocker therapy (such as rectal varices or portal hypertensive colopathy). When encountering cherry-red spots which are not obviously bleeding it is our practice to observe such patients without initiating propranolol and to repeat the endoscopy from time to time in case bleeding occurs only intermittently. Non-bleeding gastric red spots as the sole abnormality in the upper gastrointestinal tract should not be assumed to be the cause of anaemia in a patient with portal hypertension without further investigation.

The administration of propranolol to patients who are actively bleeding should be undertaken with care since such individuals may be haemodynamically unstable and β-blockade may precipitate hypotension. It is our practice to start with a single low dose of 10 mg orally and if there are no adverse effects to repeat the same dose 12 h later, and thereafter to double the propranolol at 24-h intervals until bleeding has ceased. In acutely bleeding patients this can be assessed by stabilization of the haemoglobin and by the stool returning to normal colour—reduction in resting pulse rate by 25% is not a reliable indicator under such conditions. Once a therapeutic dose of propranolol has been achieved we usually convert the patient to an equivalent once-daily dose of a long-acting preparation. In patients who are severely ill and unable to take the drug orally we have successfully used an intravenous preparation given in an infusion at a rate of 1 mg/h.

Once propranolol has arrested bleeding it usually has to be continued on a long-term basis, particularly if the bleeding was documented to occur for a period of weeks or months rather than being a single acute episode. Experience has shown that if the drug is stopped at least 50% of patients experience rebleeding (Hosking et al, 1987).

There is little or no information available on alternative drugs to propranolol. On an anecdotal basis H_2 receptor antagonists and antacids have been found to be ineffective and other β-blockers have not been evaluated. The suggestion of a deficiency of gastric PGE_2 in portal hypertensive gastropathy has prompted Urabe et al (1989) to use the oral prostaglandin analogue ornoprostil, in patients with cirrhosis. In a preliminary study they have observed it to produce a significant increase in gastric mucosal blood flow but there are no data on its clinical efficacy in portal hypertensive gastropathy. Prostaglandin analogues, however, appear to be associated with a high incidence of unwanted side-effects such as diarrhoea in cirrhotics and this may preclude their widespread use.

SUMMARY

There is now substantial clinical evidence to suggest that portal hypertensive gastropathy is an important source of gastrointestinal bleeding in patients with portal hypertension. Although a relatively uncommon presenting feature in such patients, it appears to become progressively more frequent and important the longer such patients with bleeding oesophageal varices survive after treatment by endoscopic sclerotherapy. It is now being increasingly recognized as the most important cause of haemorrhage after oesophageal varices in such patients. The endoscopic and histological characteristics of the condition are now well established but from a clinical point of view it is important to distinguish it from a number of other disorders. The pathogenesis of portal hypertensive gastropathy is poorly understood; venous congestion secondary to portal hypertension undoubtedly plays an important role but this is not thought to account entirely for the condition since abnormalities in the arterial blood supply are also observed. Many abnormalities in gastric mucosal function have been reported but it is unclear whether these are secondary disturbances or whether they play an important primary role in the development of the condition. Animal studies to date have not been helpful due to the lack of a satisfactory experimental model.

Portocaval shunt surgery cures portal hypertensive gastropathy but propranolol has been shown to be highly effective in controlling haemorrhage from this condition and should now be considered the treatment of choice. The mechanism of action is unclear, and it remains to be shown whether other β-blockers, or indeed any other drugs, are useful in treating this disorder.

REFERENCES

Adachi H, Mitsunaga A, Yokoyama S et al (1989) The study of gastric mucosal changes and their mechanism in patients with liver cirrhosis. *Journal of Gastroenterology and Hepatology* **4 (supplement 1):** 96–98.
Angerson WJ, Geraghty JG & Carter DC (1992) Taurocholate induced gastric mucosal injuries in experimental portal hypertension. *Gut* (in press).
Arakawa A, Satoh H, Fukuda T et al (1987) Endogenous prostaglandin E_2 in gastric mucosa of patients with alcoholic cirrhosis and portal hypertension. *Gastroenterology* **93:** 135–140.
Babb RR & Mitchell RL (1988) Portal decompressive surgery in haemorrhagic gastritis. *American Journal of Gastroenterology* **83:** 777–779.
Calès P, Payen JL, Pienkowski P et al (1989) Relation of congestive gastropathy of cirrhosis to hemoglobin level, hepatic function and mucosal barrier weakness. *Journal of Hepatology* **9 (supplement 1):** S15.

Calès P, Zabotto B, Meskens C et al (1990) Gastroesophageal endoscopic features in cirrhosis. *Gastroenterology* **98:** 156–162.

Chung RS, Bruch D & Dearlove J (1988) Endoscopic measurement of gastric mucosal blood flow by laser doppler velocimetry: effect of chronic oesophageal variceal sclerosis. *American Surgeon* **52:** 116–120.

Clemente C, Bosch J, Rodes J et al (1977) Functional renal failure and haemorrhagic gastritis associated with endotoxaemia in cirrhosis. *Gut* **18:** 556–560.

Dagradi AE, Mehler R, Tan DT & Stempien SJ (1970) Sources of upper gastrointestinal bleeding in patients with liver cirrhosis and large esophago-gastric varices. *American Journal of Gastroenterology* **54:** 458–463.

D'Amico G, Montalbano L, Traina M et al (1990) Natural history of congestive gastropathy in cirrhosis. *Gastroenterology* **99:** 1558–1564.

Eleftheriadis E, Kotzampassi K & Aletral H (1990) The microcirculatory status of portal hypertensive mucosa in 'normal' and post-sclerotherapy patients. *American Journal of Gastroenterology* **85:** 1538–1539.

Foster PN, Wyatt JI, Bullimore DW & Losowsky MS (1989) Gastric mucosa in patients with portal hypertension: prevalence of capillary dilatation and Campylobacter pylori. *Journal of Clinical Pathology* **42:** 919–921.

Geraghty JG, Anderson WJ & Carter DC (1988) Autoradiographic study of the regional distribution of gastric blood flow in portal hypertensive rats. *Gastroenterology* **97:** 1108–1114.

Gostout CJ, Ahlquist DA, Radford CM et al (1989) Endoscopic laser therapy for water melon stomach. *Gastroenterology* **96:** 1462–1465.

Granai F, Hood H, Walsh JT et al (1991a) Gastric acid output in portal hypertension: effect of gastropathy and treating oesophageal varices. *Gut* **32:** A553.

Granai F, Smart HL & Triger DR (1991b) Is anaemia a feature of hypertensive gastropathy? *Gut* **32:** A1211.

Groszmann RJ & Colombato LA (1988) Gastric vascular changes in portal hypertension. *Hepatology* **8:** 1708–1710.

Hashizume M, Tanaka M & Inokuchi K (1983) Morphology of gastric microcirculation in cirrhosis. *Hepatology* **3:** 1008–1016.

Haung Jie-fei (1989) Ultrastructural study of gastric mucosal capillaries in liver cirrhosis with portal hypertension. *Chinese Journal of Digestion* **9:** 17–19.

Hosking SW, Kennedy HJ, Seddon I & Triger DR (1987) The role of propranolol in congestive gastropathy of portal hypertension. *Hepatology* **7:** 437–441.

Iwao T, Toyonaga A & Tanikawa K (1990) Gastric red spots in patients with cirrhosis: subclinical condition of gastric mucosal haemorrhage? *Gastroenterologia Japonica* **25:** 685–692.

Jabbari M, Cherry R, Lough JO et al (1984) Gastric antral vascular ectasia: the watermelon stomach. *Gastroenterology* **87:** 1165–1170.

Kameyama J, Suzuki U, Suzuki A et al (1989) Gastric mucus secretion in portal hypertension. *Journal of Gastroenterology and Hepatology* **4 (supplement 1):** 126–128.

Khodadoost J & Glass GBJ (1972) Erosive gastritis and acute gastroduodenal ulcerations as source of upper gastrointestinal bleeding in liver cirrhosis. *Digestion* **7:** 129–138.

Laine L, Marin-Sorensen M & Weinstein WM (1989) Campylobacter pylori in alcoholic haemorrhagic 'gastritis'. *Digestive Diseases and Sciences* **34:** 677–680.

Laing RW, Smart HL, Hood H & Triger DR (1990) Gastric mucosal changes in portal hypertension: the value of mucosal biopsy. *Gut* **31:** A616–617.

Lam SK (1976) Hypergastrinaemia in cirrhosis of the liver. *Gut* **17:** 700–708.

Mackintosh CE & Keel L (1977) Anatomy and radiology of the areae gastricae. *Gut* **18:** 855–864.

McCormack TT, Simms J, Eyre-Brooke I et al (1985) Gastric lesions in portal hypertension: inflammatory gastritis or congestive gastropathy? *Gut* **26:** 1226–1232.

McCray RS, Martin F, Amir-Ahmedi H et al (1969) Erroneous diagnosis of haemorrhage from oesophageal varices. *American Journal of Digestive Diseases* **14:** 755–760.

Manabe T, Suzuki T & Honjo I (1978) Changes of gastric mucosal blood flow in experimentally induced cirrhosis of the liver. *Surgery, Gynecology and Obstetrics* **147:** 753–757.

Nishiwaki H, Asai T, Sowa T & Umeyama K (1990) Endoscopic measurement of gastric mucosal blood flow with special reference to the effect of sclerotherapy in patients with cirrhosis. *American Journal of Gastroenterology* **85:** 34–37.

Osler W (1898) *Principles and Practice of Medicine* 3rd edn, p 466. Edinburgh and London: Young J. Pentland.

Papazian A, Braillon A, Dupas JL et al (1986) Portal hypertensive gastric mucosa: an endoscopic study. *Gut* **27:** 1199–1203.

Perez-Ayuso RM, Pique JM, Saperas E et al (1989) Gastric vascular ectasias in cirrhosis: association with hypoacidity and related to gastric atrophy. *Scandinavian Journal of Gastroenterology* **24:** 1073–1078.

Perez-Ayuso RM, Piqué JP, Bosch J et al (1991) Propranolol in prevention of recurrent bleeding from severe portal hypertensive gastropathy in cirrhosis. *Lancet* **337:** 1431–1434.

Petrini JL & Johnston JH (1989) Heat probe treatment for antral vascular ectasia. *Gastrointestinal Endoscopy* **35:** 324–328.

Pienkowski P, Payen JL, Calès P et al (1989) Functional study, in man, of congestive gastropathy in cirrhosis by measurement of potential difference. *Gastroenterologie Clinique et Biologique* **13:** 763–768.

Piqué JM, Leung FW, Kitahora T et al (1988) Gastric mucosal blood flow and acid secretion in portal hypertensive rats. *Gastroenterology* **95:** 727–733.

Preble RB (1900) Conclusions based on 60 cases of fatal gastro-intestinal haemorrhage due to cirrhosis of the liver. *American Journal of Medical Science* **119:** 263–280.

Pretolani S, Bonvicini F, Baraldini M et al (1988) Hypertensive gastritis and Campylobacter pylori colonization in cirrhotic patients. *Hepatology* **8:** 1346.

Quintero E, Piqué JM, Bombi JA et al (1985) Antral mucosal hyperemia: characterisation of a portal hypertension related syndrome causing gastric bleeding in patients with cirrhosis. *Journal of Hepatology* **supplement 2:** S315.

Quintero E, Piqué JM, Bombi JA et al (1987) Gastric mucosal vascular ectasias causing bleeding in cirrhosis. *Gastroenterology* **93:** 1054–1061.

Sacchetti C, Capello M, Rebecchi P et al (1988) Frequency of upper gastrointestinal lesions in patients with liver cirrhosis. *Digestive Diseases and Sciences* **33:** 1218–1222.

Saperas E, Piqué JM, Perez-Ayuso R et al (1989) Comparison of snare and large biopsy forceps biopsies in the histological diagnosis of gastric vascular ectasia in cirrhosis. *Endoscopy* **21:** 165–167.

Saperas E, Perez-Ayuso RM, Poca E et al (1990) Increased gastric PGE_2 biosynthesis in cirrhotic patients with gastric vascular ectasia. *American Journal of Gastroenterology* **85:** 138–144.

Sarfeh IJ & Tarnawski A (1987) Gastric mucosal vasculopathy in portal hypertension. *Gastroenterology* **93:** 1129–1131.

Sarfeh IJ, Juler GL, Stemmer EA & Mason GR (1982) Results of surgical management of haemorrhagic gastritis in patients with gastroesophageal varices. *Surgery, Gynecology and Obstetrics* **155:** 167–170.

Sarfeh IJ, Tarnawski A, Malki A et al (1983) Portal hypertension and gastric mucosal injury in rats: effects of alcohol. *Gastroenterology* **84:** 987–993.

Sarfeh IJ, Tarnawski A, Maeda R et al (1984) The gastric mucosa in portal hypertension: effects of topical bile acid. *Scandinavian Journal of Gastroenterology* **19 (supplement 92):** 189–194.

Sarfeh IJ, Tarnawski A, Hajduczek A et al (1988) The portal hypertensive gastric mucosa: histologic, ultrastructural and functional analysis after aspirin induced damage. *Surgery* **104:** 79–85.

Sarfeh IJ, Soliman H, Waxman K et al (1989) Impaired oxygen of gastric mucosa in portal hypertension. The basis for increased susceptibility to injury. *Digestive Diseases and Sciences* **34:** 225–228.

Tarnawski AS, Sarfeh IJ, Stachura J et al (1988) Microvascular abnormalities of the portal hypertensive gastric mucosa. *Hepatology* **8:** 1488–1494.

Thomas E, Rosenthal WS, Rymer W & Katz D (1979) Upper gastrointestinal haemorrhage in patients with alcoholic liver disease and oesophageal varices. *American Journal of Gastroenterology* **72:** 623–629.

Triger DR (1989) The natural history and treatment of portal hypertensive gastropathy. *Journal of Gastroenterology and Hepatology* **4 (supplement 1):** 8–14.

Triger DR & Hosking SW (1989) The gastric mucosa in portal hypertension. *Journal of Hepatology* **8:** 267–272.

Urabe T, Murata T, Terada M et al (1989) Effects of exogenous prostaglandin E_1 derivative on portal vein blood flow and gastric mucosal blood flow in patients with liver cirrhosis. *Journal of Gastroenterology and Hepatology* **4 (supplement 1):** 221–223.

Van Vliet ACM, Ten Kate FJV, Dees J & Van Blankensteen M (1978) Abnormal blood vessels of the pre-pyloric antrum in cirrhosis of the liver as a cause of chronic gastrointestinal bleeding. *Endoscopy* **10:** 89–94.

Waldram R, Davis M, Nunnerley H & Williams R (1974) Emergency endoscopy after gastrointestinal haemorrhage in 50 patients with portal hypertension. *British Medical Journal* **iv:** 94–96.

Walsh JT, Smart HL, Tindale WB & Triger DR (1988) Gastric mucosal blood flow in portal hypertension. *Gut* **29:** A1461.

6
The role of portosystemic shunting in the management of portal hypertension

GIANPAOLO SPINA
ROBERTO SANTAMBROGIO

The first portocaval shunt established in a human was performed by Vidal de Periguez in 1903 (Vidal, 1903). The patient had an uneventful postoperative course after an end-to-side anastomosis until after the second week, when he died from pylephlebitis. After a series of reports of single cases, Blakemore and Lord (1945) reported the first successful series of five end-to-side portocaval shunts utilizing Vitallium tubes. In 1946, they used the suture technique (Blakemore, 1946), on the basis of the principles of vascular anastomosis formulated by Blalock (1947). The good results contributed to the popularity of this operation which was immediately recognized as the best procedure in preventing variceal rebleeding (Rousselot et al, 1963). After this initial enthusiasm, however, a period of critical reflection set in. During the 1960s, documentation of clinical and metabolic sequelae of shunt surgery, e.g. hepatic encephalopathy (HE), began to appear in the literature (McDermott et al, 1961). They were attributed to two factors: the diversion of the entire portal blood flow into the systemic circulation, and the loss of liver portal perfusion (Warren and Muller, 1959). Warren sought to overcome these problems with a procedure that decompressed oesophageal varices and maintained portal perfusion (Warren et al, 1967). These new prospects seemed to restore the prestige of shunt surgery.

In the last few years, other treatments have been proposed: β-blocker agents, endoscopic sclerotherapy and, more recently, liver transplantation. For this reason, we now ask: what is the role in 1992 of portosystemic shunting in the management of portal hypertension? We will try to find an answer in this chapter by examining the three circumstances in which the surgeon might consider intervention: prophylaxis, emergencies and prevention of rebleeding.

PROPHYLACTIC TREATMENT

The unquestionable ability of shunting to prevent variceal haemorrhage is the reason why surgeons used it for patients who had not had previous episodes of bleeding, to avoid the high risk of death after the first episode. In 1954, Palmer analysed a series of 50 patients in which 18 patients with no history of haemorrhage were operated on and came to the conclusion that 'The attitude that the presence of esophageal varices constitutes a proper indication for surgical portal decompression is considered justified, particularly in view of the dire results of a sizable hemorrhage in cirrhosis and the incidence of death from hemorrhage even in the first episode' (Palmer et al, 1954).

The problem, however, was evaluated scientifically only much later, when four controlled trials were performed in the USA (Conn and Lindemuth, 1968; Jackson et al, 1968; Resnick et al, 1969; Conn et al, 1972). They involved 292 patients, followed up for mean periods of 14–78 months. The meta-analysis (Collins et al, 1985) of these studies showed that prophylactic shunting significantly decreased the risk of bleeding (Figure 1). This advantage, however, did not affect survival because the risk of death for the shunted group was slightly increased (Figure 2). There are two explanations for these contrasting results: the low risk of bleeding in the controls and the high risk of liver failure in the shunted patients. For the control group, the risk of bleeding was 26% and only 50% of these patients (13%) died from haemorrhage. Shunting decreased the risk of death due to haemorrhage from 13% to 4%. This advantage is too slight to guarantee better survival and, in any case, it is cancelled by the number of deaths due to liver failure, much higher in the shunted group (33 cases) than in the controls (17 cases). In conclusion, the intervention did not accomplish its proposed aim because of the inability to identify patients at high risk of bleeding and because of

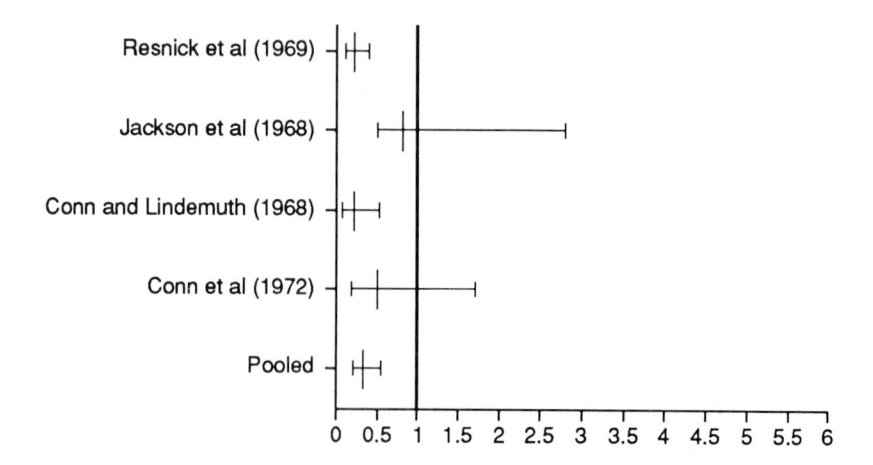

Figure 1. Meta-analysis of bleeding in trials comparing prophylactic shunt surgery with controls. Graph of the bleeding risk, with 95% confidence interval (├───┤). The vertical line indicates the boundary between reduction and increase in the risk of bleeding after shunt surgery versus controls. Horizontal axis indicates the odds ratio with 95% confidence interval. 'Pooled' represents the global bleeding risk: since the 95% intervals are all to the left of the vertical axis, it shows a significant decrease for the shunt group. Heterogeneity test: chi square 4.4; $p > 0.05$.

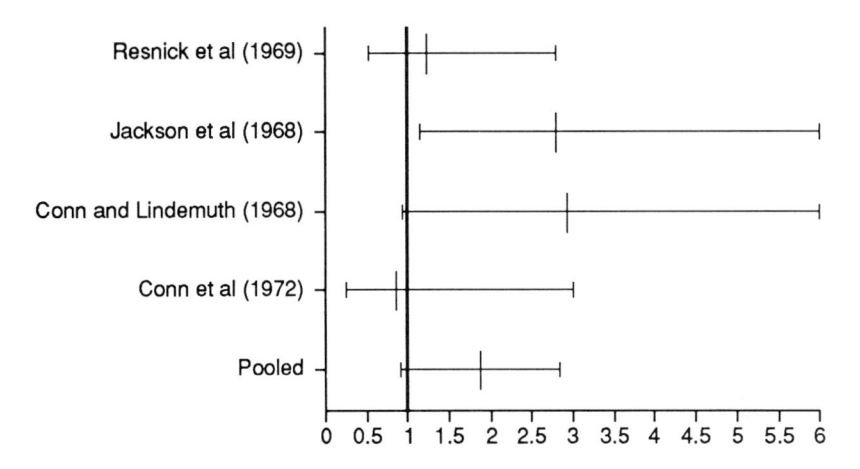

Figure 2. Meta-analysis of death in trials comparing prophylactic shunt surgery with controls. Graph of the death risk, with 95% confidence interval (├──┤). 'Pooled' represents the global death risk: it shows a favourable trend for the control group. Heterogeneity test: chi square 2.7; $p > 0.05$.

increased liver failure in the shunted group. Therefore these surgical procedures did not appear to be warranted for primary prophylaxis of variceal bleeding (Chalmers, 1974).

In the early 1980s, Beppu et al (1981) showed that 'red colour signs', variceal size and colour, as described in a Japanese Study (Japanese Research Society for Portal Hypertension, 1980), were very predictive for variceal haemorrhage. This observation opened new perspectives. In 1983, we initiated a randomized trial enrolling patients with good liver function (and, thus, at low surgical risk) and high risk of bleeding according to the Beppu criteria. In a period of 3 years 23 patients entered the study: 13 were submitted to shunt surgery and 10 treated by propranolol, which was preferred to placebo on the basis of its reported results on the prevention of rebleeding (Lebrec et al, 1980). In spite of these selection criteria, the study was closed prematurely because, in the shunt group, a slight decrease of bleeding risk (zero versus two cases) was outweighed by an increase of both deaths (four cases versus one case) and chronic HE (two versus zero cases), though these results did not reach statistical significance. This result showed once again the inability to overcome the two obstacles of prophylactic therapy, the major one being the selection of the patients at risk of bleeding. In fact, in the control group, with a mean follow-up of 36 months, only 20% of cases bled, which is 7% each year. Although it is possible that the propranolol halved the risk of bleeding, its theoretical rate (14% each year) was too low to justify prophylactic shunt surgery (Burroughs et al, 1986).

The combination of selection by Beppu risk criteria with 'non-decompression' surgery (80% direct procedures, 20% selective shunts) gave very good results in a recent randomized trial of Inokuchi and Cooperative Study Group of Portal Hypertension of Japan (1990). The surgery significantly reduced the incidence of bleeding (7% versus 35%, $p<0.01$) and significantly improved the survival at 5 years (72% versus 45%, $p<0.05$). However, some perplexity about these results has been expressed (Conn, 1990). There is a very high rate of mortality (49%) in the control group despite the relatively low rate of bleeding (35% during a follow-up period of 38 months) and the good liver function (Child's classes: A, 31; B, 21; C, 0). In the surgical group the rate of bleeding was relatively low (35%) although most were direct procedures (A Peracchia, personal communication); the operative mortality was also low (4%) although several institutions were included (22). Finally, the low total mortality (22%) did not agree with that in the previous series of the same groups (Inokuchi, 1985).

The availability of more reliable selection criteria for patients at high risk of bleeding, as recently suggested by the NIEC (North Italian Endoscopic Club, 1988) would seem to justify doing new prophylactic surgical trials. However, the patients at higher risk of bleeding, identified by this classification, are, for the most part, in Child's C class, which is *per se* a contraindication for operation. Patients in A and B classes have a low bleeding risk (about 10% per year) that does not justify so invasive a procedure as surgery. At the moment, this excludes any possibility of using prophylactic treatments as routine, especially surgical ones, since they always include a certain number of operative deaths. In exceptional cases, however, surgery might be considered for particular patients (Nagasue et al, 1988a), especially those who would not be expected to respond to medical therapy according to endoscopic and haemodynamic investigations (Conn, 1988).

EMERGENCY TREATMENT

Without prophylactic therapy, about 18% of cirrhotics with portal hypertension bleed per year and about 50% of these die of haemorrhage (D'Amico et al, 1986; North Italian Endoscopic Club, 1988; Burroughs et al, 1989). Since the efficacy of shunt surgery in stopping bleeding has been established, it is logical to expect good improvement of survival after using shunt surgery for emergencies. This was the opinion of those who did the first series of emergency portocaval shunts, despite the high mortality observed (30–50%) (Smith et al, 1974; Pezzuoli and Spina, 1986; Burroughs, 1988). These rates have improved globally during the last few years (Burroughs, 1988), but physicians, acknowledging the progress obtained with conservative treatment, especially using sclerotherapy, still greatly mistrust surgery. Considerable improvement in survival has been evident over the years (Table 1). In our experience (35 shunted patients), for example, bleeding stopped in 97% of cases and operative mortality was 9% (Spina et al, 1990a). Why this improvement? One reason is probably the more aggressive approach: our patients were operated on within a mean of 32 h after hospitalization. Procrastination before operation can exacerbate the patients' condition increasing the surgical mortality rate (Grossman and McGreevy, 1988; Langer et al, 1990). A second contribution has certainly been the improvement in resuscitation and anaesthetic techniques (Burroughs, 1988). A third

Table 1. Historical series of emergency shunt surgery.

Authors	Year	No. patients	Operative mortality (%)	Child's C (%)
Hivet	1952	65	45	NR
Leger	1973	134	69	27
Turcotte	1973	43	51	26
Prandi	1975	93	57	NR
Rueff	1975	343	47	25
Malt	1978	24	73	20
Osborne and Hunt	1981	20	35	30
Orloff and Bell	1986	21	19	27
Cello et al	1987	31	56	100
Villeneuve et al	1987	39	26	8
Teres et al	1987	16	19	0
Orloff et al	1990	21	19	52
Spina	1990	35	9	31

reason was better patient selection (Franco, 1990). Liver function, evaluated as Pugh–Child's risk (Pugh et al, 1973), was the only preoperative parameter in multivariate analysis (among 16 clinical, biochemical and haemodynamic factors evaluated) that influenced mortality (Spina et al, 1990a). The survival curves of the patients confirmed this (Figure 3). These findings suggest that great caution should be taken with Child's C patients, in whom there should not be an *a priori* rejection of operation. In fact, the shunt rescues some patients destined to die.

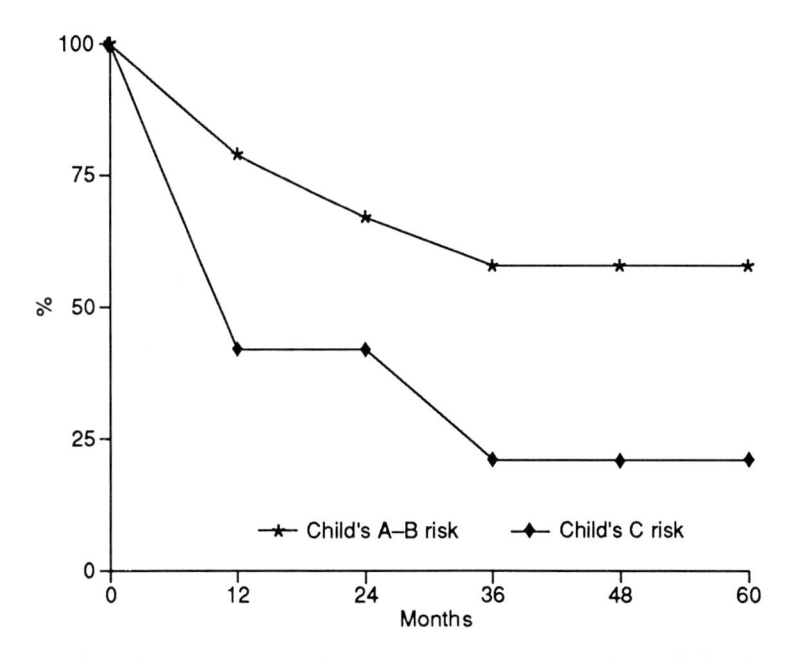

Figure 3. Actuarial survival curves after emergency portosystemic shunts divided into two classes according to the Child's classification (A–B risk combined versus C risk) ($p < 0.05$).

The idea that a more aggressive approach can improve survival stimulated us to investigate the results when the shunt was used very early (immediate treatment), instead of using it after the failure of conservative therapies (rescue treatment). The analysis of seven studies published in the last 10 years (three of rescue treatment) (Osborne and Hobbs, 1981; Teres et al, 1987a; Spina et al, 1990a) and four of immediate treatment (Orloff and Bell, 1986; Cello et al, 1987; Villeneuve et al, 1987; Orloff et al, 1990) (Table 2) did not clarify this situation, because the data are not suitable for a cumulative statistical assessment. The only significant study is that of Orloff et al (1990), in which the emergency shunt (performed within 6h of hospitalization) was compared with conservative therapy followed by elective operation. The results are very favourable for immediate shunt surgery and seem to indicate that the standard procedure, e.g. use of surgery only after the failure of sclerotherapy, is not so good. This does not mean that the standard procedure should be abandoned, at least for the present, since the results are not comparable with those of other series and, although it was randomized, have been published only in abstract form.

Table 2. Results of recently published studies of emergency shunt surgery: comparison between immediate treatment (Orloff and Bell, 1986; Cello et al, 1987; Villeneuve et al, 1987; Orloff et al, 1990) and rescue treatment (Osborne and Hobbs, 1981; Teres et al, 1987a; Spina et al, 1990a).

Authors	Year	No. patients	Operative mortality (%)	Control of bleeding (%)	Survival (%)
Osborne and Hobbs	1981	20	35	95	50 (12 months)
Orloff and Bell	1986	21	19	100	72 (60 months)
Cello et al*	1987	31	56	81	18 (18 months)
Villeneuve et al	1987	39	26	97	71 (24 months)
Teres et al	1987a	16	19	100	39 (36 months)
Orloff et al	1990	21	19	100	54 (60 months)
Spina et al	1990a	35	9	97	43 (60 months)

* Only Child's C risk.

At present, although not confirmed by randomized trials, the widely accepted view is that emergency shunt surgery should be used only after failure of sclerotherapy, which is almost as effective in stopping bleeding (Burnett and Rikkers, 1990) and less demanding. In addition, stopping the bleeding with conservative measures gives time to choose the best elective treatment, whereas emergency surgery is a road without return.

Finally, the last problem: if a shunt must be performed, do we choose a total or a selective shunt? With the first, immediate and safe stopping of haemorrhage is guaranteed; with the second, there is greater possibility of protecting liver function. On this basis, it seems logical to use the total shunt for massive haemorrhage and to reserve selective shunts for less serious haemorrhage that does not require immediate decompression of the varices. However, there are some data that contradict this approach, showing a haemostatic effect of the selective shunt (80–100% of stopping bleeding) similar to that of total shunt, with the same operative mortality (21–28%)

(Potts et al, 1984; Peterson and Giles, 1986; Nagasue et al, 1988). Without controlled studies, it is difficult at present to decide on correct management.

In conclusion, the emergency shunt should be used, except in particular cases, only after the failure of sclerotherapy. We must not forget, however, that the decision to operate on the patient must be made at the right time, because it is certain that these patients tolerate shunt surgery better if there has not been progressive deterioration due to persistent, even slight, bleeding.

ELECTIVE TREATMENT

The prevention of recurrent variceal bleeding is the real battlefield of shunt surgery and it is the area in which the most experience has accumulated. The reason is that in elective treatment, clinicians can select the patient better and operate on the selected patient better (Conn, 1974). Elective shunt surgery excited great enthusiasm initially. When in the late 1950s Child proposed a multihospital randomized study of portocaval shunts in cirrhotics with previous episodes of variceal bleeding versus patients treated medically, the study was not initiated because the department of surgery at one participating hospital believed it would be unethical to deny the patients the proven benefit of a total shunt (Donovan, 1984). However, initial enthusiasm began to weaken when four randomized studies (Jackson et al, 1971; Resnick et al, 1974; Rueff et al, 1976; Reynolds et al, 1981) comparing portocaval shunt with conservative therapy were completed and showed that, even with a decrease in variceal rebleeding (5–20% versus 64–75%), shunt surgery did not improve survival (44–55% versus 24–56%) and introduced two negative effects: deterioration of liver function (rate of deaths due to liver failure: 53–81% versus 10–48%) and increased chronic HE (20–49% versus 0–35%). These were probably due to the lack of portal perfusion and the diversion of splanchnic blood flow into the systemic circulation. As a result, shunt surgery was mainly abandoned and was not revived by the use of technical devices to regulate the calibre of the anastomosis (Marion et al, 1979).

The solution of the problem was found after major contributions from Texeira et al (1967) and Warren et al (1967) to haemodynamics and Davidson et al (1967) to metabolic areas. The new procedure was called the 'distal splenorenal shunt' (DSRS). The idea of the DSRS, initially proposed by Texeira on the basis of autopsy studies and tried unsuccessfully in the human being, was made practical in 1967 by Warren, who was inspired by observing the splenoportogram of a patient with a spontaneous splenorenal shunt: he did not have oesophagogastric varices, but did have portal hypertension with hepatopedal portal flow (Warren et al, 1967). The procedure is based on the fact that by ligating the splenic, coronary, gastroepiploic and pyloric veins and the other major tributaries, it is possible to separate the abdomen into two areas, so that the high pressure in the portomesenteric area maintains portal perfusion of the liver while the relatively low pressure in the gastrosplenic area guarantees, through the anastomosis, the decompression of gastro-oesophageal varices. The validity of this approach has been gradually confirmed by the improving results in numerous controlled studies.

Selective versus total shunts

To date, the results of six controlled trials, all randomized, have been published comparing the DSRS with a variety of portosystemic shunts (PSS)—portocaval (Langer et al, 1985; Harley et al, 1986), splenorenal (Fischer et al, 1981), mesocaval (Reichle et al, 1979)—in pure or mixed series (Millikan et al, 1985; Grace et al, 1988). Against variceal rebleeding the DSRS showed similar efficacy as PSS in five of six studies (6–18% versus 0–17%). The higher incidence of variceal rebleeding (30%) in the DSRS group in the last study (Harley et al, 1986) has been ascribed to high incidence of shunt thrombosis (13%) and haemorrhage in patients with patent shunts (17%).

Four of the six studies showed a trend to better survival for the DSRS patients than for PSS patients (Langer et al, 1985; Millikan et al, 1985; Harley et al, 1986; Grace et al, 1988), one showed similar survival (Fischer et al, 1981) and the last showed an unfavourable trend (Reichle et al, 1979). In no study was the difference large enough to be statistically significant. These data contrast, at least in part, with the results for non-randomized series, which seem to show better survival after DSRS (Henderson et al, 1984).

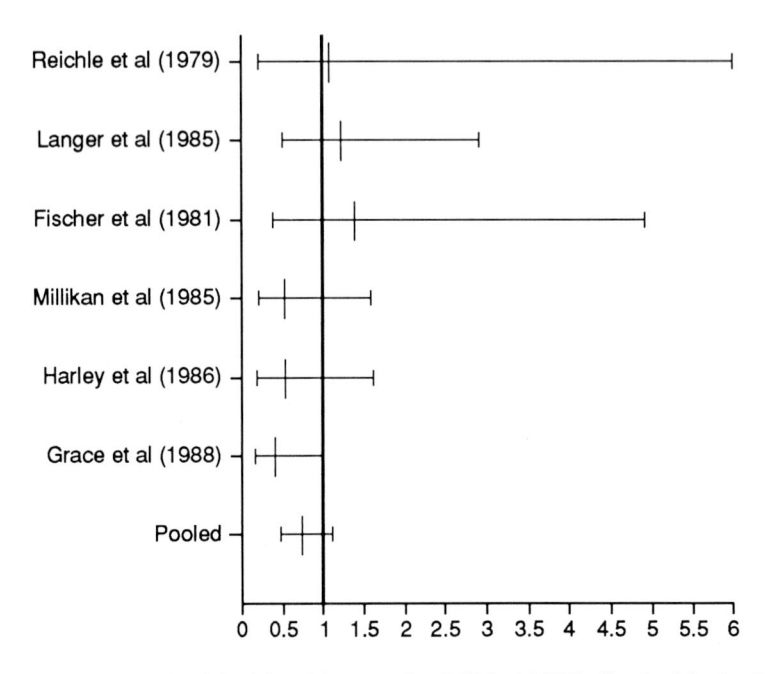

Figure 4. Meta-analysis of death in trials comparing DSRS with PSS. Graph of the death risk, with 95% confidence interval (|—|). 'Pooled' represents the global death risk: it shows a favourable trend for the DSRS. Heterogeneity test: chi square 7.73; $p > 0.05$.

Why is the trend not confirmed by randomized studies? The first reason is probably the small number of cases enrolled in each group: for these numbers the average survival at 5 years would become statistically significant if there were a difference of 25–35%, which is an impossible goal for present treatments (Lebrec et al, 1980; Westaby et al, 1985). Not even meta-analysis obviates this disadvantage: it shows only a favourable trend for the DSRS in reducing the pooled risk of death (Figure 4). We must add to this the fact that in some trials the recruitment period was very long, from 5 to 11 years. There could have been inserted into the protocol of study several new factors which might cause large changes in patient outcome. One negative factor could have been the participation of many surgeons with varying skills. Finally, the aetiology of the cirrhosis of the patients was not homogeneous (Zeppa et al, 1978; Henderson et al, 1983).

Chronic HE has always been the Achilles heel of shunt surgery and, therefore, it is a very important element in comparison. After DSRS, the incidence of HE was lower in four studies (Fischer et al, 1981), significantly so in three (Reichle et al, 1979; Langer et al, 1985; Millikan et al, 1985) and higher in two (Harley et al, 1986; Grace et al, 1988). How is it possible to explain these contrasting results? In part, probably, they are due to differences in the haemodynamic results of the DSRS in the various studies. Alcohol abuse, frequent in some subgroups of these patients, could be implicated, because the outcome of the DSRS seems to be affected more than that of PSS (Harley et al, 1986). The variation in evaluating HE is certainly a factor of great importance. It was assessed in only three trials (Langer et al, 1985; Millikan et al, 1985; Harley et al, 1986) by objective criteria (rate of hospitalization for HE, duration of chronic HE episodes, actuarial curves) or semiquantitative methods (HE index). Finally, the small number of patients can accentuate the apparent differences in results. However, when meta-analysis is used to solve this problem, the pooled risk of chronic HE is significantly lower in the DSRS group (Figure 5). What is more, an accurate evaluation of HE can reveal other important differences (Spina et al, 1988a,b). After DSRS, severe HE is no longer a problem (9% versus 0%; $p = 0.049$). HE reaches its maximum rate (18% in the actuarial curve) later (27 versus 4 months). Its duration, assessed as a sum of single episodes of HE, lasts less during the follow-up period (18% versus 46%). Consequently, the risk of hospital admission for HE was almost one-half (0.42 admissions per patient versus 0.83%; $p = 0.037$). In conclusion, haemostatic efficacy, with a favourable trend to better survival and, above all, a significantly improved quality of life after DSRS, are the reasons why we believe that selective shunts are preferable for the prevention of variceal rebleeding.

The results reported for HE after DSRS seem to be further improved by the recent modification of the operation devised by Warren (Warren et al, 1986). The importance of the collateral pathways in determining HE has been widely documented (Henderson et al, 1985; Maffei-Faccioli et al, 1990; Spina et al, 1990b). We ourselves have found 4% of chronic HE in patients who have little or no collateral circulation versus 21% in those with widespread pathways (Spina et al, 1990c). In our recent multivariate analysis,

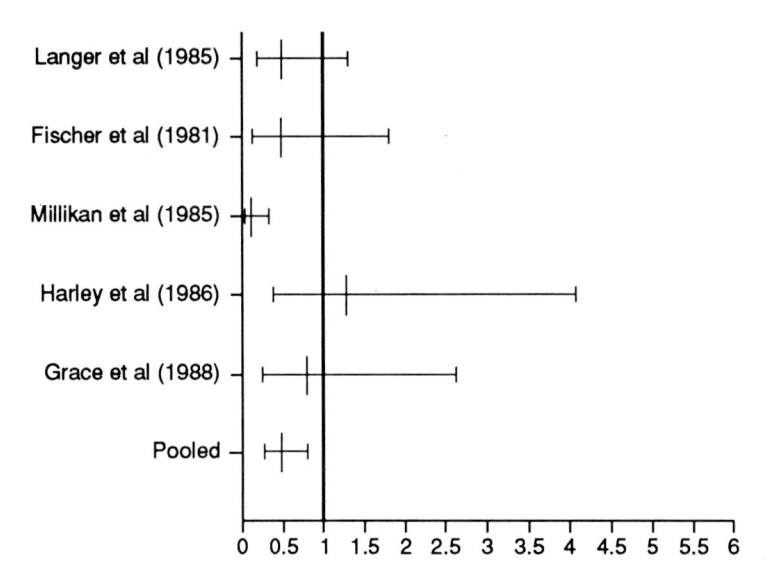

Figure 5. Meta-analysis of chronic encephalopathy (HE) in trials comparing DSRS with PSS. Graph of the risk of chronic HE, with 95% confidence interval (⊢——⊣). 'Pooled' represents the HE risk: it shows a significant decrease after DSRS. Heterogeneity test: chi square 1.88; $p > 0.05$.

collateral pathways were found to be, together with portal perfusion and splanchnic pressure, the only independent variables of HE. To improve the surgical disconnection, Warren et al (1986) suggested that the splenocolic ligament should be taken down and a complete dissection of the splenic vein should be performed from the pancreas to its bifurcation at the splenic hilum, the so-called 'splenopancreatic disconnection' (SPD). The operation improves portal perfusion and could have consequences for survival (Ashida et al, 1989; Henderson et al, 1989; Maffei-Faccioli et al, 1990; Spina et al, 1990c). It is evident that this extension of the shunt surgery increases the difficulties of operation. It must be attempted, nevertheless, obviously taking into account the need for safety: the operative risk must never be neglected. It is important to note that, although it is not possible to perform complete SPD on every occasion, partial improvement of the disconnection should give more favourable results (Spina et al, 1990b).

In consideration of the technical difficulties of the DSRS with or without SPD, the use of the prosthetic portocaval H-graft (PCHG) has also been proposed again recently, but using a small-diameter graft, to maintain the portal perfusion (Johansen, 1989; Rypins and Sarfeh, 1988; Capussotti et al, 1990; Chabert et al, 1990; Rosemurgy et al, 1991). It has become possible because new prosthetic materials (Goretex) seems to prevent the old problem of the alloplastic graft: thrombosis formation (Rypins and Sarfeh, 1988). The results of the first experience (Table 3) seem promising, but we must wait for the publication of randomized studies before definitive judgement (Shah et al, 1989).

Table 3. Results after small-diameter portocaval H-grafts.

Authors	Year	No. patients	Survival (%)	Rebleeding (%)	HE (%)	Portal perfusion (%)
Rypins and Sarfeh	1988	43	32 (60 months)	3	—	59
Johansen	1989	50	88*	2	6	0
Chabert et al	1990	38	60 (48 months)	3	16	25
Capussotti et al	1990	29	76*	7	7	76
Rosemurgy et al	1991	36	83*	3	11	52

* No actuarial data.

While awaiting these studies, we think that at present, the DSRS, with or without the SPD, should be proposed for the elective treatment of all cases in which it can be achieved technically with low operative mortality. This statement requires caution, since it is well known that, when there are unfavourable anatomical situations, which become fewer with experience, formation of a selective shunt can be followed by failure.

Shunt surgery versus sclerotherapy

The good results of surgery obtained in recent years must be compared with conservative therapy. At present we have the results of five randomized trials, all versus endoscopic sclerotherapy. In four studies, the shunt was a DSRS (Rikkers et al, 1987; Teres et al, 1987b; Henderson et al, 1990; Spina et al, 1990d), and in the last, it was a portocaval shunt (Planas et al, 1991). The results of the first four studies, in addition to those published, were obtained from a questionnaire sent by us to the investigators. The data from all the trials were analysed by meta-analysis.

Table 4. Prevention of rebleeding due to portal hypertension in the trials comparing shunt surgery with sclerotherapy.

Authors	Year	Shunt (%)	Sclerosis (%)	p
Henderson et al	1990	3	59	<0.001
Teres et al	1987b	14	37	<0.02
Rikkers et al	1987	17	60	<0.001
Spina et al	1990d	3	38	<0.003
Planas et al	1991	6	51	<0.01

All the studies confirmed that the shunt is more effective than sclerotherapy in preventing rebleeding (Table 4). This advantage is in part due to the fact that in the sclerosis group some of the haemorrhages were due to congestive gastropathy, whereas it almost disappeared in the shunted group. However, this efficacy in preventing rebleeding was not accompanied by an evident improvement of survival (Figure 6). The reason is that the trend was for a low mortality after shunts in four studies, but in one study there was also significant improvement in the sclerotherapy group (Henderson et al, 1990). The latter seemed to be due to two factors not encountered in the other studies: the large number of sclerotherapy failures operated on

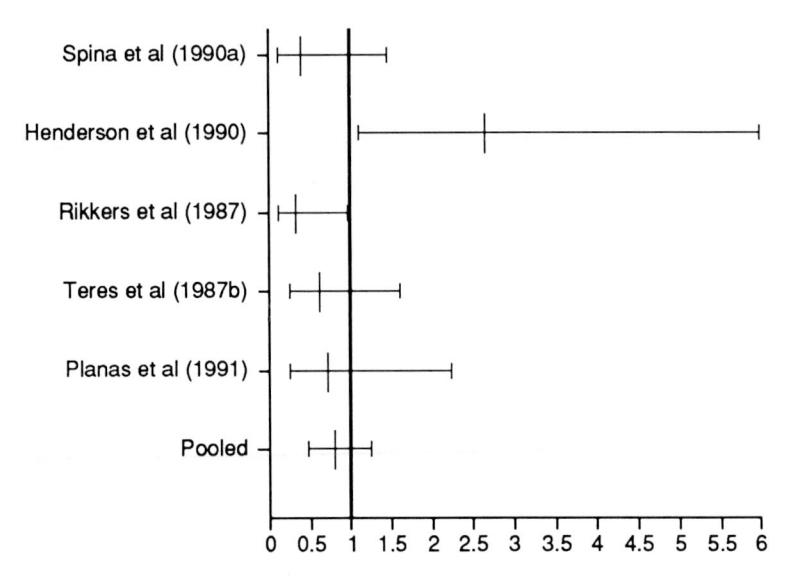

Figure 6. Meta-analysis of death in trials comparing shunt surgery with sclerotherapy. Graph of the death risk, with 95% confidence interval (⊢——⊣). 'Pooled' represents the global death risk: it shows a slightly favourable trend for shunt group. Heterogeneity test: chi square 10.48; $p < 0.05$.

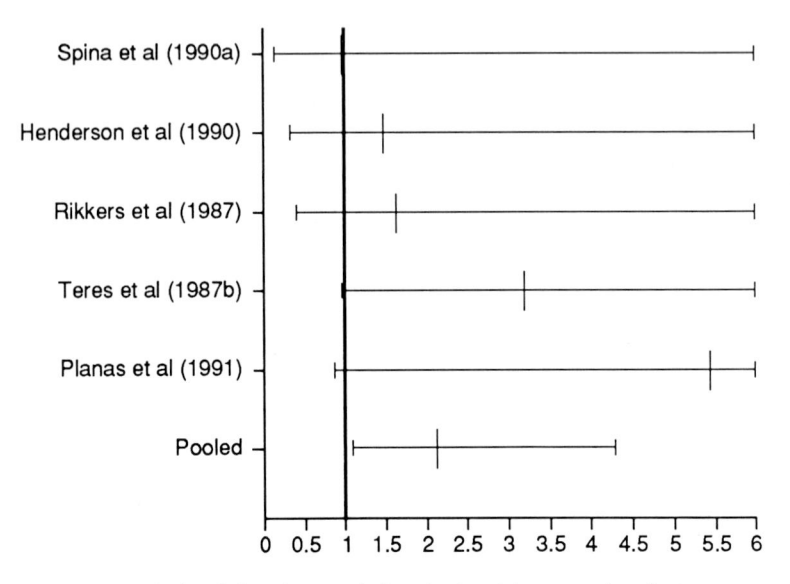

Figure 7. Meta-analysis of chronic encephalopathy in trials comparing shunt surgery with sclerotherapy. Graph of the encephalopathy risk, with 95% confidence interval (⊢——⊣). 'Pooled' represents the global encephalopathy risk: it shows a significant decrease in sclerotherapy group. Heterogeneity test: chi square 2.82; $p > 0.05$.

successfully (12 out of 37) and the bad results for the alcoholic patients operated on versus those for non-alcoholics (Kawasaki et al, 1991).

It is evident that the shunt increases significantly the risk of development of HE (Figure 7). However, in confirmation of the results of the studies already described, this increase was significant only for total shunts (Planas et al, 1991) and less selective shunts (Teres et al, 1987b). There were no significant differences in the studies using the DSRS (Spina et al, 1990c).

Therefore, at present we think that both therapies produce similar results, at least in the short term, and, in making a choice, the acceptability to the patient of the two therapies must be relevant: the shunt is a more traumatic but definitive treatment, with a small risk of HE; sclerotherapy has a minimal impact, but it must be repeated and is less effective, at least initially, in preventing variceal rebleeding. The study of Henderson et al (1990) also suggests a need to ensure a shunt rescue for the patient when sclerotherapy fails. At present, efforts must be made to identify the subgroups of patients who can benefit best from one or the other procedure.

Shunt and liver transplantation

Recently, a new therapy has become very important for treatment of variceal haemorrhages in cirrhotics: liver transplantation (LT), the only way to cure both the complication and the disease. In Pittsburgh, 302 patients with severe hepatic failure were submitted to LT after episodes of variceal haemorrhage. The survival at 5 years was 71% (Iwatsuki et al, 1988).

LT is probably the treatment of the future, but it is not yet possible to advise the procedure for all patients with variceal bleeding and severe liver disease (Bismuth et al, 1990). For some time yet, the patients who do not stop bleeding will have to have shunts. This approach gives rise to two problems: (1) which patient with previous variceal bleeding should have a shunt and which an LT; (2) if the LT must be delayed, which shunt has less effect on subsequent LT.

There are a number of diseases that result in portal hypertension and oesophageal varices for which LT is inappropriate and for which the shunt is the best indication: to cite the most common, prehepatic blocks, schistosomiasis, congenital hepatic fibrosis, and hepatic artery–portal vein fistula (Bismuth et al, 1987). The candidate for LT is certainly the patient with such advanced liver disease that he cannot tolerate the effects of the shunt (Wood et al, 1990). The indications are more difficult for cirrhotics with good hepatic reserve (Child's classes A and B). For them, survival at 4 years after LT is similar to that after DSRS (87% versus 74%) (Wood et al, 1990). The two therapies differ in the slopes of the two curves: after LT, it is flat after the first year, in which there is the major mortality, whereas after DSRS, survival continuously declines with time. However, it is easy to forecast a decrease in early mortality after LT as more are performed and experience increases; moreover new immunosuppressive therapies will prevent rejection better.

As regards the second question (Esquivel et al, 1987; Brems et al, 1989; Crass et al, 1989; Mazzaferro et al, 1990), from the technical point of view, the least compromising shunts for subsequent LT are H-graft mesocaval or mesorenal shunts. However, if there is fear of early shunt thrombosis (with high risk with the use of prosthetic materials), and a portocaval shunt is chosen, some investigators prefer an end-to-side portocaval shunt (Wood et al, 1990) because it does not risk compromising the length of extrahepatic portal vein. The DSRS should be reserved for those patients who will have LT in the long term and, therefore, can take advantage of this technically more difficult operation.

CONCLUSIONS

In this chapter, we have tried to indicate the role of PSS in treatment of portal hypertension. The conclusions are evident: shunt surgery has undergone some important technical changes: from the Vitallium tube used in the first shunts it has been transformed into a surgery with functional purposes. In spite of this evolution, it lost its role as leader in the treatment of portal hypertension. It is not possible now to agree with the statement of Orloff at the International Symposium on Medical and Surgical Problems of Portal Hypertension, held in Rome in 1979: 'Portal-systemic shunt is the only definitive treatment that has been devised for bleeding esophageal varices in patients with cirrhosis. To my knowledge, there is no alternative form of therapy of proven long-term effectiveness' (Orloff, 1980). Choices must be made from the new medical therapies, endoscopic sclerotherapy and LT. Our duty is to select the best treatment for each patient and, when a shunt is chosen, to use the best shunt (Conn, 1974). It can be affirmed that:

1. The selective shunt is a solution that provides both good variceal decompression and satisfactory maintenance of liver function. Its results in great part depends on the skill of the surgeon.
2. Only a patient with good liver function (Child's classes A and B) is a candidate for shunt surgery, with, very occasionally, a patient with severe disease (class C).
3. In prophylaxis, except for particular cases, shunt surgery is not advisable and will not be until good candidates at high risk of bleeding can be identified for shunt surgery.
4. In an emergency, the operation is used only after failure of sclerotherapy, but it must be used at the right time before the patient's condition has deteriorated.
5. In the prevention of variceal rebleeding, the DSRS is the alternative solution to sclerotherapy as a routine measure. The choice between the two treatments depends on the patient's willingness and the ability of the institution to perform both procedures successfully. If sclerotherapy is chosen, the institution must be able to rapidly rescue a sclerotherapy failure by shunt surgery.

We hope that in the near future patients can be selected better and the best treatment for each can be performed.

SUMMARY

In this chapter, we have tried to indicate the role of the portosystemic shunt in the treatment of portal hypertension. The conclusions are evident: in the last 10 years it has lost its role as leader in the treatment of portal hypertension. However, some firm statements can be made. The selective shunt is an operation that provides both good variceal decompression and satisfactory maintenance of liver function. Its results in great part depend on the skill of the surgeon. Only a patient with good liver function (Child's classes A and B) is a candidate for shunt surgery, with, very occasionally, a patient with severe disease (class C). In an emergency, the operation is used only after failure of sclerotherapy, but it must be used at the right time before the patient's condition has deteriorated. In the prevention of variceal rebleeding, the selective shunt or sclerotherapy can be routine measures. The choice between the two treatments depends on the patient's willingness and the ability of the institution to perform both procedures successfully. If sclerotherapy is chosen, the institution must be able to rapidly rescue a sclerotherapy failure by shunt surgery. Liver transplantation is probably the treatment of the future, but it is at present impossible to suggest that the procedure is feasible for all patients with variceal bleeding and severe liver disease.

REFERENCES

Ashida H, Utsunomiya J, Kotoura Y et al (1989) Results of distal splenorenal shunt with versus without splenopancreatic disconnection. *Journal of Clinical Gastroenterology* **11:** 658–662.
Beppu K, Inokuchi K, Koyanagi N et al (1981) Prediction of variceal hemorrhage by esophageal endoscopy. *Gastrointestinal Endoscopy* **27:** 213–218.
Bismuth H, Castaing D, Ericzon BG et al (1987) Hepatic transplantation in Europe. *Lancet* **1:** 674–676.
Bismuth H, Adam R, Mathur S & Sherlock S (1990) Options for elective treatment of portal hypertension in cirrhotic patients in the transplantation era. *American Journal of Surgery* **160:** 105–110.
Blakemore AH (1946) Portacaval anastomosis: report on fourteen cases. *Bulletin of the New York Academy of Medicine* **22:** 254–259.
Blakemore AH & Lord JW (1945) The technique of using Vitallium's tubes in establishing porta-caval shunts for portal hypertension. *Annals of Surgery* **122:** 476–489.
Blalock A (1947) The use of shunt or by-pass operations in the treatment of certain circulatory disorders, including portal hypertension and pulmonic stenosis. *Annals of Surgery* **125:** 129–137.
Brems JJ, Hiatt JR, Klein AS et al (1989) Effect of a prior portasystemic shunt on subsequent liver transplantation. *Annals of Surgery* **209:** 51–56.
Burnett DA & Rikkers LF (1990) Nonoperative emergency treatment of variceal hemorrhage. *Surgical Clinics of North America* **70:** 291–306.
Burroughs AK (1988) The management of bleeding due to portal hypertension. Part I. The management of acute bleeding episodes. *Quarterly Journal of Medicine* **254:** 447–458.
Burroughs AK, D'Heygere F & McIntyre N (1986) Pitfalls in studies of prophylactic therapy for variceal bleeding in cirrhotics. *Hepatology* **6:** 1407–1413.
Burroughs AK, Mezzanotte G, Phillips A et al (1989) Cirrhotics with variceal hemorrhage: the importance of the time interval between admission and the start of analysis for survival and rebleeding rates. *Hepatology* **9:** 801–807.

Capussotti L, Aricò S, Bouzary H et al (1990) Do partial porto-systemic shunts reduce postoperative encephalopathy rate? *International Journal of Gastroenterology* **22:** 166.

Cello JP, Grendell JH, Crass RA et al (1987) Endoscopic sclerotherapy versus portacaval shunt in patients with severe cirrhosis and acute variceal hemorrhage. Long-term follow-up. *New England Journal of Medicine* **316:** 11–15.

Chabert M, Page Y, Cadi F et al (1990) L'anastomose porto-cave latéro-latérale calibrées dans le traitement des hémorragies par rupture de varices oesophagiennes. *Gastroenterologie Clinique et Biologique* **14:** 698–704.

Chalmers TC (1974) Prophylactic shunts. In Child CG (ed.) *Portal Hypertension*, 3rd edn, pp 121–126. Philadelphia: WB Saunders Company.

Collins R, Yusuf S & Peto R (1985) Overview of randomized trials of diuretics in pregnancy. *British Medical Journal* **290:** 17–23.

Conn HO (1974) Therapeutic portacaval anastomosis: to shunt or not to shunt. *Gastroenterology* **67:** 1065–1073.

Conn HO (1988) Prophylactic propranolol: the first big step. *Hepatology* **8:** 167–170.

Conn HO (1990) Why is prophylactic portal nondecompression surgery effective in preventing hemorrhage from esophageal varices? *Hepatology* **12:** 166–169.

Conn HO & Lindemuth WW (1968) Prophylactic portacaval anastomosis in cirrhotic patients with esophageal varices. Interim results, with suggestions for subsequent investigations. *New England Journal of Medicine* **279:** 725–732.

Conn HO, Lindemuth WW, May CJ & Ramsby GR (1972) Prophylactic portacaval anastomosis. A tale of two studies. *Medicine* **51:** 27–40.

Crass RA, Keefe EB & Wright Pinson C (1989) Management of variceal hemorrhage in the potential liver transplant candidate. *American Journal of Surgery* **157:** 476–478.

D'Amico G, Morabito A, Pagliaro L et al (1986) Six-week prognostic indicators in upper gastrointestinal hemorrhage in cirrhosis. *Frontiers of Gastrointestinal Research* **9:** 247–257.

Davidson F, Denize A, Hurwitt ES & Laufman H (1967) Reverse splenocaval anastomosis for prevention of postshunt ammonia intoxication. *Surgery, Gynecology and Obstetrics* **125:** 815–818.

Donovan AJ (1984) Surgical treatment of portal hypertension: an historical perspective. *World Journal of Surgery* **8:** 626–645.

Esquivel CO, Klintmalm G, Iwatsuki S et al (1987) Liver transplantation in patients with patent splenorenal shunts. *Surgery* **101:** 430–432.

Fischer JE, Bower RH, Atamian S & & Welling BAR (1981) Comparison of distal and proximal spleno-renal shunts. *Annals of Surgery* **194:** 531–542.

Franco D (1990) Traitement d'urgence des hémorragies digestives hautes de l'hypertension portale: chirurgie. *Gastroenterologie Clinique et Biologique* **14:** 58B–62B.

Grace ND, Conn HO, Resnick RH et al (1988) Distal spleno-renal vs. portal-systemic shunts after hemorrhage from varices: a randomized controlled trial. *Hepatology* **8:** 1475–1481.

Grossman MD & McGreevy JM (1988) Effect of delayed operation for bleeding esophageal varices on Child's class and indices of liver function. *American Journal of Surgery* **156:** 502–505.

Harley HAJ, Morgan T & Redeker G (1986) Results of a randomized trial of end-to-side portacaval shunt and distal splenorenal shunt in alcoholic liver disease and variceal bleeding. *Gastroenterology* **91:** 802–809.

Henderson JM, Millikan WJ, Wright-Bacon L et al (1983) Hemodynamic differences between alcoholic and non-alcoholic cirrhotics following distal spleno-renal shunt. Effect on survival? *Annals of Surgery* **198:** 325–334.

Henderson JM, Millikan WJ & Warren WD (1984) The distal spleno-renal shunt: an update. *World Journal of Surgery* **8:** 722–732.

Henderson JM, Gong-Liang J, Galloway J et al (1985) Portaprival collaterals following distal splenorenal shunt. Incidence, magnitude and associated portal perfusion changes. *Journal of Hepatology* **1:** 649–661.

Henderson JM, Warren WD, Millikan WJ et al (1989) Distal splenorenal shunt with splenopancreatic disconnection. A 4-year assessment. *Annals of Surgery* **210:** 332–339.

Henderson JM, Kutner MH, Millikan WJ et al (1990) Endoscopic variceal sclerosis compared with distal splenorenal shunt to prevent recurrent variceal bleeding in cirrhosis. A prospective, randomized trial. *Annals of Internal Medicine* **112:** 262–269.

Hivet M, Lagadec B & Poilleux J (1972) 65 derivations porto-caves en urgence chez les cirrhotiques (abstract). *Biologie et Gastroenterologie* **5**: 616c.

Inokuchi K (1985) Present status of surgical treatment of esophageal varices in Japan: a nationwide survey of 3588 patients. *World Journal of Surgery* **9**: 171–180.

Inokuchi K & Cooperative Study Group of Portal Hypertension of Japan (1990) Improved survival after prophylactic portal nondecompression surgery for esophageal varices: a randomized clinical trial. *Hepatology* **12**: 1–6.

Iwatsuki S, Starzl TE, Todo S et al (1988) Liver transplantation in the treatment of bleeding esophageal varices. *Surgery* **104**: 697–705.

Jackson FC, Perrin EB, Smith AG et al (1968) A clinical investigation of the portacaval shunt. II. Survival analysis of the prophylactic operation. *American Journal of Surgery* **115**: 22–42.

Jackson FC, Perrin EB, Felix R et al (1971) A clinical investigation of the portacaval shunt. V. Survival analysis of the therapeutic operation. *Annals of Surgery* **174**: 672–701.

Japanese Research Society for Portal Hypertension (1980) The general rules for recording endoscopic findings on esophageal varices. *Japanese Journal of Surgery* **10**: 84–87.

Johansen K (1989) Partial portal decompression for variceal hemorrhage. *American Journal of Surgery* **157**: 479–482.

Kawasaki S, Henderson JM, Hertzler G & Galloway JR (1991) The role of continued drinking in loss of portal perfusion after distal splenorenal shunt. *Gastroenterology* **100**: 799–804.

Langer B, Taylor BR, Mackenzie DR et al (1985) Further report of a prospective randomized trial comparing distal spleno-renal shunt with end-to-side portacaval shunt. *Gastroenterology* **88**: 424–429.

Langer BF, Greig PD & Taylor BR (1990) Emergency surgical treatment of variceal hemorrhage. *Surgical Clinics of North America* **70**: 307–317.

Lebrec D, Nouel O, Corbic M et al (1980) Propranolol—a medical treatment for portal hypertension? *Lancet* **2**: 180–182.

Leger L, Delaitre B & Nicodeme JP (1973) Hemorragies digestives chez le cirrhotique. Notre attitude therapeutique à propos de 134 observations. *Journal de Chirurgie* **106**: 45–56.

McDermott WV Jr, Palazzi H, Nardi GL & Mondet A (1961) Elective portalsystemic shunt: an analysis of 237 cases. *New England Journal of Medicine* **264**: 419–431.

Maffei-Faccioli A, Gerunda GE, Neri D et al (1990) Selective variceal decompression and its role relative to other therapies. *American Journal of Surgery* **160**: 60–66.

Malt RA, Abbott WM, Warshaw AL, Vander Salm TJ & Smead WL (1978) Randomized trial of emergency mesocaval and portacaval shunts for bleeding esophageal varices. *American Journal of Surgery* **185**: 584–588.

Marion P, George M, Vacca C & Vadot L (1979) L'anastomose porto-cave latéro-latérale à débit minimum réglé pour cirrhose hémorragique. *Lyon Chirurgicales* **75**: 235–243.

Mazzaferro V, Todo S, Tzakis AG et al (1990) Liver transplantation in patients with previous portasystemic shunt. *American Journal of Surgery* **160**: 111–116.

Millikan JN, Warren WD, Henderson JM et al (1985) The Emory prospective randomized trial: selective versus non-selective shunt to control variceal bleeding. Ten year follow-up. *Annals of Surgery* **201**: 712–722.

Nagasue N, Ogawa Y, Yukaya H et al (1988a) Prophylactic distal splenorenal shunt for Child's class A and B patients at high risk of bleeding. *Zentralblatt für Chirurgie* **113**: 1329–1337.

Nagasue N, Ogawa Y, Yakaya H, Tamada R, Chang Y & Nakamura T (1988b) Emergency distal spleno-renal shunt for medically uncontrollable variceal hemorrhage. *Zentralblatt für Chirurgie* **113**: 446–454.

North Italian Endoscopic Club (1988) Prediction of the first variceal hemorrhage in patients with cirrhosis of the liver and esophageal varices. A prospective multicenter study. *New England Journal of Medicine* **319**: 983–989.

Orloff MJ (1980) Elective therapeutic portacaval shunt. In Orloff MJ, Stipa S & Ziparo V (eds) *Medical and Surgical Problems of Portal Hypertension*, pp 127–136. London: Academic Press.

Orloff MJ & Bell RH (1986) Long-term survival after emergency portacaval shunting from bleeding varices in patients with alcoholic cirrhosis. *American Journal of Surgery* **151**: 176–183.

Orloff MJ, Bell RH, Hardison WG & Greenburg AG (1990) Randomized clinical comparison of emergency portacaval shunt versus medical therapy for bleeding varices in cirrhosis. *Gastroenterology* **98**: A618 (abstract).

Osborne DR & Hobbs KEF (1981) The acute treatment of hemorrhage from esophageal varices: a comparison of esophageal transection and staple gun anastomosis with mesocaval shunt. *British Journal of Surgery* **68**: 734–737.

Palmer ED, Brick IB & Jahnke EJ (1954) Esophageal varices without hemorrhage in cirrhosis. *New England Journal of Medicine* **250**: 863–865.

Peterson K & Giles GR (1986) Distal spleno-renal (Warren) shunt in the management of actively bleeding esophageal varices. *British Journal of Surgery* **73**: 618–620.

Pezzuoli G & Spina GP (1986) La complicanza emorragica. In Pezzuoli G & Spina GP (eds) *Progressi Clinici: Chirurgia. L'ipertensione portale*, pp 225–290. Padova: Piccin Pub.

Planas R, Boix J, Broggi M et al (1991) Portacaval shunt versus endoscopic sclerotherapy in the elective treatment of variceal hemorrhage. *Gastroenterology* **100**: 1078–1086.

Potts JR, Henderson JM, Millikan WJ & Warren WD (1984) Emergency distal spleno-renal shunts for variceal hemorrhage refractory to non-operative control. *American Journal of Surgery* **148**: 813–816.

Prandi D, Rueff B & Roche-Sicot J et al (1976) Life threatening hemorrhage of the digestive tract in cirrhotic patients. *American Journal of Surgery* **131**: 204–209.

Pugh RNH, Murray-Lyon IM, Dawson JL et al (1973) Transection of the oesophagus for bleeding oesophageal varices. *British Journal of Surgery* **60**: 646–648.

Reichle FA, Fahmy WF & Golsorkhi M (1979) Prospective comparative clinical trial with distal spleno-renal and meso-caval shunts. *American Journal of Surgery* **137**: 13–21.

Resnick RH, Chalmers TC, Ishihara AM et al (1969) A controlled study of the prophylactic portacaval shunt. A final report. *Annals of Internal Medicine* **70**: 675–688.

Resnick RH, Iber FL, Ishihara AM et al (1974) A controlled study of the therapeutic portacaval shunt. *Gastroenterology* **67**: 843–857.

Reynolds TB, Donovan AJ, Mikkelsen WP et al (1981) Results of a 12-year randomized trial of porta-caval shunt in patients with alcoholic liver disease and bleeding varices. *Gastroenterology* **80**: 1005–1011.

Rikkers LF, Burnett DA, Volentine GD et al (1987) Shunt surgery versus endoscopic sclerotherapy for long-term treatment of variceal bleeding. Early results of a randomized trial. *Annals of Surgery* **206**: 261–271.

Rosemurgy AS, McAllister EW & Kearney RE (1991) Prospective study of a prosthetic H-graft portacaval shunt. *American Journal of Surgery* **161**: 159–164.

Rousselot LM, Panke WF, Bono RF & Moreno AH (1963) Experiences with portacaval anastomosis: analysis of 104 elective end-to-side shunts for prevention of recurrent hemorrhage from esophago-gastric varices (1952–1961). *American Journal of Medicine* **34**: 297–309.

Rueff B & Benhamou JP (1975) Management of gastrointestinal bleeding in cirrhotic patients. *Clinics in Gastroenterology* **4**: 425–438.

Rueff B, Prandi D, Degos F et al (1976) A controlled study of therapeutic portacaval shunt in alcoholic cirrhosis. *Lancet* **i**: 655–659.

Rypins EB & Sarfeh IJ (1988) Influence of portal hemodynamics on long-term survival of alcoholic cirrhosis after small-diameter portacaval H grafts. *American Journal of Surgery* **155**: 152–158.

Shah DM, Chang BB, White TZ et al (1989) Comparison between selective distal splenorenal shunt and small diameter H-graft portosystemic shunt. *Journal of Cardiovascular Surgery* **30**: 459–461.

Smith GW, Maddrey WC & Zuidema GD (1974) Portal hypertension as we see it. In Child CG (ed.) *Portal Hypertension*, pp 1–35. Philadelphia: WB Saunders Company.

Spina GP, Galeotti F, Opocher E et al (1988a) Selective distal spleno-renal shunt (DSRS) vs. side-to-side porta-caval shunt (PCS): clinical results of a prospective matched control study. *American Journal of Surgery* **155**: 564–571.

Spina GP, Galeotti F, Opocher E et al (1988b) Improved quality of life after splenorenal shunt. A prospective comparison with side-to-side portocaval shunt. *Annals of Surgery* **208**: 104–109.

Spina GP, Santambrogio R, Opocher E et al (1990a) Emergency portosystemic shunt in patients with variceal bleeding. *Surgery, Gynecology and Obstetrics* **171**: 456–464.

Spina GP, Santambrogio R, Opocher E et al (1990b) Early hemodynamic changes following

selective distal splenorenal shunt for portal hypertension: comparison of surgical techniques. *World Journal of Surgery* **14**: 115–122.
Spina GP, Santambrogio R, Opocher E et al (1990c) The distal spleno-renal shunt. In Dianzani MU & Gentilini P (eds) *Chronic Liver Damage*, pp 273–288. Amsterdam: Science Publishers BV.
Spina GP, Santambrogio R, Opocher E et al (1990d) Distal splenorenal shunt versus endoscopic sclerotherapy in the prevention of variceal rebleeding. First stage of a randomized controlled trial. *Annals of Surgery* **211**: 178–186.
Teres J, Baroni R, Bordas JM et al (1987a) Randomized trial of portacaval shunt, stapling transection and endoscopic sclerotherapy in uncontrolled variceal bleeding. *Journal of Hepatology* **4**: 159–167.
Teres J, Bordas JM, Bravo D et al (1987b) Sclerotherapy vs distal spleno-renal shunt in the elective treatment of variceal hemorrhage: a randomized controlled trial. *Hepatology* **7**: 430–436.
Texeira ED, Yu H & Bergan JJ (1967) Nova técnica na cirurgia da hipertensão portal: estudo experimental. *Revista Brasileira de Cirurgia* **53**: 443–448.
Turcotte JG & Lambert MJ (1973) Variceal hemorrhage, hepatic cirrhosis and portacaval shunts. *Surgery* **73**: 810–817.
Vidal M (1903) Traitement chirurgical des ascites dans les cirrhoses du foie. *16th Cong. Franc. Chir.* **16**: 294–301.
Villeneuve JP, Pomier-Layrargues G & Duguay L (1987) Emergency portacaval shunt for variceal hemorrhage. A prospective study. *Annals of Surgery* **206**: 48–52.
Warren WD & Muller WH (1959) A clarification of some hemodynamic changes in cirrhosis and their surgical significance. *Annals of Surgery* **150**: 413–427.
Warren WD, Zeppa R & Fomon JJ (1967) Selective trans-splenic decompression of gastroesophageal varices by distal splenorenal shunt. *Annals of Surgery* **166**: 437–455.
Warren WD, Millikan WJ, Henderson JM et al (1986) Spleno-pancreatic disconnection. Improved selectivity of distal spleno-renal shunt. *Annals of Surgery* **204**: 346–354.
Westaby D, MacDougall BRD & Williams R (1985) Improved survival following injection sclerotherapy for esophageal varices: final analysis of a controlled trial. *Hepatology* **5**: 827–830.
Wood RP, Shaw BW & Rikkers LF (1990) Liver transplantation for variceal hemorrhage. *Surgical Clinics of North America* **70**: 449–461.
Zeppa R, Hensley GT, Levi JU et al (1978) The comparative survivals of alcoholics versus non-alcoholics after distal spleno-renal shunt. *Annals of Surgery* **187**: 510–514.

7
Liver transplantation in the management of bleeding oesophageal varices

SHUNZABURO IWATSUKI
THOMAS E. STARZL

The vast majority of patients who require liver transplants have significant portal venous hypertension, and their liver replacement is specifically aimed to treat three major complications of portal hypertension, namely, bleeding oesophageal varices, refractory ascites and encephalopathy (liver failure).

Variceal haemorrhage and ascites can be treated effectively by various types of portal decompression surgery, but these procedures invariably decrease hepatic blood flow and hence worsen the function of an already compromised liver. The enthusiasm for treating oesophageal varices and ascites with non-selective portosystemic shunting started to wane more than two decades ago when it became apparent that the price of preventing haemorrhage from oesophageal varices and intractable ascites in this manner was dehumanizing encephalopathy and progressive hepatic dysfunction (Jackson et al, 1971; Resnick et al, 1974).

With the development of potent and specific diuretic drugs, truly intractable ascites is extremely uncommon. When it does occur, more appropriate therapy than portosystemic shunt will often be a peritoneojugular shunt. Chronic hepatic encephalopathy can rarely be managed by medical means, and it is effectively treated only with liver transplantation. Thus, the principal problem in portal hypertension for which therapeutic planning must be done is the haemorrhage from oesophageal varices.

Prophylactic and therapeutic uses of anti-β-adrenergic agents and endoscopic sclerotherapy play a significant role in the management of oesophageal varices. Various types of portosystemic venous shunting have been evaluated as to their efficacy in preventing both haemorrhage from varices and accelerated decline of hepatic function.

In our centre, where there is a chronic shortage of organs, Child's A patients who have had variceal bleeding are systemically screened for selective splenorenal shunts, performed electively. The procedure is being used on a trial basis because it is attended by a lower incidence of encephalopathy than is seen after non-selective shunts. Forty patients have been entered with no perioperative deaths but longer follow-up will be necessary to assess the validity of this approach. Five of the 40 have come to successful transplantation during the first 12 months after their Warren shunts, which caused no technical difficulties at the time of grafting. In most cases, the shunt is removed by splenectomy.

Liver transplantation has emerged as a safe and preferred treatment of many patients with end-stage liver diseases, the vast majority of which resulted in portal hypertension (Starzl et al, 1982). Whether the graft is placed in the natural location (orthotopic) or ectopic site (heterotopic or auxiliary), liver transplantation invariably corrects the portal hypertension and treats most effectively bleeding varices, intractable ascites and encephalopathy.

Except in isolated cases or small series, auxiliary transplantation has not provided satisfactory results. Consequently, we will concentrate in this chapter on the role of orthotopic liver transplantation in the management of portal hypertension, particularly of bleeding oesophageal varices. Also, we will examine the relationship of transplantation to other therapeutic modalities.

INCIDENCE OF PORTAL HYPERTENSION, BLEEDING OESOPHAGEAL VARICES AND PORTAL VEIN THROMBOSIS AMONG LIVER TRANSPLANT RECIPIENTS

The liver diseases of the first 1000 patients who received liver transplants under cyclosporin-steroid therapy (March 1980 to July 1987) are listed in Table 1 with the incidences of bleeding from oesophageal varices.

More than 90% of the patients had end-stage chronic liver disease with significant portal hypertension. Furthermore, 22 patients had undergone non-selective shunt, 15 patients had undergone selective shunt, and five

Table 1. Liver diseases of 1000 patients who received liver transplants between March 1980 and July 1987 and the incidences of bleeding from oesophageal varices.

Diseases	No. of patients	No. of oesophageal bleeders
Cirrhosis	319	115 (36%)
(postnecrotic, cryptogenic, alcoholic)	(41)	(15) (37%)
Biliary atresia	180	38 (21%)
Primary biliary cirrhosis	166	63 (38%)
Liver-based inborn metabolic errors	98	35 (36%)
(α_1-antitrypsin deficiency, Wilson's disease, etc.)		
Primary sclerosing cholangitis	82	32 (39%)
(with bile duct cancer)	(8)	
Hepatobiliary malignancy	45	0
Fulminant hepatic failure	37	0
Secondary biliary cirrhosis	21	8 (38%)
Budd–Chiari syndrome	15	2 (13%)
Familial cholestatic syndrome	15	4 (27%)
Congenital hepatic fibrosis	6	5 (83%)
Others	16	0
Total	1000	302 (30%)

patients had undergone non-shunt operations for treatment of bleeding oesophageal varices at an earlier time. Thus, the total incidence of previous splanchnic intervention was 16% of which 12% were shunts. Two hundred and nineteen patients had received endoscopic sclerotherapy for the treatment of oesophageal varices.

It is worthwhile noting that nearly a third (302 out of 1000) of the patients with various end-stage chronic liver diseases had bled from oesophageal varices before the transplantation for hepatic failure (Table 1). The incidence was low (13%) among the patients with Budd–Chiari syndrome. This was due in part to the fact that three patients (of the 15 with this diagnosis) had had side-to-side portocaval shunts for intractable ascites. The incidence of 21% among the children with biliary atresia was falsely low because haemorrhage from the varices around the enterostomy stoma was not counted. A high incidence of variceal haemorrhage among the children with congenital hepatic fibrosis merely reflected the far advanced disease of those six children. Many children with this disease have good hepatic function when they bleed, and they often have been managed either by sclerotherapy or by a shunt operation rather than by liver transplantation.

The case mix has changed only slightly as the years have gone by. Among a subsequent series of 885 patients who received their first liver allografts between January 1989 and December 1990, 341 (40%) patients had a history of bleeding from oesophageal varices prior to transplantation. The frequency of their liver diseases and the incidences of variceal bleeding were similar to those reported earlier (Table 1).

Thirty-six (11%) of the 341 oesophageal bleeders had been treated with various types of shunt operation and 204 (60%) patients were managed by a series of endoscopic sclerotherapy. Thus, the incidence of these interventions was similar between the first series (1980–1987) and the more recent series (1989–1990) of patients.

Among the more recent 849 patients (1989–1990) without prior portosystemic shunt, 49 (6%) patients had a complete obstruction and 27 (3%) patients had a partial obstruction of the portal vein trunk at the time of liver transplantation.

Portal vein thrombosis is a well-recognized complication of end-stage liver disease, and it has been a formidable challenge in orthotopic liver transplantation. If known in advance, the portal vein thrombosis was formerly a relative contraindication to orthotopic liver transplantation (Van Thiel et al, 1982). However, the need to treat unexpected thrombosis discovered during surgery led to the development of vein graft procedures and further evolved into the increasingly sophisticated techniques to deal with this problem (Shaw et al, 1985; Lerut et al, 1987; Tzakis et al, 1989; Stieber et al, 1991). Currently, almost all patients with portal vein thrombosis can be treated with orthotopic liver transplantation, and increasing numbers of patients with portal vein thrombosis have received orthotopic liver transplantation in recent years. The incidence of portal vein thrombosis among the 1585 liver transplant recipients between April 1986 and October 1989 was 2% (Stieber et al, 1991), but it has risen to 6% in the 885 recipients between January 1989 and December 1990.

With these technical improvements, all types of portal hypertension (prehepatic, intrahepatic and posthepatic) or any combination of them can be effectively treated by orthotopic liver transplantation. This has widened the indications for treatment.

RESULTS OF LIVER TRANSPLANTATION FOR PATIENTS WITH END-STAGE LIVER DISEASE AND BLEEDING FROM OESOPHAGEAL VARICES

The overall survival rates of the first 1000 consecutive patients after liver transplantation with cyclosporin-steroid therapy (March 1980 to July 1987) were 74% at 1 year, 71% at 2 years, 67% at 3 years, 65% at 4 years, and 64% at 5 years, when they were calculated by the method of Kaplan–Meier as of September 1987 (Iwatsuki et al, 1988a). The overall survival rates under cyclosporin-steroid therapy were unchanged when they were re-examined in the consecutive 1469 recipients as of July 1989 (Starzl and Demetris, 1990) and in the consecutive 1583 recipients as of July 1990 (Gordon et al, 1991). However, the survival rates appeared to be improved starting in August 1989 when a novel immunosuppressive drug, FK-506, was introduced to our clinical trial (Starzl et al, 1989; Todo et al, 1990, 1991; Fung et al, 1991). The 1-year survival rate of 409 liver recipients treated with FK-506 has risen to 85% as of July 1991.

The survival rates of 302 variceal bleeders among the first 1000 consecutive liver recipients under cyclosporin-steroid therapy were 79% at 1 year, 74% at 2 years, and 71% at 3, 4 and 5 years as of February 1988 (Iwatsuki et al, 1988b). There was no statistically significant difference in the survival rates among the patients with the five most common liver diseases shown in Table 1.

The survival rates of the first consecutive 1000 liver recipients under cyclosporin-steroid therapy were updated as of September 1991, with a minimum follow-up of 4 years. One- to 5-year survival rates of the 1000 patients were 73%, 69%, 67%, 65% and 64%, respectively. Those of the 302 variceal bleeders were 80%, 77%, 75%, 74% and 71%, respectively. Thus, the actuarial survival rates calculated in 1987 and 1988 precisely predicted the actual survival rates in 1991.

LIVER TRANSPLANTATION FOR ALCOHOLIC CIRRHOSIS

Alcoholic liver disease is the most common form of liver disease in the USA and other Western countries. However, the use of liver transplantation to treat patients with end-stage alcoholic cirrhosis has long been debated. We have been treating some of the patients with end-stage alcoholic liver disease by orthotopic liver transplantation. During the pre-cyclosporin era between 1963 and 1979, 15 patients (18% of adult recipients) with alcoholic cirrhosis were transplanted. The first eight alcoholic recipients died peroperatively. However, four of the next seven patients survived more than 4 years. Three of the four patients are still alive and in good health after 17, 15 and 14 years, respectively. None has returned to drinking. During the cyclosporin era between 1980 and 1989, 134 alcoholic patients (12% of adult recipients) received liver transplants. One- to 4-year survival rates were 81%, 75%, 73% and 73%, respectively, as of July 1990 (Gordon et al, 1991). These survival rates were better than those of patients with viral hepatitis B and those with hepatic malignancy. Moreover, nearly 90% of the transplant survivors remained alcohol abstinent.

Although abstinence was considered to be a favourable factor, a 'dry' period of specific duration was not required before transplantation since this would invite systematic falsification of the medical history and because death would often be the price of a significant wait. Instead, acknowledgement of the alcoholism problem is expected and commitments not to drink in the future are obtained from the patient and family. Going through a trauma of such magnitude as liver transplantation seemingly has been the starting point for long and permanent abstinence and usually for rehabilitation. For the last several years, however, extensive psychiatric and social support has been systematically provided, as the number of alcoholic liver transplant candidates has been increasing. The fact that relapses into alcoholism have been uncommon after liver transplantation weakens the potential objection that provision of a new liver is a futile gesture as well as a waste of an organ.

ROLE OF LIVER TRANSPLANTATION IN THE MANAGEMENT OF BLEEDING OESOPHAGEAL VARICES

The survival rates after liver transplantation for patients with advanced liver disease (Child's class C) who had had bleeding from oesophageal varices are quite satisfactory as presented earlier, and there is little doubt of the value of liver transplantation in this situation. Nevertheless, the results achieved by liver transplantation were compared with those reported in nine well-studied control trials of therapeutic shunt operations (Table 2). All of these well-designed studies failed to show the survival superiority of non-selective shunt over medical management (Jackson et al, 1971; Resnick et al, 1974; Reynolds et al, 1981), that of selective shunt over non-selective shunt (Conn et al, 1981; Langer et al, 1985; Millikan et al, 1985), or that of selective shunt over chronic endoscopic sclerotherapy (Warren et al, 1986; Rikkers et al, 1987; Teres et al, 1987).

As the outcomes of shunt operations, sclerotherapy or medical management are highly influenced by the hepatic functional reserve of the patients, the results of one study cannot be simply compared with those of another. More than 75% of the patients in each report listed in Table 2 had good hepatic function or moderately impaired hepatic function (Child's class A and B), and fewer than 25% of them had advanced hepatic dysfunction (Child's class C). On the other hand, all the patients who received liver transplants had advanced or far-advanced hepatic dysfunction; many of them had been rejected for shunt operation and some of them had already had a shunt operation. Despite this severe disadvantage in preoperative condition, the survival rates of liver transplant recipients who had had variceal bleeding were better than or similar to those of patients who had other kinds of conventional therapy (Table 2).

Because surgical therapy for oesophageal varices is usually withheld from the patients with advanced hepatic dysfunction (Child's class C), the literature contains few survival data for these patients. In Table 3 the results obtained by liver transplantation are compared with those achieved in patients with advanced hepatic dysfunction after conventional surgical therapy (Turcotte and Lambert, 1973; Yamamoto et al, 1976; Warren et al, 1982; Rikkers et al, 1984; Chandler et al, 1985; Spence and Johnston, 1985;

Table 2. Survival comparison among various treatments for bleeding oesophageal varices (Child's classes A, B, and C).

Treatment	No. of patients	1 yr	2 yr	3 yr	4 yr	5 yr
Jackson et al (1971)						
Non-selective shunt	67	80*	73*	62*	58*	55*
Medical	77	80	66	43*	35*	32*
Resnick et al (1974)						
Non-selective shunt	54	70*	58*	50*	48*	48*
Medical	25	67*	52*	40*	40*	40*
Reynolds et al (1981)						
Non-selective shunt	41	—	72*	64*	52*	44
Medical	37	—	60*	44*	36*	22
Conn et al (1981)						
Selective shunt	24	76*	70*	—	—	—
Non-selective shunt	29	70*	67*	—	—	—
Langer et al (1985)						
Selective shunt	38	80*	76*	63*	54*	51*
Non-selective shunt	40	90*	85*	70*	56*	56*
Millikan et al (1985)						
Selective shunt	26	85*	77*	65*	60*	55*
Non-selective shunt	29	80*	72*	70*	65*	60*
Warren et al (1986)						
Sclerotherapy†	36	90*	84	82*	82*	—
Selective shunt	35	70*	59	45*	45*	—
Rikkers et al (1987)						
Sclerotherapy	30	77*	61	60*	50*	—
Selective shunt‡	27	75*	65	60*	39*	—
Teres et al (1987)						
Selective shunt	57	90*	90*	82*	70*	70*
Sclerotherapy	55	81*	75*	65*	65*	65*
Iwatsuki et al (1988b)						
Liver transplantation	302	79	74	71	71	71
Iwatsuki et al						
Liver transplantation (update 1991)	302	80	77	75	74	71

* Value estimated from survival curve.
† Sclerotherapy failures were rescued by surgical therapy.
‡ Twenty-three selective shunts and four non-selective shunts.

Iwatsuki et al, 1988b). It is obvious that the survival rates of liver transplant recipients are far better than those achieved by conventional types of surgical therapy when the liver disease is advanced.

Should all the cirrhotic patients be treated with liver transplantation when they have significant episodes of variceal haemorrhage? The answer is obviously no, because chronic endoscopic sclerotherapy is quite effective in controlling the haemorrhage from oesophageal varices, and the survival rates after sclerotherapy are superior or equal to those of shunt operations providing the sclerotherapy failures are rescued by surgical intervention (Warren et al, 1986; Rikkers et al, 1987; Teres et al, 1987).

The role of endoscopic sclerotherapy in the treatment of bleeding oesophageal varices has been well established. However, the sclerotherapy cannot be effectively applied to gastric varices, and has its own special complications, such as oesophageal perforation or stricture of the distal oesophagus. The incidence of these complications rises astronomically when sclerotherapy is used during a crisis such as exists during active bleeding and especially if hepatic failure is a co-factor.

Portosystemic shunt operations should be limited to those who have failed endoscopic sclerotherapy but who still have excellent hepatic function. Although the survival rates after transplantation are not jeopardized by previous portosystemic shunt operations, the actual liver transplant

Table 3. Survival comparison among various treatments for bleeding oesophageal varices (Child's class C, poor liver function).

Treatment	No. of patients	1 yr	2 yr	3 yr	4 yr	5 yr
Turcotte and Lambert (1973)						
Non-selective shunt	50	36	32	22	20	17
Yamamoto et al (1976)						
Non-shunt operation	13	39	30	22	22	18
Warren et al (1982)						
Selective shunt	?	60*	53*	45*	40*	35
Non-selective shunt	?	50*	40*	37*	20*	15*
Rikkers et al (1984)						
Shunt and non-shunt operation†	24	45	35*	30*	20*	17*
Chandler et al (1985)						
Shunt‡	30	36	30	25	20	13
Spence and Johnston (1985)						
Non-shunt operation	25	70	53	38	38	35
Iwatsuki et al (1988b)						
Liver transplantation	302	79	74	71	71	71
Iwatsuki et al						
Liver transplantation (update 1991)	302	80	77	75	74	71

* Value estimated from survival curve.
† Fifteen non-selective shunts, seven selective shunts, and two non-shunt operations.
‡ Both selective and non-selective operations.

procedures for those patients are quite challenging even with recently developed sophisticated methods of portal vein reconstruction (Lerut et al, 1987; Tzakis et al, 1989; Mazzaferro et al, 1990; Stieber et al, 1991). Among the various types of portosystemic shunt operations, the shunts created without hepatic hilum dissection (distal splenorenal shunt and mesocaval H-graft shunt) are more convenient for liver transplantation. However, the incidence of complete portal vein thrombosis after distal splenorenal shunt is approximately 10%, and that of partial thrombosis is approximately 15% (Henderson et al, 1982; Orozco et al, 1988; Spina et al, 1990; Jin and Rikkers, 1991). The thrombosis appears to develop early in the post-shunt period.

Early reports of percutaneous transjugular portosystemic stent shunt (or transjugular intrahepatic portosystemic shunt, TIPS) are promising (Vinel et al, 1985; Richter et al, 1989; Zemel et al, 1991). In this radiological procedure a balloon-expandable, self-expanding metallic stent is placed between the portal vein and the hepatic vein through the hepatic parenchyma. The technical success rate (75% or more) of TIPS and the patency rate (80% or more) of the stent at 1 year are incentives for further clinical trials.

Although further experience and follow-up are needed to confirm the early results of this new technique, TIPS will further diminish the need for a surgical portosystemic shunt, and may revolutionize the treatment of bleeding oesophageal varices.

REFERENCES

Chandler JG, VanMeter CH, Kaiser DL et al (1985) Factors affecting immediate and long-term survival after emergent and elective splanchnic-systemic shunts. *Annals of Surgery* **201**: 476–487.

Conn HO, Resnick RH & Grace ND (1981) Distal splenorenal shunt versus portal-systemic shunt: current status of a controlled trial. *Hepatology* **1**: 151–160.

Fung J, Todo S, Tzakis A et al (1991) Current status of FK 506 in liver transplantation. *Transplantation Proceedings* **23**: 1902–1905.

Gordon RD, Todo S, Tzakis AG et al (1991) Liver transplantation under cyclosporine: a decade of experience. *Transplantation Proceedings* **23**: 1393–1396.

Henderson JM, Millikan WJ, Chipponi J et al (1982) The incidence and natural history of thrombosis in the portal vein following distal splenorenal shunt. *Annals of Surgery* **196**: 1–7.

Iwatsuki S, Starzl TE, Todo S et al (1988a) Experience in 1,000 liver transplants under cyclosporine-steroid therapy: a survival report. *Transplantation Proceedings* **20**: 498–504.

Iwatsuki S, Starzl TE, Todo S et al (1988b) Liver transplantation in the treatment of bleeding esophageal varices. *Surgery* **104**: 697–705.

Jackson FC, Perrin EB, Felix WR et al (1971) A clinical investigation of the porta-caval shunt. V. Survival analysis of the therapeutic operation. *Annals of Surgery* **174**: 672–701.

Jin G & Rikkers LF (1991) The significance of portal vein thrombosis after distal splenorenal shunt. *Archives of Surgery* **126**: 1011–1016.

Langer B, Taylor BR, Mackenzie DR et al (1985) Further report of a prospective randomized trial comparing distal splenorenal shunt with end-to-side portalcaval shunt: an analysis of encephalopathy, survival, and quality of life. *Gastroenterology* **88**: 424–429.

Lerut J, Tzakis A, Bron K et al (1987) Complications of venous reconstruction in human orthotopic liver transplantation. *Annals of Surgery* **205**: 404–414.

Mazzaferro V, Iwatsuki S & Starzl TE (1990) Liver transplantation in patients with previous portosystemic shunt. *American Journal of Surgery* **160**: 111–116.

Millikan WJ, Warren WD, Henderson JM et al (1985) The Emory prospective randomized trial: selective versus nonselective shunt to control variceal bleeding. Ten year follow-up. *Annals of Surgery* **201:** 712–722.

Orozco H, Juarez F, Santillan P et al (1988) Ten years of selective shunts for hemodynamic portal hypertension. *Surgery* **103:** 27–31.

Resnick RH, Iber FL, Ishihara AM et al (1974) A controlled study of the therapeutic portacaval shunt. *Gastroenterology* **67:** 843–857.

Reynolds TB, Donovan AJ, Mikkelsen WB et al (1981) Results of a 12 year randomized trial of portalcaval shunt in patients with alcoholic liver disease and bleeding varices. *Gastroenterology* **80:** 1005–1111.

Richter GM, Palmaz JC, Noldge G et al (1989) Der transjugulare intrahepatic portosystemische stent-shunt (TIPSS). *Radiologe* **29:** 406–411.

Rikkers LF, Soper NJ & Cormier RA (1984) Selective operative approach for variceal hemorrhage. *American Journal of Surgery* **147:** 89–96.

Rikkers LF, Burnett DA, Volentine GD et al (1987) Shunt surgery versus endoscopic sclerotherapy for long-term treatment of variceal bleeding: early results of a randomized trial. *Annals of Surgery* **206:** 261–271.

Shaw BW, Iwatsuki S, Bron K & Starzl TE (1985) Portal vein grafts in hepatic transplantation. *Surgery, Gynecology and Obstetrics* **161:** 67–68.

Spence RAJ & Johnston GW (1985) Results in 1000 consecutive patients withg stapled esophageal transection for varices. *Surgery, Gynecology and Obstetrics* **160:** 323–329.

Spina GP, Santambrogio R, Opocher E et al (1990) Early hemodynamic changes following distal splenorenal shunt for portal hypertension: comparison of surgical techniques. *World Journal of Surgery* **14:** 115–122.

Starzl TE & Demetris AJ (1990) Liver transplantation: a 31 year perspective (Part III). *Current Problems in Surgery* **27:** 187–240.

Starzl RE, Iwatsuki S, Van Thiel DH et al (1982) Evolution of liver transplantation. *Hepatology* **2:** 614–636.

Starzl TE, Todo S, Fung J et al (1989) FK 506 for liver, kidney and pancreas transplantation. *Lancet* **2:** 1000–1004.

Stieber AC, Zetti G, Todo S et al (1991) The spectrum of portal vein thrombosis in liver transplantation. *Annals of Surgery* **213:** 199–206.

Teres J, Bordas JM, Bravo D et al (1987) Sclerotherapy vs. distal splenorenal shunt in the elective treatment of variceal hemorrhage: a randomized controlled trial. *Hepatology* **7:** 430–436.

Todo S, Fung JJ, Starzl TE et al (1990) Liver, kidney, and thoracic organ transplantation under FK 506. *Annals of Surgery* **212:** 295–305.

Todo S, Fung JJ, Tzakis A et al (1991) 110 consecutive primary orthotopic liver transplantations under FK-506 in adults. *Transplantation Proceedings* **23:** 1397–1402.

Turcotte JG & Lambert ML (1973) Variceal hemorrhage, hepatic cirrhosis, and portalcaval shunts. *Surgery* **73:** 810–817.

Tzakis A, Todo S, Stieber AC & Starzl TE (1989) Venous jump grafts for liver transplantation in patients with portal vein thrombosis. *Transplantation* **48:** 530–531.

Van Thiel D, Schade RR, Starzl TE et al (1982) Liver transplantation in adults. *Hepatology* **2:** 637–640.

Vinel JP, Scotto JM, Levade M et al (1985) Transjugular embolization of esophageal varices in severe variceal bleeding in cirrhosis. Results of a prospective study. *Gastroenterologie Clinique et Biologique* **9:** 814–818.

Warren WD, Millikan WJ, Henderson JM et al (1982) Ten years' portal hypertensive surgery at Emory: results and new perspectives. *Annals of Surgery* **195:** 530–542.

Warren WD, Henderson JM, Millikan WJ et al (1986) Distal splenorenal shunt versus endoscopic sclerotherapy for long-term treatment of variceal bleeding: preliminary report of a prospective, randomized trial. *Annals of Surgery* **203:** 454–467.

Yamamoto S, Hidemura R, Sawada M et al (1976) The late results of terminal esophago-proximal gastrectomy (TEPG) with extensive devascularization and splenectomy for bleeding esophageal varices in cirrhosis. *Surgery* **80:** 106–114.

Zemel G, Katzen BT, Becker GJ et al (1991) Percutaneous transjugular portosystemic shunt. *Journal of the American Medical Association* **226:** 390–391.

8
Management of gastric varices

S. K. SARIN
D. LAHOTI

It was nearly 80 years ago that Stadelmann (1913) described gastric varices (GV) as an accompaniment of portal hypertension. It is, however, only in the last decade that specific attention has been paid to their study. By logic, any varix present in the stomach should be termed a gastric varix. Over the years, differences in the nomenclature and semantics of GVs (Evans and Delany, 1953; Yasumoto, 1971; Hosking and Johnson, 1988; Sarin and Kumar, 1989) have resulted in considerable confusion. Terms like gastric varices, fundal varices, lesser curve varices (Hosking and Johnson, 1988), isolated gastric varices (Rosch, 1974), true gastric varices (Snady, 1987), junctional varices (Korula et al, 1991), gastro-oesophageal varices, etc. have been used, often with different connotations. Moreover, the pathogenesis and natural history of GVs which may have an important bearing on overall management have received little attention. Therefore, before the management of GVs can be discussed, it is necessary to understand their classification, origin and natural history. This information has become all the more important because the success of endoscopic sclerotherapy and development of newer techniques significantly decreased the need for shunt surgery (Achord, 1992). In fact, the indications for shunt surgery need to be redefined (Wood et al, 1990).

CLASSIFICATION OF GASTRIC VARICES

At present, GVs can be satisfactorily classified only by endoscopy. Several classifications of GVs have been proposed based on their location, size and endoscopic features (Yasumoto, 1971; Hosking and Johnson, 1988; Hashizume et al, 1990). However, due to considerable overlap in the different types of GVs or because of the complexity of the grading systems, these classifications have not been very helpful. We had proposed a simple classification based on the location of GVs and their relation to oesophageal varices (Sarin and Kumar, 1989). This classification was evaluated in a prospective manner in a series of 568 patients (Sarin et al, 1991) and was found to be quite useful in defining the natural history and outlining the management of GVs. According to this classification (Figure 1), we divide GVs into two main types, as follows.

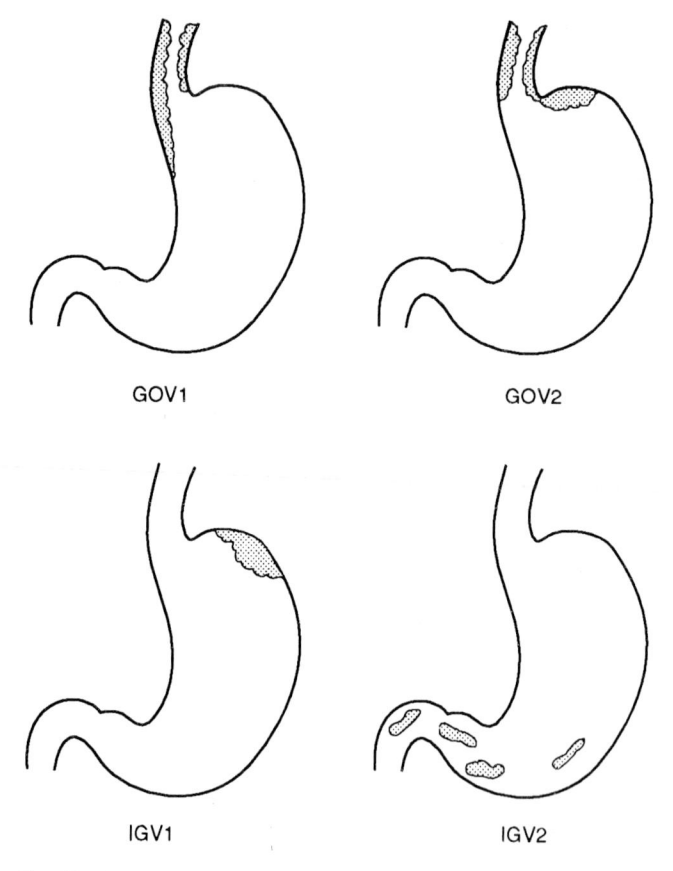

Figure 1. Classification of gastric varices. GOV, gastro-oesophageal, type 1 and 2; IGV, isolated gastric varices, type 1 and 2.

Gastro-oesophageal varices (GOV)

These varices extend beyond the gastro-oesophageal junction and are always associated with oesophageal varices. They can be further subdivided into:

1. *Type 1 (GOV1)*. These appear as continuations of oesophageal varices and extend for 2–5 cm below the gastro-oesophageal junction, along the lesser curve of the stomach. These varices are more or less straight.
2. *Type 2 (GOV2)*. These varices extend beyond the gastro-oesophageal junction towards the fundus of the stomach. They appear as long, tortuous and nodular elevations at the cardia.

Isolated gastric varices (IGV)

GVs in the absence of oesophageal varices are termed 'isolated' GVs (Rosch, 1974). Depending on their location, they can be subdivided into:

1. *Type 1 (IGV1)*. These varices are located in the fundus of the stomach and fall short of the cardia by a few centimetres.
2. *Type 2 (IGV2)*. These include isolated ectopic varices present anywhere in the stomach, such as in the antrum, pylorus or body.

FREQUENCY OF DIFFERENT TYPES OF GASTRIC VARICES

The exact incidence of GVs in patients with portal hypertension is not known. An incidence of 2–100% has been reported (Evans and Delany, 1953; Feldman and Feldman, 1956; Karr and Wohl, 1960; Yasumoto, 1971; Trudeau and Prindiville, 1985; Hosking and Johnson, 1988; Watanabe et al, 1988; Sarin et al, 1991). Possibly, the reasons for wide discrepancies in the incidence of GVs are related to difficulties in the diagnosis and differences in the techniques for confirming their diagnosis.

In our experience of 568 consecutive patients with portal hypertension (Sarin et al, 1991), primary GVs (varices detected at the initial presentation) were seen in 114 (20%) patients; they were significantly more common in those who bled than in those who did not (27% versus 4%, $p<0.001$). The incidence of different types of GVs is shown in Figure 2. GOV1, or the lesser curve varices, are the commonest variety. Hosking and Johnson (1988) have also reported similar observations.

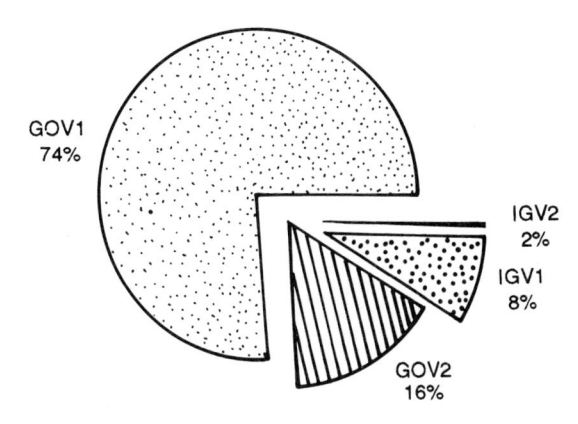

Figure 2. Relative frequency (%) of different types of primary gastric varices.

PATHOGENESIS AND ORIGIN OF GASTRIC VARICES

To understand the development of GVs it is necessary to recall the venous drainage of the stomach and spleen (Figure 3). The fundus of the stomach has a rich venous plexus in its submucosa. This plexus drains into the splenic vein via the short gastric veins and into the portal vein via the coronary vein. GVs can develop in patients with either generalized (e.g. in cirrhosis) or segmental (e.g. in splenic vein thrombosis) portal hypertension.

Haemodynamically, an increase in portal pressure in a patient with *generalized portal hypertension* would be transmitted by the left gastric vein to oesophageal varices and via the short and posterior gastric veins to the fundic plexus and cardiac veins. GOV1, or lesser curve varices, are formed by the dilatation of the left gastric veins at the cardia (Takashi et al, 1985).

Hashizume et al (1988) have shown that GOV1 develop because one of the branches of the left gastric vein perforates the gastric wall perpendicularly and joins the deep submucosal veins about 2 cm below the gastro-oesophageal junction. These deep gastric submucosal veins connect directly with the

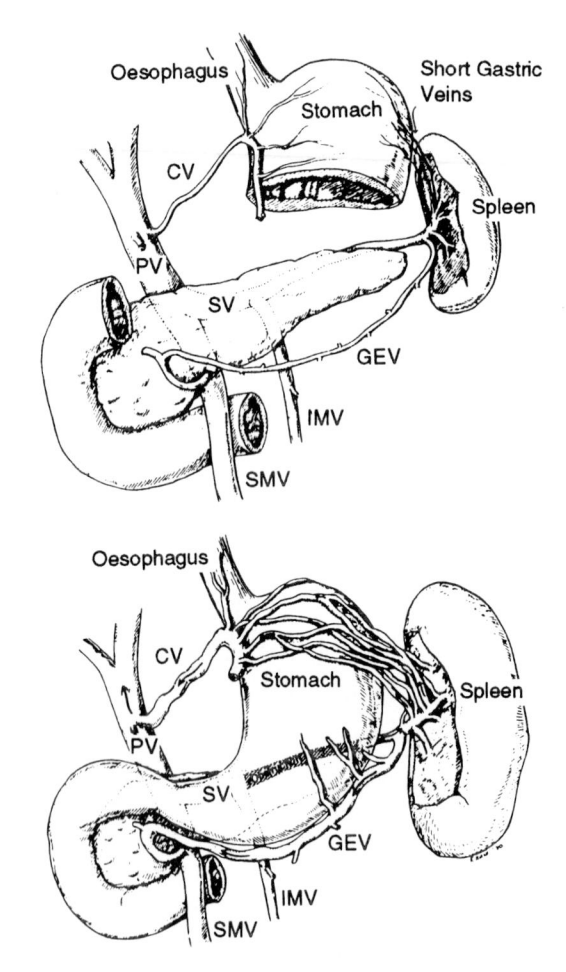

Figure 3. Normal venous anatomy of the stomach (top). Splenic vein (SV) thrombosis leads to reversed flow distribution. Left-sided portal hypertension leads to gastric varices and dilatation of short gastric veins, gastroepiploic vein (GEV) and coronary vein (CV). The portal vein (PV) is patent. IMV and SMV, inferior and superior mesenteric vein. From Little and Moosa (1981) with permission.

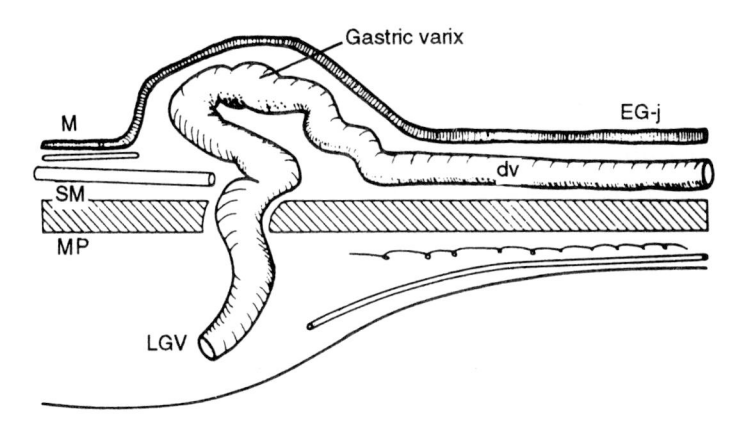

Figure 4. Gastric varices form in the submucosa where branches of the left gastric vein (LGV) penetrate the gastric wall perpendicularly. M, mucosa; SM, submucosa; MP, muscularis propria; EG-j, oesophagogastric junction; dv, deep submucosal vein. From Hashizume et al (1988) with permission.

oesophageal deep submucosal veins (Figure 4). These varices are almost always present with grade 3 or 4 oesophageal varices and not with small varices (Sarin et al, 1988). It suggests that GOV1 develop as a manifestation of advanced portal hypertension. While none of the patients with IGV1 have oesophageal varices, about 50% of patients with GOV2 have associated large oesophageal varices.

In *segmental portal hypertension*, GVs develop in the absence of oesophageal varices. They commonly result from splenic vein obstruction leading to an increase in splenic venous pressure with normal portal pressure. Increase in splenic venous pressure leads to opening up of a number of splenoportal collaterals (see Figure 3) taking the blood in a reverse manner; away from the spleen into the portal vein, bypassing the splenic vein. There is retrograde flow through the short and posterior gastric veins into the submucous space and subsequently varices develop in the fundus and the cardia region, from which blood flows hepatopetally through the coronary vein to the portal vein. Retrograde flow through the left to the right gastroepiploic vein and superior mesenteric vein also occurs. The lower oesophageal veins are bypassed so that oesophageal varices need not develop (Marshall et al, 1977).

Isolated GVs could also develop in generalized portal hypertension. Nine of the 17 cases reported by Rice et al (1977) had cirrhosis of the liver. In patients with patent splenic vein it is difficult to explain development of fundal varices. Fleming and Seaman (1968) suggested that this could occur because of direct anastomosis between the gastric and retroperitoneal veins.

What determines the route by which major portosystemic collaterals develop when portal pressure increases is not known. The size and length of the potential collateral vein probably determines whether a patient develops oesophageal or gastric varices, and, in the latter case, which type (Watanabe et al, 1988).

NATURAL HISTORY OF DIFFERENT TYPES OF GASTRIC VARICES

Before management strategies can be planned, it is important to know the natural history of GVs. Patients with GVs generally present either with recurrent episodes of upper gastrointestinal bleeding or with hepatic encephalopathy.

Profile of gastric variceal bleeding

A proportion of patients with gastric variceal bleeding present as a diagnostic problem. In fact, Madsen et al (1986) have shown that the cause of bleeding may remain obscure in up to 50% of patients with GVs at the time of their first bleed. It is only with a high index of suspicion and a careful search that a correct diagnosis of GVs can be established.

Bleeding should be considered to have arisen from GVs if (1) an active bleed, or ooze, is seen from the GV, (2) a clot or blackish ulcer is seen over the GV, and (3) in the presence of distinct large GVs and absence of oesophageal varices, no other cause of upper gastrointestinal bleeding is detectable (Ramond et al, 1989).

The exact *mechanism* of rupture of GVs is not known. Unlike oesophageal varices, where a decrease in the wall thickness and an increase in the diameter of the varix predisposes to rupture (Mahal and Groszmann, 1990), GVs are covered with relatively thick gastric mucosa. Furthermore, the pressure in the GVs is relatively lower than in the oesophageal varices (Watanabe et al, 1988). Hence, an erosion or an ulcer over the varix probably precipitates bleeding from GVs.

There is little information available in the literature regarding how severely and often GVs bleed. Teres et al (1978) have reported an incidence of 14–16% bleeding from GVs. Paquet (1982) observed GVs in 60–70% of patients with portal hypertension and bleeding from fundal varices in 3% of patients. Weissberg et al (1984) found bleeding from GVs to be milder and less common. While 52% of patients bleeding from oesophageal varices died in their series, only 20% with bleeding from GVs, died ($p<0.03$). Bretagne et al (1986), on the other hand, found bleeding from gastro-oesophageal varices to be more severe and more frequently fatal than from oesophageal varices. Korula et al (1991) also reported a significantly higher bleeding risk, and transfusion need, in patients with GVs compared to those with oesophageal varices.

We prospectively studied the bleeding profile in patients with gastric and oesophageal varices in 393 consecutive variceal bleeders (Sarin et al, 1991) (Figures 5 and 6). The number of bleeding episodes, the bleeding risk factor (total number of bleeding episodes/time interval between the first and the last bleed) and the severity of bleeding (as assessed by the blood transfusion requirements) were determined in patients with gastric and oesophageal varices. The mean number of bleeding episodes before presentation in patients with gastric and oesophageal varices were comparable (2.1 ± 1.0 versus 2.3 ± 1.8). The bleeding risk factor for oesophageal varices was

4.3±0.4 compared with 2.0±0.6 for GVs, the difference being significant ($p<0.01$). The mean blood transfusion requirements in gastric variceal bleeds were significantly more than for oesophageal variceal bleeds (4.8±0.6 versus 2.9±0.3 transfusion units, $p<0.01$) (Figure 6). These data suggest that GVs bleed less frequently but more severely than oesophageal varices. It is also important to understand the profile of bleeding of different types of GVs. Figure 5 depicts the frequency of bleeding in various types of GVs. It is clear that IGV1 and GOV2 have a high incidence of bleeding and

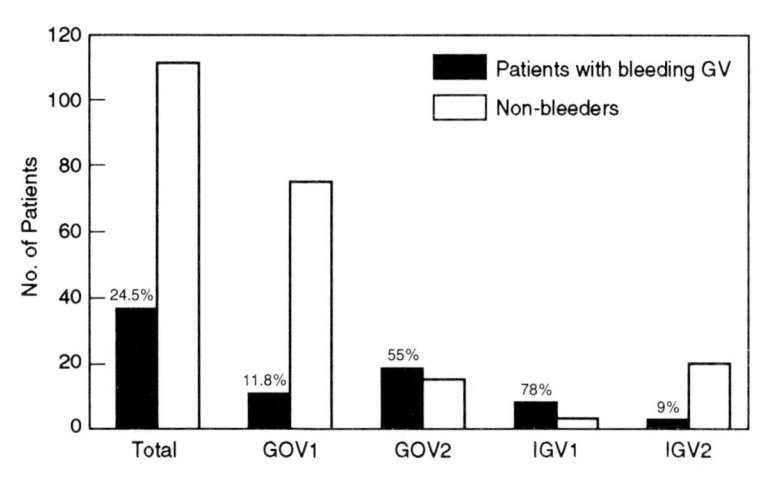

Figure 5. Frequency of bleeding from different types of gastric varices. The percentages shown indicate the proportion of total patients with GVs which bled.

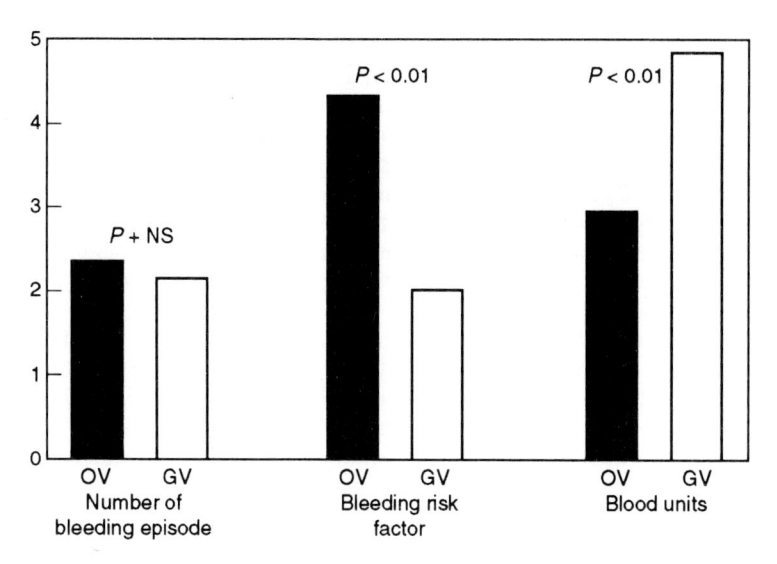

Figure 6. Comparison of the bleeding profile of oesophageal and gastric varices. OV, oesophageal varices; GV, gastric varices.

hence require careful management. A higher incidence of bleeding from fundic varices has been reported by other workers (Little and Moossa, 1981; Mathur et al, 1990; Korula et al, 1991).

Influence of oesophageal variceal sclerotherapy

Certain factors are likely to influence the natural history and subsequent management of GVs. These include:

1. The influence of sclerotherapy for oesophageal varices on coexisting GVs.
2. Development of GVs following obliteration of oesophageal varices (secondary GVs).
3. Bleeding from GVs while sclerotherapy for oesophageal varices is being done.
4. Influence of coexisting GVs on the development of portal hypertensive gastropathy.

Fate of coexisting gastric varices

Only GOVs are likely to be influenced by sclerotherapy for oesophageal varices. MacDougall et al (1982) have reported persistence of GVs after disappearance of oesophageal varices in two patients. On the contrary, Terblanche et al (1979) have described disappearance of GVs after sclerotherapy. However, both these series consisted of only a small number of patients with GVs.

Gastro-oesophageal varices type 1 (GOV1). In our prospective study, 78 patients with GOV1 presenting with oesophageal variceal bleeding underwent sclerotherapy. GVs disappeared concurrently or within 6 months (mean ± SEM 4.6 ± 0.42 months) of obliteration of the oesophageal varices in 46 (59%) patients. However, in 32 (41%) patients, GOV1 persisted. A similar disappearance of gastro-oesophageal junctional varices with oesophageal variceal sclerotherapy has also been reported by other workers (Graham and Smith, 1981; Hedberg et al, 1982). In fact, Takase et al (1982) and Jorge et al (1983) have recommended injecting a large volume of sclerosant into the oesophageal varices to achieve obliteration of these veins.

In patients in whom the GVs persist for more than 6 months after obliteration of oesophageal varices, the clinical course is generally more eventful. Bleeding was seen significantly more often in patients in whom GVs persisted than in those in whom the GVs were to disappear (28% versus 2%, $p < 0.01$) (Sarin et al, 1991). Similar high rates of bleeding from persisting GVs are reported by Korula et al (1991).

The exact mechanism of disappearance of GVs after obliteration of oesophageal varices is not clear. Kitano et al (1986) have shown that large oesophageal varices arise from deep intrinsic veins of the oesophageal wall and communicate with the GV directly. Contrast venographic studies have shown that, in a proportion of cases, the sclerosant injected into the oesophageal varix flows in a caudal direction, towards the GV (Grobe et al, 1984), possibly leading to its obliteration.

Gastro-oesophageal varices type 2 (GOV2). Oesophageal variceal sclerotherapy only marginally influences the treatment of GOV2. Of our 18 patients who received sclerotherapy, GOV2 disappeared in only three (17%) patients within 6 months.

Thus in our experience, three out of five patients with GOV1 do not require any treatment except sclerotherapy for oesophageal varices. A close endoscopic observation is, however, advisable to see if the GOV1 persist, because such patients would require gastric variceal sclerotherapy. Most of the patients with GOV2 do require direct and specific therapy. In general, we recommend that in a patient with GOV, be it GOV1 or GOV2, initially only oesophageal varices should be injected.

Development of secondary gastric varices

Do GVs develop as a complication after successful sclerotherapy for oesophageal varices? Hosking and Johnson (1988) observed development of secondary GVs at the lesser curve in 20 of 208 (10%) patients within 1 week to 3 years after injection of oesophageal varices. Mathur et al (1990) observed secondary GVs in 57% of patients during or after sclerotherapy for oesophageal varices. Korula et al (1991) found recurrence as GVs in 15% of patients after sclerotherapy.

In our experience, GVs were seen to develop in about 9% of patients after sclerotherapy during a mean follow-up of 24.6 ± 5.3 months (Sarin et al, 1991). In the majority of our patients, secondary GVs were GOV2 or IGV2 in type. While the secondary GOV1 and IGV2 types of varices rarely bleed, frequency of bleeding in patients with secondary GOV2 was similar to that in patients with primary GOV2. These patients therefore require specific therapy.

Induction of bleeding from gastric varices

Gastric bleeding after sclerotherapy for oesophageal varices could be from varices, gastric ulcer, gastritis or portal hypertensive gastropathy (Snady, 1987; Sarin et al, 1992). In their experience of 36 patients undergoing sclerotherapy for oesophageal varices, Clark et al (1980) from the King's College Hospital, London, observed bleeding in nine patients from oesophageal varices and in three patients from GVs. Schubert et al (1989) have indicated a 1–10% incidence of bleeding from GVs during sclerotherapy for oesophageal varices. It has been suggested that sclerotherapy blocks the shunting veins which are present in the palisade zone. This leads to increased blood flow in the gastric veins (Ohnishi et al, 1987) and a rise in portal pressure (Korula and Ralls, 1991), possibly leading to dilatation and rupture of these veins. In our own experience, this complication is rather rare.

The influence of coexisting GVs on the development of portal hypertensive gastropathy

Endoscopic sclerotherapy has been shown by several workers, including ourselves, to increase the incidence of gastropathy (McCormack et al, 1985; Papazian et al, 1986; Sarin et al, 1992). In our prospective study of 107 patients, 36 had coexisting GVs and the rest had only oesophageal varices prior to sclerotherapy. Forty-two per cent of the former group of patients developed portal hypertensive gastropathy (PHG) compared with only 11% who had no GVs prior to sclerotherapy ($p<0.01$), suggesting that the chances of development of PHG are quite high (nearly four times more) if a patient presents with gastro-oesophageal varices rather than with oesophageal varices alone.

The higher association of PHG with GVs could be explained by redistribution and an increase in gastric blood flow after obliteration of oesophageal varices. However, Eleftheriadis et al (1990), using an endoscopic laser doppler technique, did not find any increase after sclerotherapy in the gastric microcirculation in the fundic area where gastropathy is more common, but only in the pyloric area.

Hepatic encephalopathy

GVs could lead to development of chronic portosystemic encephalopathy. Watanabe et al (1988) showed that patients with GVs develop encephalopathy significantly more often than patients with only oesophageal varices (25% versus 3%, $p<0.01$). This phenomenon could be due to the blood leaving the superior mesenteric vein and flowing retrogradely into the splenic vein and bypassing the liver (type B and C in Figure 7). As a result nitrogenous substances from the gut enter the systemic circulation directly

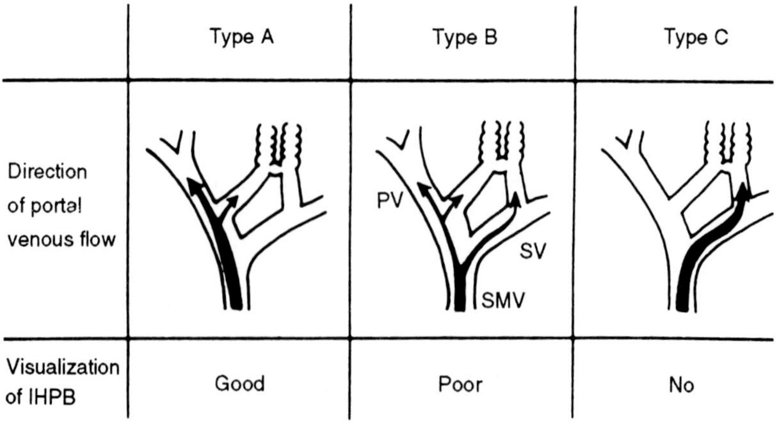

	Type A	Type B	Type C
Direction of portal venous flow		PV, SV, SMV	
Visualization of IHPB	Good	Poor	No

Figure 7. Schematic representation of the types of portal haemodynamics with respect to the flow of superior mesenteric venous blood flow (SMV). IHPB, intrahepatic portal vein branches; PV, portal vein; SV, splenic vein. From Watanabe et al (1988) with permission.

through the shunts. This explanation may not be true in all cases, especially in those with non-cirrhotic portal hypertension, who, despite having a higher reported incidence of GVs, do not have an increased incidence of hepatic encephalopathy (Sarin and Nundy, 1985).

MANAGEMENT OF GASTRIC VARICES

The management of GVs is predominantly the management of their bleeding. The rationale and the methods for controlling the gastric variceal bleeding at present are empirical and far from satisfactory. Except for a subset of patients with persisting GOV1, there is little role for prophylactic therapy in GVs. Spontaneous regression of GVs has been rarely reported (Goldberg et al, 1984). The various treatment modalities employed for the control of gastric variceal bleeding include the following.

Balloon tamponade

Two types of tubes are available for controlling bleeding from GVs; namely, the Sengstaken–Blakemore tube and the Linton–Nachlas tube. The conventional Sengstaken–Blakemore tube has an oesophageal balloon and a gastric balloon with a capacity of 200–250 ml. The Linton–Nachlas tube, on the other hand, has a single gastric balloon with a capacity of 600 ml (Figure 8). Teres et al (1978), in a series of 79 patients, had 12 patients with only gastric bleeding, two with both gastric and oesophageal bleeding, and the

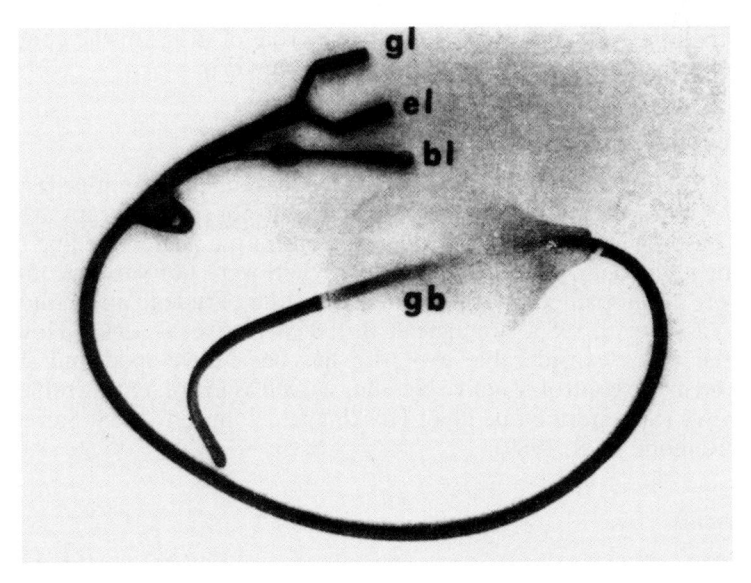

Figure 8. Linton–Nachlas tube modified by Bertand and Michel. gb, gastric balloon; gl, gastric lumen; el, oesophageal lumen; bl, balloon tamponade. From Teres et al (1978) with permission.

rest with only oesophageal variceal bleeding. Whereas balloon tamponade with the Sengstaken–Blakemore tube did not succeed in controlling bleeding from GVs in any patient, the Linton–Nachlas tube could achieve primary haemostasis in four out of nine (44%) patients and permanent haemostasis in three (33%) patients. This finding indicates that a direct compression of the bleeding site required for controlling gastric variceal bleeding is achievable only through a large-capacity gastric bulb, as in the Linton–Nachlas tube. Besides direct compression, the traction on the tube exerts pressure against the cardia and interrupts the submucosal venous flow. The same workers recently reported balloon tamponade to be superior to vasopressin ($P = 0.009$) in the control of bleeding oesophagogastric varices (Terés et al, 1990). Although the overall experience with the Linton–Nachlas tube is limited, we recommend that this tube should be readily available.

Embolization

There are occasional case reports of treating bleeding GVs with embolization of the splenic artery by catheterization (Jones and Koos, 1984). After embolization with gel-foam, part of the splenic tissue may be infarcted. This method could be chosen in a patient with high risk, especially with marked hypersplenism. Alwmark et al (1981) successfully treated a case of actively bleeding GVs by embolization. Menu et al (1987) similarly treated a patient with bleeding duodenal varix (IGV2).

Pharmacotherapy

There is little information available on the role of drugs in the control of acute bleeding or prophylaxis of bleeding from GVs.

Gastric variceal sclerotherapy (GVS)

Due to the success of oesophageal variceal sclerotherapy, enthusiasm was generated to attempt sclerosis of GVs. The goals for sclerotherapy are same as for oesophageal variceal bleeding; to control the acute bleeding and to prevent rebleeding. The initial results of GVS were not very encouraging and were accompanied by a high rebleeding rate (Trudeau and Prindiville, 1985; Yassin et al, 1985; Bretagne et al, 1986; Crotty et al, 1986). However, over the years considerable expertise has been developed and success achieved in the control of active bleeding as well as in preventing rebleeding from GVs (Sohendra et al, 1986; Hosking and Johnson, 1988; Sarin et al, 1988; Ramond et al, 1989).

Sclerosants

A potent sclerosant with properties of thrombosis of the blood with minimum tissue necrosis would be ideal for sclerotherapy of GVs. It is also desirable that the sclerosant should act instantaneously at the site of the injection with negligible flow to the portal vein. Sodium tetradecyl sulphate

(STD) (Trudeau and Prindiville, 1985), absolute alcohol (Sarin et al, 1988) and a glue, butyl cyanoacrylate (Sohendra et al, 1986; Ramond et al, 1989), have all been successfully used by different workers.

Technique of GVS

GVS can be done with a flexible fibreoptic endoscope using either a straight end-on technique (i.e. by keeping the endoscope straight) (Figure 9) or by

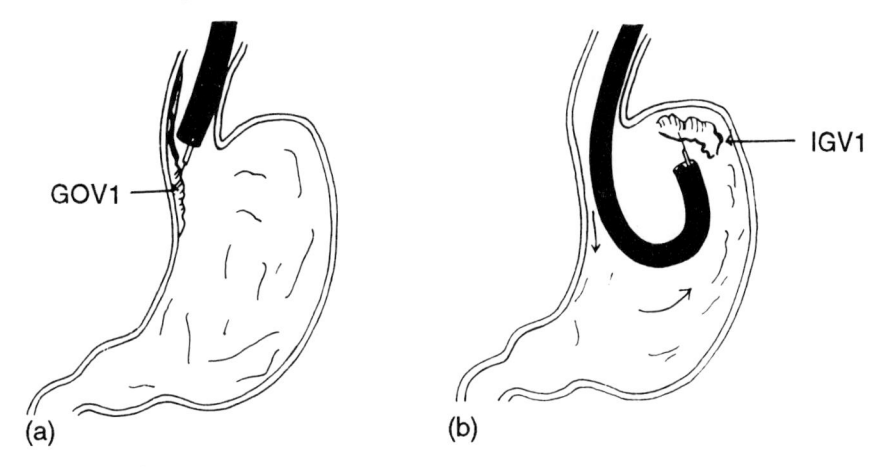

Figure 9. Technique of gastric variceal sclerotherapy: (a) straight-end technique for GOV1; (b) retroflexion technique for injecting GOV2 and IGV1.

retroflexion (i.e. by retroverting the endoscope at the incisura angularis) for better visualization of the fundus. The former technique is employed for lesser curve varices (GOV1) while the latter method was used for varices situated at cardia (GOV2) and deep-seated fundal varices (IGV1). We prefer using a 5–6-mm-long needle (3–4 mm long for oesophageal variceal sclerotherapy) and a transparent teflon injector (Olympus 11 and 14L) for GVS. A transparent injector helps in proper intravariceal placement of the injector needle.

Different modes of injection, including paravariceal, intravariceal or a combination of the two methods, have been employed for GVS. While Stray et al (1982) employed a paravariceal technique, Ramond et al (1989) found an intravariceal technique effective. We, however, observed a high rebleeding rate with the latter. We have therefore been using a combination technique in which initially 0.5–1.0 ml sclerosant is injected at multiple sites, raising blebs along the entire course of the GV (Figure 10). On average, four injections (range two to nine) are given paravariceally. Thereafter, the sclerosant is injected intravariceally into the GV. Usually one to three injections are given intravariceally into each GV. Attainment of an area of 0.5–1.0 cm of blanching around the injection site is considered desirable for adequate sclerotherapy as this criterion has been found useful in sclerotherapy for oesophageal varices (Sarin et al, 1987). The most prominent

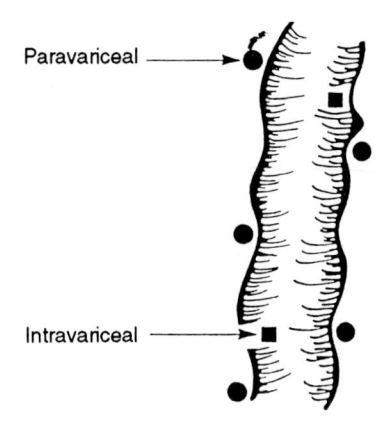

Figure 10. Combination of paravariceal and intravariceal techniques for gastric variceal sclerotherapy. First, paravariceal injections (●) are given 1–3 cm apart; then intravariceal injections (■) are placed on the side walls of the gastric varix. From Sarin et al (1988) with permission.

point of the GV is avoided during intravariceal injection and an attempt is made to give the injection on the side wall of the GV (Figure 10). The endoscope is withdrawn only after adequate haemostasis has been achieved and air and secretions have been sucked out of the stomach to decompress it. The patients are given nothing by mouth for half an hour and are carefully observed for the next week for any evidence of rebleeding.

Gastric variceal obturation

Gotlib et al (1984) proposed the use of adhesive butyl cyanoacrylate for obturation of oesophagogastric varices. Subsequently, Sohendra et al (1986), Ramond et al (1989) and Feretis et al (1990) have used isobutyl 2-cyanoacrylate (Bucrylate) or n-butyl cyanoacrylate (Histoacryl) and mixed it with Lipiodol. Lipiodol, besides making the mixture radio-opaque, lengthens the butyl cyanoacrylate polymerization. The injection needle is rinsed with Lipiodol before and after each injection. One to two sessions of one to eight intravariceal injections are given in each patient. In case of leakage of the mixture into the gastric lumen, the endoscope is withdrawn and cleaned; otherwise polymerization of the glue leads to obstruction of the needle and the endoscope channel.

Emergency GVS

GVS has been attempted by a few endoscopists during active gastric variceal bleeding. The procedure is technically difficult, especially in patients with fundal varices, since much blood accumulates in the area and proper visualization of the bleeding spot and the varix becomes difficult.

In a small study, Stray et al (1982) reported successful control of acute variceal bleeding in three patients using the paravariceal technique. Using an intravariceal injection technique and 1.5% STD, Trudeau and Prindiville

Table 1. Results of emergency gastric variceal sclerotherapy.

Author	Year	Agent	No. of patients	Successful control (no. (%))	Rebleeding rate (%)
Bretagne	1986	PD	10	6 (60)	63
Trudeau	1986	STD	9	9 (100)	89
Ramond	1989	BC	6	6 (100)	33
Sarin	1990	AA	16	14 (88)	19

PD, Polidocanol; STD, sodium tetradecyl sulphate; AA, absolute alcohol; BC, butyl cyanoacrylate.

(1985) were able to successfully control gastric variceal bleeding in all nine of their patients (Table 1). The rebleeding rate was, however, extremely high (eight out of nine patients), with a total of 25 rebleeding episodes. In our initial study, we had reported successful control of acute bleeding from GVs in six of the eight patients (Sarin et al, 1988). We have been successful in arresting acute bleeding in all subsequent eight cases, with an overall success in 15 (88%) cases. Three patients rebled. One of these and four other patients went for semi-emergency surgery. Seven went for chronic GVS; in two, varices were obliterated after the first injection. Good success in emergency control of gastric variceal bleeding has also been reported by Ramond et al (1989) and Feretis et al (1990) using cyanoacrylate glue.

Elective GVS

Repeated GVS has been used to obliterate GVs (Table 2). Obliteration of GOV1 is often possible with a single session of GVS and was achieved in 16 of our 20 patients. Hosking et al (1988) also treated 24 patients with lesser curve varices by intravariceal injection sclerotherapy at the squamocolumnar junction. This treatment is effective even if the blood flow is cephalad. Korula et al (1991) also observed successful obliteration of these varices with a single injection.

Fundal varices (GOV2 and IGV1) generally require three or more sclerotherapy sessions. Trudeau et al (1985) were not able to achieve obliteration of GV despite five or six injection courses. They observed a high incidence of rebleeding which could partly be due to rather slow and incomplete obliteration achieved by 1.5% STD. Using absolute alcohol, we were able to achieve obliteration in 25 (68%) out of 37 patients with a mean of three sessions per patient. Of the 12 remaining patients, obliteration could not be

Table 2. Elective gastric variceal sclerotherapy.

Author	Year	No. of patients	Successful obliteration (no. (%))	Rebleeding (no. (%))
Yassin	1985	35	6 (17)	8 (23)
Ramond	1989	27	19 (70)	6 (22)
Sarin	1990	37	25 (68)	9 (24)

achieved in two, and rebleeding occurred in ten. Six of the latter patients had fundal (GOV2–4, IGV1–2) varices. In their series of 27 patients, Ramond et al (1989) had three patients with isolated fundal varices and the rest with gastro-oesophageal varices. They were able to achieve obturation of GVs in 19 (70%) patients with one to two sessions of one to eight injections each. After injection of bucrylate, GVs appear as a hard cord. Bucrylate sheds out from the GV within 2 weeks to 3 months and finally the GV disappears, leaving a depressed area. The use of a glue appears to be particularly useful for treating GVs since the incidence of post-sclerotherapy ulcers is quite low. Since bucrylate is not a sclerosant and does not cause thrombosis, obturation is often incomplete. For occlusion of left gastric vein, a combination of alcohol followed by injection of bucrylate has been found to be quite effective (Connor et al, 1989). It remains to be seen whether a similar combination could improve the efficacy of GVS.

Complications

Besides rebleeding (Tables 1 and 2), the commonest complication of GVS is gastric mucosal ulcerations. Occasionally these could be the site of rebleeding. In our experience (Singal et al, 1988), while sucralphate is of little advantage in oesophageal variceal ulcers, it is effective in accelerating the healing of gastric variceal ulcers. Other complications like pain, dysphagia and fever are similar to that seen with oesophageal variceal sclerotherapy. Although, theoretically, there is a reasonable chance of splenic or portal vein thrombosis occurring after GVS, this complication has rarely been documented.

Complications associated with tissue adhesive injection appear to be similar in sclerotherapy (Steigmann and Yamamoto, 1992). Besides nearly identical rebleeding rates (Tables 1 and 2) oesophageal stenosis has been reported in 4–6.5% of cases (Ramond et al, 1989; Sohendra et al, 1986). Three deaths directly related to the technique (Ramond et al, 1986) and two deaths to stroke developing immediately after bucrylate injection (See et al, 1986) have been reported. In the later cases, the tissue glue had disseminated into the cerebral arterial system.

In summary, GVS is effective in (1) controlling acute gastric variceal bleeding, (2) obliteration of GOV1 in the majority of patients, (3) obliteration of GOV2 in 54% and IGV1 in 22% of patients, and (4) prophylactic sclerotherapy of GOV1.

Surgery for gastric variceal bleeding

Surgical management of GVs could be broadly divided into management of GVs due to (1) segmental portal hypertension in the absence of liver disease, and (2) generalized portal hypertension.

Segmental portal hypertension

Splenectomy effectively cures most patients with segmental portal hypertension without liver disease. Madsen et al (1986) reviewed the literature and described the course of 72 patients followed-up for up to 24 years after splenectomy for segmental portal hypertension. Only two patients rebled after splenectomy (Yale and Crummy, 1971; Stone et al, 1978); one requiring total gastrectomy. In another patient mesocaval shunt was done but was found ineffective in controlling the rebleeding (Larmi et al, 1976). Sutton et al (1970), in their review of 53 cases, recorded rebleeding in 9% of patients after splenectomy. Mortality after splenectomy has been reported to be around 7.3% (Roder, 1984).

Splenectomy effectively reduces the flow of venous blood and the pressure in the varices and other collaterals. To decrease the perioperative loss of blood, a ligature of the splenic artery is recommended before mobilizing the spleen, which may have a great number of collaterals in the ligaments. Some surgeons prefer to treat the underlying pancreatic disease by performing cystojejunostomy simultaneously (Salam et al, 1973; Keith et al, 1982).

Generalized portal hypertension

There is abundant information available on the surgical management of GOVs. Little, however, is mentioned specifically about the management of GVs. There are no clear guidelines available on the selection of patients for a given surgical procedure. In fact, for most, treatment of GVs is the treatment of generalized portal hypertension.

For patients with generalized portal hypertension and isolated GVs, a definitive treatment is advisable. Hosking and Johnson (1988) advocate variceal ligation with gastric devascularization for the control of active bleeding from such varices. However, they suggest that if GOV1 are associated, a shunt procedure may be better. Alternatively, for patients with acute gastric variceal bleeding, an emergency shunt could be equally effective. According to Wood et al (1990), the shunt of choice is a large-bore H-graft mesocaval or mesorenal shunt. This shunt effectively controls the acute bleeding, is relatively simple to perform, does not hinder the subsequent transplant, and can be ligated after the transplant is completed. For an elective procedure, a distal splenorenal shunt is preferred by many surgeons because it maintains hepatic portal perfusion and does not require dissection of the porta hepatis.

In the 1980s and 1990s, the indications for shunt surgery for portal hypertension have changed considerably. Today, shunt surgery is recommended for (1) patients who bleed from GVs, (2) patients bleeding from portal hypertensive gastropathy, (3) failures of sclerotherapy or non-compliant patients, and (4) individuals living in remote areas with limited medical facilities (Rikkers et al, 1987).

Transjugular intrahepatic portosystem shunt (TIPS)

With this technique a communication is created between the hepatic and portal venous system within the liver parenchyma. A transjugular liver

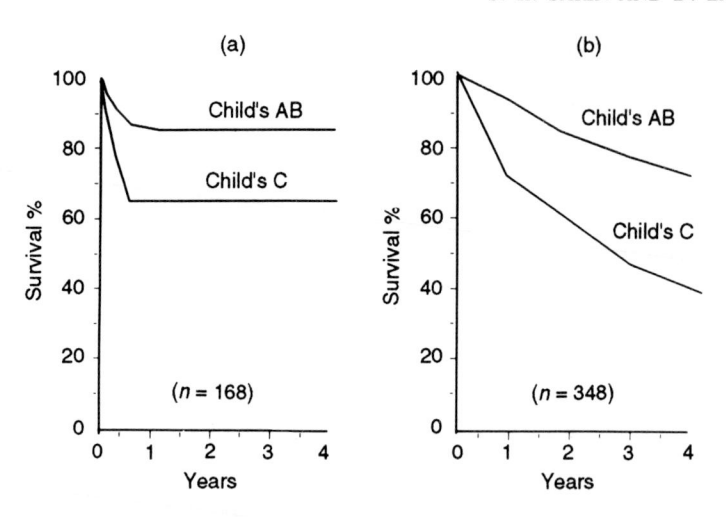

Figure 11. Survival curves for 168 adult Child's class A/B and C patients receiving liver transplantation at the University of Nebraska Medical Center (a) compared with 348 adult Child's A/B and C patients receiving selective shunts at Emory University (b). From Wood et al (1990) with permission.

biopsy needle is passed into the main hepatic veins through a sheath, introduced via the right internal jugular vein. The needle is advanced through the liver parenchyma, until a large portal vein branch is punctured. The tract is then dilated to the required size, using a balloon catheter and a stent is placed to maintain shunt patency. Preliminary results suggest that it can successfully decompress the portal venous system with minimal morbidity (Zemel et al, 1991). The effectiveness of the procedure and its role in the management of patients with portal hypertension have still to be assessed. However, it has particular application to patients bleeding from gastric varices, in whom the long-term results suggest that it would be a more promising alternative to operation.

Liver transplantation

Liver transplantation has emerged as an alternative to sclerotherapy and shunt surgery. The survival rates for patients undergoing chronic sclerotherapy range from 50% to 90% at 1 year and from 40% to 80% at 5 years, compared to 70–90% at 1 year and 40–60% at 5 years for patients undergoing portosystemic shunts (Terblanche et al, 1983; Warren et al, 1986; Rikkers et al, 1987; Garrett et al, 1988; Wood et al, 1990). The survival rates in transplanted patients are 79% at 1 year and 71% at 5 years (Iwatsuki, 1987). The differences in the survival rates became more prominent when Child's class C patients who received liver transplants (79% 1-year and 71% 5-year survival rates) were compared with Child's C patients who were treated with shunts (30–70% 1-year and 13–35% 5-year survival rates).

Almost similar conclusions are reached if the data of shunt surgery from Emory University and the transplant data from Nebraska University are compared (Figure 11) (Wood et al, 1990).

These results bring a ray of hope for the large number of patients with cirrhosis and portal hypertension, including those having GVs. At present, however, for a significant proportion of patients transplant remains an expensive and difficult option, especially in the developing countries. It is encouraging to know that a previous shunt operation, especially one not involving the hepatic hilum, does not reduce the chances of successful transplantation in the future.

SUMMARY

Gastric varices (GV) are a common (20%) accompaniment of portal hypertension; they are more often seen in those patients who bleed than in those who do not (27% versus 4%, $p < 0.01$). They can develop in both segmental and generalized portal hypertension. Depending on their location and relation with oesophageal varices, GVs can be classified as gastro-oesophageal varices (GOV) and isolated gastric varices (IGV); each of these can be further subdivided as follows: GOV1 (extension of oesophageal varices along lesser curve) and GOV2 (extension of oesophageal varices towards fundus); and IGV1 (varices in the fundus) and IGV2 (isolated varices anywhere in the stomach). The common presentation of GVs is variceal bleeding and encephalopathy. In comparison with oesophageal varices, GVs bleed significantly less often (64% versus 25%, $p < 0.01$) but more severely (2.9 ± 0.3 versus 4.8 ± 0.6 transfusion units, $p < 0.01$). Patients with GOV2 and IGV1 bleed more often than patients with other types of GVs. Sclerotherapy for oesophageal varices can significantly influence the natural history of GVs. GOV1, or lesser curve varices, disappear in the majority of cases (59%) after obliteration of oesophageal varices. In those with persisting GOV1, the incidence of bleeding and mortality is high and these patients require gastric variceal sclerotherapy (GVS). During oesophageal variceal sclerotherapy, bleeding can occasionally be induced from GVs. After obliteration of oesophageal varices, recurrence as GVs (secondary GVs) can occur in about 9% of patients. Emergency GVS is quite effective in controlling acute bleeding from GVs, more so than balloon tamponade. Potent sclerosants like tetradecyl sulphate and alcohol and a glue, bucrylate, have been quite effective. Elective GVS can achieve obliteration of GVs in nearly 70% of patients. Rebleeding and ulceration are common complications of GVS; probably related to incomplete obliteration and mucosal injury respectively. Splenectomy is quite effective in treating GVs due to segmental portal hypertension. For GV bleeding due to generalized portal hypertension, a shunt operation is often effective. TIPS procedure appear to be a very promising therapy for GV bleeding. Liver transplantation may be a superior alternative to sclerotherapy and shunt surgery for gastric varices.

REFERENCES

Achord JL (1992) Has another surgical procedure been replaced? *Gastroenterology* **102**: 1080–1081.
Alwmark A, Gullstrand P, Ihse I et al (1981) Regional portal hypertension in chronic pancreatitis. *Acta Chirurgica Scandinavica* **147**: 155–157.
Bretagne JF, Dudicourt JC, Morisot D et al (1986) Is endoscopic variceal sclerotherapy effective for the treatment of gastric varices? (Abstract) *Digestive Diseases and Sciences* **31**: 505S.
Clark AW, Westaby D, Silk DBA et al (1980) Prospective controlled trial of injection sclerotherapy in patients with cirrhosis and recent variceal haemorrhage. *Lancet* **ii**: 552–554.
Connor KW, Lehman G, Yune H et al (1989) Comparison of three non-surgical treatments for bleeding esophageal varices. *Gastroenterology* **96**: 899–906.
Crotty B, Wood LJ, Willett IR et al (1986) The management of acutely bleeding varices by injection sclerotherapy. *Medical Journal of Australia* **145**: 130–133.
Eleftheriadis E, Kotzampassi K & Aletras H (1990) The influence of sclerotherapy on gastric mucosal blood flow distribution. *American Surgeon* **56**: 593–595.
Evans JA & Delany F (1953) Gastric varices. *Radiology* **60**: 46–52.
Feldman M & Feldman MR (1956) Gastric varices. *Gastroenterology* **30**: 318–321.
Feretis C, Tabakopoulos D, Benakis P et al (1990) Endoscopic hemostasis of esophageal and gastric variceal bleeding with histoacryl. *Endoscopy* **22**: 282–284.
Fleming RJ & Seaman WB (1968) Roentgenographic demonstration of unusual extra-esophageal varices. *American Journal of Roentgenology Radium Therapy Nuclear Medicine* **103**: 281–290.
Garrett K, Reilly JJ, Schade RR et al (1988) Sclerotherapy of esophageal varices: long term results and determinants of survival. *Surgery* **104**: 813–818.
Goldberg S, Katz S, Naidich J & Waye J (1984) Isolated gastric varices due to spontaneous splenic vein thrombosis. *American Journal of Gastroenterology* **79**: 304–307.
Gotlib JP, Demma I, Fonsecca A et al (1984) Resultats a 1 an du traitement endoscopique electif des hemorragies par rupture de varices oesophagiennes chez le cirrhotique. *Gastroenterologie Clinique et Biologique* **8**: 133A (abstract).
Graham D & Smith J (1981) The course of patients after variceal haemorrhage. *Gastroenterology* **80**: 800–809.
Grobe JI, Kozarek RA, Sanowski RA et al (1984) Venography during endoscopic injection sclerotherapy of oesophageal varices. *Gastrointestinal Endoscopy* **30**: 6–8.
Hashizume M, Kitano S, Sugimachi K & Sueishi K (1988) Three-dimensional view of the vascular structure of the lower oesophagus in clinical portal hypertension. *Hepatology* **8**: 1482–1487.
Hashizume M, Kitano S, Yamaga H et al (1990) Endoscopic classification of gastric varices. *Gastrointestinal Endoscopy* **36**: 276–280.
Hedberg SE, Fowler DL & Ryan RLR (1982) Injection sclerotherapy of oesophageal varices using ethanolamine oleate. *American Journal of Surgery* **143**: 426–431.
Hosking SW & Johnson AG (1988) Gastric varices: a proposed classification to management. *British Journal of Surgery* **75**: 195–196.
Iwatsuki S, Starzel TE, Todo S et al (1987) Liver transplantation in the treatment of bleeding oesophageal varices. *Surgery* **104**: 697–705.
Jones KB & Koos PTD (1984) Post embolization splenic abscess in a patient with pancreatitis and splenic vein thrombosis. *Southern Medical Journal* **77**: 390–393.
Jorge AD, Adam J, Seittert L & Segal E (1983) Sclerotherapy of oesophageal varices—an Argentinian experience. *Endoscopy* **15**: 141–143.
Karr S & Wohl GT (1960) Clinical importance of gastric varices. *New England Journal of Medicine* **263**: 665–669.
Keith RG, Mustrad RA & Saibil EA (1982) Gastric variceal bleeding due to occlusion of splenic vein in pancreatic disease. *Canadian Journal of Surgery* **25**: 301–304.
Kitano S, Terblanche J, Khan D & Bornman PC (1986) Venous anatomy of the lower oesophagus in portal hypertension: practical implications. *British Journal of Surgery* **73**: 525–531.
Korula J & Ralls P (1991) The effects of chronic endoscopic variceal sclerotherapy on portal pressure in cirrhosis. *Gastroenterology* **101**: 800–806.

Korula J, Chin K, Ko Y & Yamada S (1991) Demonstration of two distinct subsets of gastric varices: observations during a seven year study of endoscopic sclerotherapy. *Digestive Diseases and Sciences* **36:** 303–309.

Larmi TKI, Mokka REM, Kairaluoma MI et al (1976) Gastric bleeding due to segmental portal hypertension: a case report. *Acta Chirurgica Scandinavica* **142:** 609–610.

Little AG & Moossa AR (1981) Gastrointestinal hemorrhage from left sided portal hypertension; an unappreciated complication of pancreatitis. *American Journal of Surgery* **141:** 153–158.

McCormack TT, Sims J, Eyre-Brook I et al (1985) Gastric lesions in portal hypertension: inflammatory gastritis or congestive gastropathy? *Gut* **26:** 1226–1232.

MacDougall BRD, Theodossi A, Westaby D et al (1982) Increased long-term survival in variceal haemorrhage using injection sclerotherapy. *Lancet* **i:** 124–127.

Madsen MS, Patersen TH & Sommer H (1986) Segmental portal hypertension. *Annals of Surgery* **204:** 72–77.

Mahal TC & Groszmann RJ (1990) Pathophysiology of portal hypertension and variceal bleeding. *Surgical Clinics of North America* **70:** 251–266.

Marshall JP, Smith PD, Hoyumpa AM Jr (1977) Gastric varices, problems in diagnosis. *Digestive Diseases and Sciences* **22:** 947–955.

Mathur SK, Dalvi AN, Someshwar V et al (1990) Endoscopic and radiological appraisal of gastric varices. *British Journal of Surgery* **77:** 432–435.

Menu Y, Gayet B & Naham H (1987) Bleeding duodenal varices: diagnosis and treatment by percutaneous portography and transcatheter embolization. *Gastrointestinal Radiology* **12:** 111–113.

Ohnishi K, Nahate H, Terabayashi H et al (1987) The effects of endoscopic sclerotherapy combined with transhepatic variceal obliteration on portal hemodynamics. *American Journal of Gastroenterology* **82:** 1138–1142.

Papazian A, Braillon A, Dupas JL et al (1986) Portal hypertensive gastric mucosa: an endoscopic study. *Gut* **27:** 1199–1203.

Paquet KH (1982) Open discussion on technical aspects of injection sclerotherapy. In Westaby D, McDougall BRD & Williams R (eds) *Variceal Bleeding*, pp 215–217. London: Pitman Press.

Ramond MJ, Valla D, Gotlib JP et al (1986) Obturation endoscopique des varices oesophagastriques par le bucrylate. *Gastroenterologie Clinique et Biologique* **36:** 572–574.

Ramond MJ, Valla D, Mosnier JF et al (1989) Successful endoscopic obliteration of gastric varices with butyl cyanoacrylate. *Hepatology* **10:** 488–493.

Rice RP, Thompson WM, Kelvin FM et al (1977) Gastric varices without oesophageal varices. *Journal of the American Medical Association* **237:** 1976–1979.

Rikkers LF, Burnett DA, Volentine GD et al (1987) Shunt surgery versus endoscopic sclerotherapy for long-term treatment of variceal bleeding. Early results of a randomized controlled trial. *Annals of Surgery* **206:** 261–271.

Roder O Chr (1984) Splenic vein thrombosis with bleeding gastroesophageal varices: report of 2 splenectomized cases and review of the literature. *Acta Chirurgica Scandinavica* **150:** 265–268.

Rosch W (1974) Isolated gastric varices: a hint to pancreatic disorders. *Endoscopy* **6:** 217–220.

Salam AA, Warren WD & Tyras DH (1973) Splenic vein thrombosis: a diagnosable and curable form of portal hypertension. *Surgery* **74:** 961–962.

Sarin SK & Kumar A (1989) Gastric varices: profile, classification and management. *American Journal of Gastroenterology* **84:** 1244–1249.

Sarin SK & Nundy S (1985) Subclinical encephalopathy after portasystemic shunts in patients with non-cirrhotic portal fibrosis. *Liver* **5:** 142–146.

Sarin SK, Nanda R & Sachdev G (1987) Intravariceal versus paravariceal sclerotherapy, a randomized, prospective controlled trial. *Gut* **28:** 657–662.

Sarin SK, Sachdev G, Nanda R et al (1988) Endoscopic sclerotherapy in the treatment of gastric varices. *British Journal of Surgery* **75:** 747–750.

Sarin SK, Lahoti D, Saxena SP et al (1991) Gastric varices: incidence, classification and natural history of gastric varices: a study in 568 patients with portal hypertension. *Hepatology* **14:** 242A.

Sarin SK, Sreenivas DV, Lahoti D & Saraya A (1992) Factors influencing development of portal hypertensive gastropathy; role of sclerotherapy, severity of liver disease, variceal pressure, etiology of portal hypertension and presence of gastric varices. *Gastroenterology* (in press).

Schubert TT, Schnell GA & Walden JM (1989) Bleeding from varices in the gastric fundus complicating sclerotherapy. *Gastrointestinal Endoscopy* **35:** 268–269.

See A, Florent C, Larny P et al (1986) Accidents vasculaire cerebraux après obturation endoscopique des varices oesophagiennes par l'isobutyl-2-cyanoacrylate chez deux malades. *Gastroenterologie Clinique et Biologique* **10:** 604–607.

Singal AK, Sarin SK, Misra SP & Broor SL (1988) Ulceration after esophageal and gastric variceal sclerotherapy—significance of sucralfate and other factors on healing. *Endoscopy* **20:** 238–240.

Snady H (1987) The role of sclerotherapy in the treatment of oesophageal varices: personal experience and a review of the randomized trials. *American Journal of Gastroenterology* **28:** 657–662.

Sohendra N, Nam VC, Grimm H et al (1986) Endoscopic obliteration of large esophagogastric varices with Bucrylate. *Endoscopy* **18:** 25–26.

Stadelmann E (1913) Ueber seltene Formenvon Blutungen im Tractus gastrointestinalis. *Beri Klin Wochenscher* **50:** 825–829.

Stone RT, Wilson SE & Passaro E (1978) Gastric portal hypertension. *American Journal of Surgery* **136:** 73–79.

Stray N, Jacobsen CD & Rosseland A (1982) Injection sclerotherapy of bleeding oesophageal and gastric varices using a flexible endoscope. *Acta Medica Scandinavica* **211:** 125–129.

Sutton JP, Yarborough DY & Richards JT (1970) Isolated splenic vein occlusion. *Archives of Surgery* **100:** 623–626.

Takase Y, Ozak A, Orii R et al (1982) Injection sclerotherapy of oesophageal varices for patients undergoing emergency and elective surgery. *Surgery* **92:** 474–479.

Takashi M, Igarashi M, Hino S et al (1985) Esophageal varices: correlation of left gastric venography and endoscopy in patients with portal hypertension. *Radiology* **154:** 327–331.

Terblanche J (1990) Has sclerotherapy altered the management of patients with variceal bleeding? *American Journal of Surgery* **160:** 37–42.

Terblanche J, Northover JMA, Bornman P et al (1979) A prospective controlled trial of sclerotherapy in the long-term management of patients after oesophageal variceal bleeding. *Surgery, Gynecology and Obstetrics* **148:** 323–333.

Terblanche J, Bornman PC, Khan D et al (1983) Failure of repeated injection sclerotherapy to improve long-term survival after oesophageal variceal bleeding: a five year prospective controlled clinical trial. *Lancet* **ii:** 1328–1333.

Terés J, Cecilia A, Bordas JM et al (1978) Oesophageal tamponade for bleeding varices. Controlled trial between the Sengstaken Blakemore tube and the Linton–Nachlas tube. *Gastroenterology* **75:** 566–569.

Terés J, Planas R, Panés J et al (1990) Vasopressin nitroglycerin infusion vs. esophageal tamponade in the treatment of acute variceal bleeding: randomized controlled trial. *Hepatology* **11:** 964–968.

Trudeau W & Prindiville T (1985) Endoscopic injection sclerosis in bleeding gastric varices. *Gastrointestinal Endoscopy* **32:** 264–268.

Warren WD, Henderson JM, Millikan WJ et al (1986) Distal splenorenal shunt versus endoscopic sclerotherapy for long term management of variceal bleeding. *Annals of Surgery* **203:** 454–462.

Watanabe K, Kimura K, Matsutani S et al (1988) Portal hemodynamics in patients with gastric varices. A study in 230 patients with oesophageal and or gastric varices using portal vein catheterization. *Gastroenterology* **95:** 434–440.

Weissberg J, Stein DT, Fogel M et al (1984) Variceal bleeding: does it matter to the patient whether his gastric or esophageal varices bleed? *Gastroenterology* **86:** 1296 (abstract).

Wood RP, Shaw BW Jr & Rikkers LF (1990) Liver transplantation for variceal hemorrhage. *Surgical Clinics of North America* **70:** 449–461.

Yale CE & Crummy AB (1971) Splenic vein thrombosis and bleeding esophageal varices. *Journal of the American Medical Association* **217:** 317–320.

Yassin YM, Eita MS & Hussein AMT (1985) Endoscopic sclerotherapy for bleeding gastric varices. *Gut* **26:** A1105 (abstract).

Yasumoto M (1971) Clinical observations on 100 cases of gastric varices. *Japanese Journal of Gastroenterology* **68:** 721–739.

Zemal G, Katzen BT, Becker GJ et al (1991) Percutaneous transjugular portosystemic shunt. *Journal of the American Medical Association* **266:** 390–393.

9

Transection and devascularization procedures for bleeding from oesophagogastric varices

YASUO IDEZUKI

OESOPHAGEAL TRANSECTION AND DEVASCULARIZATION PROCEDURES

Oesophageal transection and devascularization in Japan was started in our institution in 1964, modifying Walker's transthoracic oesophageal transection (Walker, 1960), the main difference from the original Walker's procedure being more extensive devascularization of the lower oesophagus (Idezuki et al, 1967). This operation has been perfected as the University of Tokyo method (Sugiura procedure), where transabdominal splenectomy and devascularization of the upper half of the stomach were performed in addition to the transthoracic devascularization and transection of the oesophagus (Sugiura and Futagawa, 1973). This thoracoabdominal transection and devascularization procedure (the Sugiura procedure, more popularly known in Japan as the University of Tokyo method) has proven to be very effective for the treatment of oesophagogastric varices (Sugiura and Futagawa, 1977). However, it is a very extensive operation and often could not be tolerated by patients with advanced stages of liver cirrhosis. It should be performed in two stages (transthoracic devascularization and transection of the oesophagus as the first-stage operation, followed by transabdominal splenectomy and devascularization of the upper half of the stomach approximately one month later as the second-stage operation). More recently, transabdominal stapler transection of oesophagus and devascularization have been introduced (Johnston, 1977; Cooperman et al, 1980; Wexler, 1980; Kuzmak, 1981) and become more popular. Transection of the oesophagus is performed using staples, and devascularization of the stomach and the lower third (8–10 cm) of the oesophagus is performed transabdominally in one stage (Idezuki et al, 1990). Although the extent of devascularization of the oesophagus is less (8–10 cm) than in the transthoracic approach, where 15–16 cm of the lower oesophagus is devascularized, in 80% of the patients varices disappeared completely after transabdominal transection and devascularization. Patients in whom some of the varices remained after operation can easily be treated by adjuvant sclerotherapy. This transabdominal approach is currently preferred by many surgeons in Japan to the Sugiura procedure (Inokuchi, 1985; Idezuki, 1991).

INDICATIONS FOR TRANSECTION AND DEVASCULARIZATION PROCEDURES

Until the recent development of endoscopic sclerotherapy, surgical treatment was the only reliable method of controlling variceal bleeding, and operations were performed even in patients of Child C category or as an emergency measure. However, operative mortality and morbidity in Child C patients were high and now we consider that surgery should not be performed in Child C patients; emergency operations are only indicated after all other emergency measures to control acute bleeding have failed. More than 90% of acute massive bleeding from oesophagogastric varices could be controlled either by balloon tamponade or by sclerotherapy, and emergency operations are now performed mainly for patients bleeding from gastric varices where these conservative methods are not as effective as in the case of oesophageal variceal bleeding.

Factors which should be taken into consideration in selecting the optimal method of controlling bleeding from varices are: patient's age, severity of hepatic failure and clinical symptoms, location and grade of varices, developing pattern of portal collaterals, associated hypersplenism, associated hepatocellular carcinoma, associated diseases of other important organ systems, history of laparotomy or thoracotomy, timing and aggressiveness of the operation. Our indications for devascularization and transection procedures are listed in Table 1. Indications for surgical treatment have

Table 1. Indications for devascularization and transection procedures.

	Before 1986	After 1986
Age	70 year old or younger	65 year old or younger
History	History of bleeding	
Endoscopic findings	Red colour sign positive, moderate (F_2) to severe (F_3) varices, blue-coloured varices	No change
Clinical symptoms	No encephalopathy No ascites No cachexia	No change
Liver function tests		
Albumin	$2.8\,g\,dl^{-1}<$	$3.0\,g\,dl^{-1}<$
Bilirubin	$3.5\,mg\,dl^{-1}>$	$2.0\,mg\,dl^{-1}>$
S-GOT	200 units >	100 units >
S-GPT	200 units >	100 units >
Antipyrin clearance	$0.10\,ml\,min^{-1}\,kg^{-1}<$	No change
Prothrombin time	50% <	No change
Hepaplastin test	50% <	No change
Indocyanine green clearance at 15 min	40% >	No change
Disappearance rate constant of ICG from the blood	$0.04\,min^{-1}<$	$0.06\,min^{-1}<$
	No severe complications in other organs	No change

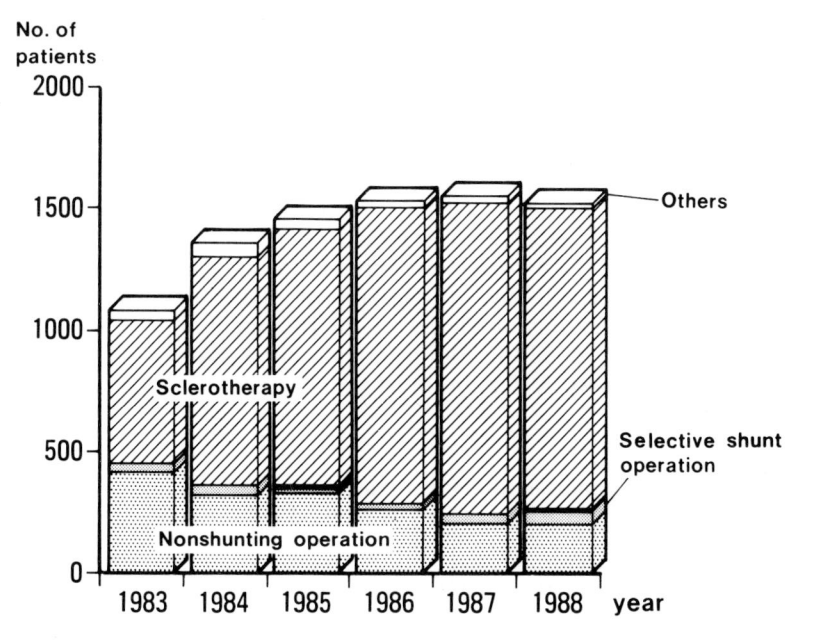

Figure 1. The changing trend of treatment of oesophagogastric varices.

become more strict and limited in our institution since 1986 when the technique of endoscopic sclerotherapy was established. The changing trend of treatment during the last six years in Japan is shown in Figure 1.

OPERATIVE PROCEDURES

The objective of transection and devascularization procedures is to block and obliterate all the blood inflow to the varices in the oesophagocardiac region. This is achieved by extensive devascularization of the upper half of the stomach and the lower oesophagus up to the level of the left pulmonary vein and transection of the oesophagus a few centimetres above the oesophagocardiac junction. Complete devascularization of the lower oesophagus up to the level of the left pulmonary vein can only be achieved by a transthoracic approach, that is, the thoracoabdominal approach used in the original University of Tokyo method (Sugiura procedure) (Idezuki et al, 1967). However, the thoracoabdominal operation is a very extensive operation, and while it may be tolerated in good risk patients (Child A category), in many of the higher risk patients (Child B category) it should be carried out in two stages (usually the transthoracic procedure first, followed by the transabdominal procedure approximately one month later). Moreover, in most of the patients in Child C category the second stage of the operation had to be abandoned because of the deterioration of the liver function after the first-stage procedure.

At present, in most of the patients transabdominal devascularization and transection using EEA stapler (modified Sugiura procedure) is carried out. This transabdominal approach results in some compromise in the extent of devascularization of the lower oesophagus, since only 8–10 cm of the lower oesophagus can be devascularized from the abdomen. Although this compromise in oesophageal devascularization may eventually result in a slightly higher postoperative recurrence of oesophageal varices, a long-term follow-up after these procedures reveals that bleeding had not been observed in 80% of the patients. Patients with residual or recurrent varices can easily be treated with one or two series of adjuvant endoscopic sclerotherapy. A recent nationwide survey on the treatment of oesophagogastric varices in Japan revealed that the transabdominal stapler transection and devascularization was by far the most popular operation for oesophagogastric varices.

Transthoracoabdominal oesophageal transection and devascularization (University of Tokyo method or Sugiura procedure)

The left thoracic cavity is entered by the sixth or seventh intercostal space as a posterolateral thoracotomy. Fifteen to sixteen centimetres of the distal oesophagus (up to the level of the left pulmonary vein) and 2–3 cm of the cardia below the oesophagocardiac junction are completely devascularized. The oesophagus is then transected approximately 3 cm above the oesophagocardiac junction and reanastomosed by hand using absorbable 4-0 or 5-0 sutures.

In a one-stage procedure, the abdominal cavity is then opened

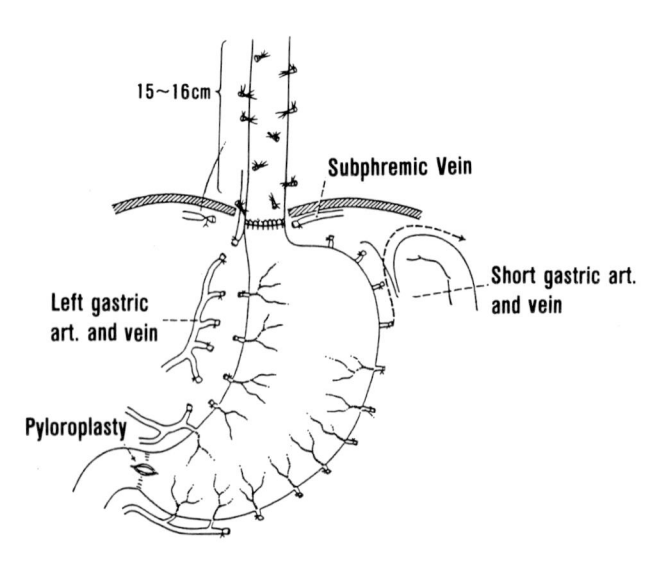

Figure 2. Thoracoabdominal devascularization and transection (University of Tokyo method).

transdiaphragmatically, and splenectomy and complete devascularization of the proximal half of the stomach are carried out. In a two-stage procedure, approximately one month after the thoracic procedure, the abdomen is entered by a separate upper midline incision, and splenectomy and devascularization of the proximal half of the stomach are performed. Pyloroplasty is usually added (Figure 2).

Transabdominal stapler (EEA) transection and devascularization (modified Sugiura procedure)

The transabdominal oesophageal transection and devascularization procedures consist of seven components: (1) devascularization of the greater curvature of the stomach; (2) splenectomy; (3) devascularization of the lesser curvature; (4) devascularization of the retrocardiac region; (5) devascularization of the lower oesophagus; (6) transection of the oesophagus using the stapler (EEA); (7) pyloroplasty.

The abdomen is opened through a long midline incision, or by an L incision when the spleen is markedly enlarged or adhesions around the spleen are very extensive. Devascularization of the greater curvature of the stomach is started at a point opposite to the incisura angularis on the lesser curvature, by doubly ligating close to the gastric wall and then dividing the branches of the right gastroepiploic vessels. Devascularization of the greater curvature is continued cephalad until all the branches of the left gastroepiploic vessels and many of the short gastric vessels are also ligated and divided. In the presence of a marked splenomegaly, the uppermost branches of the short gastric vessels are difficult to ligate and divide at this stage. This part of the operation may be postponed until the splenic artery is ligated.

The splenic artery is located along the superior border of the pancreas, carefully dissected free and then ligated with a suture. This interrupts the main splenic inflow, thereby causing the enlarged spleen to shrink considerably. This manoeuvre facilitates safer dissection of the upper pole of the spleen and also mobilization of the spleen from the retroperitoneum. Care should be taken not to tear the capsule of the spleen, which may bleed massively until the spleen is removed, necessitating a blood transfusion. Massive bleeding (more than 1000 ml) during operation is known to cause postoperative deterioration of the liver function; therefore haemostasis should be meticulous and complete. Ligaments attached to the spleen (splenocolic ligament, lienorenal ligament, lienogastric ligament and phrenicolienal ligament) often house abundant portal collaterals, so that these collaterals should be carefully ligated before division. After mobilizing the spleen from the retroperitoneum, the splenic artery and vein are doubly ligated with transfixing sutures close to the splenic hilum and then divided. The spleen is removed. After removal of the enlarged spleen, there is an easy working space and the remaining operative procedures may be carried out without much difficulty or significant bleeding.

The posterior gastric vessels are dissected, ligated and then divided. The upper gastric fundus with its apical fat pad are severed from diaphragmatic attachments.

Devascularization of the lesser curvature of the stomach is carried out very close to the gastric wall, starting from just inferior to the incisura angularis and extending cephalad to the oesophagus. The collaterals behind the stomach (innominate or retrogastric vessels) should also be completely devascularized since these minute veins also communicate with the gastro-oesophageal varices.

After completely devascularizing the upper half of the stomach, devascularization is continued cephalad along the oesophagus. Opening the oesophageal hiatus facilitates devascularization of the oesophagus. Usually 8–10 cm of the oesophagus is devascularized. Usually, the fundic portion of the stomach becomes ischaemic after complete devascularization of these regions.

After completion of devascularization, a 2-cm incision is made in the anterior wall of the gastric body for insertion of the EEA (End to End Autosuture, US Surgical) staplers. The small gastrotomy should be made in the lower portion of the gastric body, where circulation is least altered by the devascularization. The EEA stapler is introduced into the oesophagus through this gastrotomy and transection is carried out at a level 2–3 cm above the oesophagocardiac junction. Usually, a 25- or 28-mm disposable cartridge is used in oesophageal transection. The gastrotomy is closed in two layers, using interrupted sutures for both layers. A nasogastric tube is passed across the line of transection into the stomach. Bleeding from the anastomotic line is checked by gastric lavage using cold saline.

Finally, pyloroplasty is performed to prevent postoperative gastric retention since the vagal nerves are usually divided in the process of oesophageal devascularization (Figure 3). A silicone rubber drain is inserted in the left subdiaphragmatic space and the abdomen is closed.

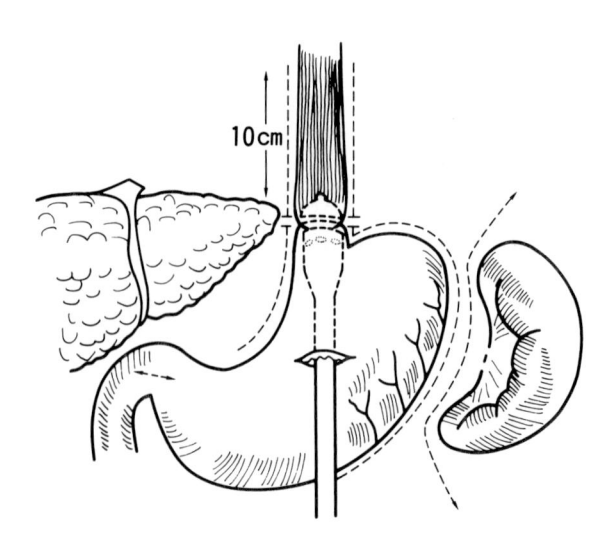

Figure 3. Transabdominal oesophageal transection and devascularization.

The patient is maintained on parenteral nutrition for 9–10 days after operation, and the oral intake of fluid meal is usually started on the 10th postoperative day after confirming by fluoroscopy that anastomotic leakage is absent.

RESULTS

Since 1964 we have performed more than 500 transection and devascularization procedures in our department, of which 287 were transthoracoabdominal transection and devascularization (University of Tokyo method or Sugiura procedure), and 52 were transabdominal transection and devascularization using the EEA stapler (Table 2). Of the 287 transthoracoabdominal transection and devascularization procedures, 127 were performed in one stage and 160 were performed in two stages. Overall operative mortality rate in transthoracoabdominal transection and devascularization was only 2.4% (7 out of 287) and 0% (0 out of 52). It should be noted that in earlier days transthoracic oesophageal transection and devascularization was routinely selected as the emergency operation for controlling acute bleeding from varices and many of the patients who received emergency transthoracic transection and devascularization could not proceed to the second-stage transabdominal procedures because of further deterioration of hepatic function.

Overall operative mortality rate in these patients was 5.0%, but operative deaths were observed only in patients with liver cirrhosis. Operative mortality rate for emergency procedures in patients with cirrhosis was 23.3% (14 out of 60) and it was also high in patients of Child C category (17.1%) (Tables 3 and 4). It is recommended that emergency operation be avoided and cirrhotic patients of Child C category be treated conservatively.

Transection and devascularization procedures were effective in the treatment of oesophagogastric varices. Varices disappeared completely in almost all patients after a transthoracoabdominal procedure and in approximately 80% of patients after transabdominal transection and devascularization. The remaining varices could easily be treated by a session or two of endoscopic sclerotherapy. The effect of transection and devascularization was most prominent and also long lasting after the thoracoabdominal procedure where devascularization of the distal oesophagus was extensive and more complete than after the transabdominal approach. Recurrence of varices was observed endoscopically in approximately 30% of the patients who received transabdominal transection and devascularization procedure after five years, but bleeding from these recurrent varices was rare. Late deaths caused from bleeding were 6.6% (33 out of 496).

The common complications after transection and devascularization were stricture or stenosis at the lower end of the oesophagus, minor leakage at the anastomosis, abdominal discomfort, and portal hypertensive gastropathy. Stricture or stenosis at the lower end of the oesophagus was observed in approximately 10% of patients after oesophageal transection and devascularization. Most of these stenoses were achalasia-like functional stenoses,

Table 2. Operative mortality of non-shunting operations.

Operation	Liver cirrhosis	Idiopathic portal hypertension	Extrahepatic portal obstruction	Schistosomiasis	Others	Total
University of Tokyo method (one stage)	77 (3)	36	14	0	0	127 (3)
University of Tokyo method (two stages)	127 (4)	24	5	3	1	160 (4)
Walker's operation	16 (1)	13	2	0	0	31 (1)
Transthoracic oesophageal transection	77 (15)	11	6	0	0	94 (15)
Transabdominal oesophageal transection	40 (0)	8	3	0	1	52 (0)
Hassab's operation	38 (2)	12	0	0	1	51 (2)
Others	3 (1)	0	8	1	0	12 (1)
Total	378 (26)	104 (0)	38 (0)	4 (0)	3 (0)	527 (26)

Operative deaths in parentheses.

Table 3. Results of non-shunting operations (1).

Disease	Operation	No. of cases	Operative death (%)	Hepatoma	Late death Liver failure	Bleeding	Others
Liver cirrhosis	Emergency	60	14 (23.3)	12	10	2	2
	Elective	192	7 (3.6)	32	46	15	11
	Prophylactic	126	5 (4.0)	19	24	8	8
Idiopathic portal hypertension	Emergency	13	0 (0)	0	2	1	2
	Elective	51	0 (0)	1	3	5	3
	Prophylactic	40	0 (0)	1	4	0	7
Extrahepatic portal obstruction	Emergency	5	0 (0)	0	0	1	0
	Elective	26	0 (0)	0	0	1	2
	Prophylactic	7	0 (0)	0	0	0	0
Total		520	26 (5.0)	65	89	33	35

Table 4. Results of non-shunting operations (2).

Disease	Child's classification	No. of cases	Operative death (%)	Hepatoma	Late death Liver failure	Bleeding	Others
Liver cirrhosis	A	76	0 (0)	12	15	2	3
	B	173	4 (2.3)	24	32	13	9
	C	129	22 (17.1)	27	33	10	9
Idiopathic portal hypertension	A	69	0 (0)	1	5	4	6
	B	30	0 (0)	1	2	1	5
	C	5	0 (0)	0	2	1	1
Extrahepatic portal obstruction	A	36	0 (0)	0	0	2	2
	B	2	0 (0)	0	0	0	0
	C	0	0 (0)	0	0	0	0
Total		520	26 (5.0)	65	89	33	35

probably caused by extensive devascularization of the lower oesophagus, which lasted for one to three months but disappeared spontaneously within three months in most of the cases. Anastomotic stricture caused by web formation or scar tissue formation was also observed in approximately 10% of patients after EEA stapler transection. This was usually treated successfully by endoscopic dilatation or bouginage.

Minor anastomotic leakages were observed in about 10% of the patients by fluoroscopy which was performed routinely between the 8th and the 10th postoperative day. Minor leakage was usually treated successfully by conservative measures (parenteral nutrition and antibiotics). A major leak was observed in two patients in Child C category which triggered a deterioration in hepatic function and finally resulted in the death of the patients.

Abdominal discomfort after meals and a feeling of gastric fullness were frequently observed in patients after transection and devascularization procedures. Gastric retention of meals was also frequently observed even in patients with pyloroplasty. In most of the patients, the abdominal discomfort and gastric retention spontaneously disappeared after three months.

Minor or major haematemesis was observed in approximately 20% of patients during 10 years of follow-up. Emergency endoscopic examination in these patients revealed that many of the bleedings were from haemorrhagic gastritis; variceal bleeding was rare.

The number and causes of late deaths are listed in Tables 3 and 4. Hepatic failure caused by advanced liver cirrhosis and hepatocellular carcinoma in posthepatitic liver cirrhosis were the most common causes of late death in patients with cirrhosis. Recurrent bleeding either from recurrent varices or gastritis was the cause of death in 33 patients. The overall cumulative survival rate of the patients after transection and devascularization procedures was 66.2% at five years and 45.2% at ten years. Further analysis revealed that cumulative survival rates of the patients differed markedly

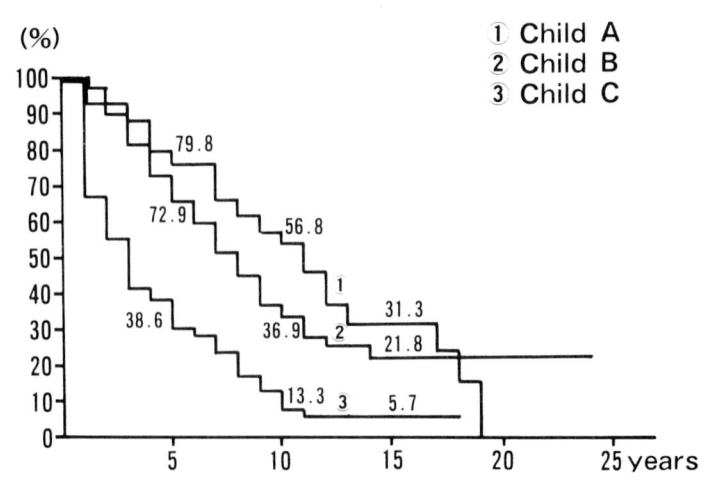

Figure 4. Cumulative survival rate of non-shunting operations (1).

(%)

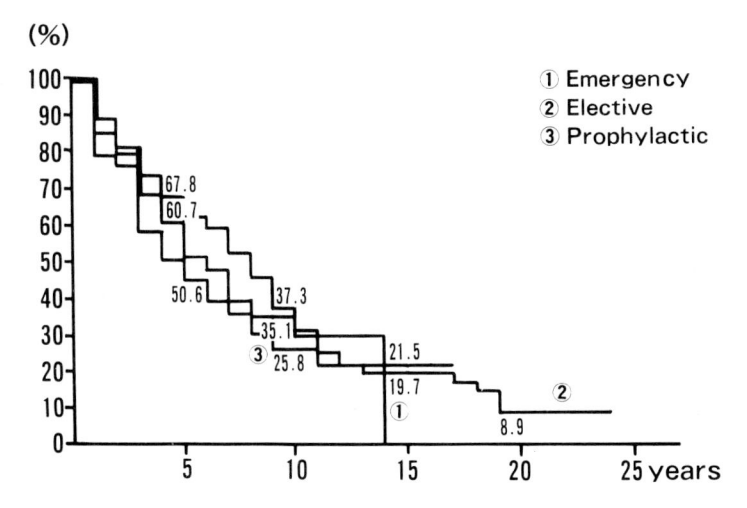

Figure 5. Cumulative survival rate of non-shunting operations (2).

according to the nature of the original disease, and severity of liver damage at the time of operation, but was not affected by the timing of the operation (Figures 4 and 5).

DISCUSSION

The reintroduction and recent development of endoscopic sclerotherapy has greatly changed the management strategy for oesophageal varices. In most institutions in Japan, emergency operations have been completely abandoned, or are seldom performed now, and acute bleeding from oesophageal varices is initially treated by endoscopic sclerotherapy. A nationwide survey performed on the treatment of oesophageal varices in 1990 jointly by the Japanese Research Society for Portal Hypertension and the Japanese Research Society for Sclerotherapy of Esophageal Varices (Idezuki, 1991) revealed that sclerotherapy is currently much more popular than surgery. Emergency operation was considered as the first treatment of choice in surgical institutions in 24% of Child A cases, in 17% of Child B cases but in no Child C cases. In medical institutions operation was not considered at all as the initial treatment for any Child category. This nationwide survey also revealed that the strategy in elective cases greatly differed between surgical and medical institutions; surgical procedures were indicated more frequently in surgical institutions than in medical institutions in patients of Child A and B categories. However, in Child C cases, operation was indicated only in a few surgical institutions.

According to this survey, the mortality rates of oesophageal transection and devascularization procedures and sclerotherapy were respectively 27.8% and 2.6% in emergency cases, and 5.8% and 1.5% in elective cases, indicating that sclerotherapy was superior to operation in terms of the risk of treatment. In contrast, the bleeding rates from varices following transection and devascularization procedures and sclerotherapy were respectively 7.6% and 22.3% in emergency cases, and 11.1% and 15.7% in elective cases. The difference in rebleeding rates in emergency cases may have resulted from the fact that sclerotherapy was undertaken also in Child C cases or emergency cases in which emergency operations were not indicated because of the poor risk.

Although endoscopic sclerotherapy enjoys a greater popularity, recurrence of varices after sclerotherapy is not rare and close follow-up of the patient is mandatory. Multiple sessions of sclerotherapy are often required to prevent recurrence of varices and bleeding and quality of life in these patients is often poor. An operative procedure may still be recommended in a certain group of elective cases, especially in patients under the age of 50 and with a good liver function.

Moreover, the multiplicity of the grades and location of varices, the various types of underlying liver diseases and liver function, and the variety of development patterns of portal collaterals suggest that no single treatment can be ideal for all patients in all clinical circumstances. Surgery should be indicated in those patients who can expect superior results by operation or who do not respond well to sclerotherapy. Our long experiences with transection and devascularization procedures (Idezuki and Sanjo, 1989) suggest that, in selected cases, especially in patients under the age of 60 and without severe deterioration of the liver function in elective situations, transabdominal oesophageal transection using EEA stapler and devascularization are to be recommended.

SUMMARY

Transection and devascularization procedures (Sugiura procedure and transabdominal transection of oesophagus and devascularization) had been the most popular modality of treatment for oesophagogastric varices until the 1970s but the trends of treatment for varices have changed drastically during the last decade. This is partly due to the recent development of endoscopic sclerotherapy and partly due to the patient's increasing demand for less invasive treatment. Recently most patients with oesophagogastric varices are treated initially by endoscopic sclerotherapy and surgical treatment is only called for after sclerotherapy has failed.

REFERENCES

Cooperman M, Fabri PJ, Martin EW et al (1980) EEA esophageal stapling for control of bleeding esophageal varies. *American Journal of Surgery* **140**: 821–824.
Idezuki Y (1991) Current status of treatment for esophageal varices in Japan. A national study. *Japan Medical Journal* **3517**: 23–29.
Idezuki Y & Sanjo K (1989) Twenty-five-year experiences with esophageal transection for esophageal varices. *Journal of Thoracic and Cardiovascular Surgery* **98**: 876–883.

Idezuki Y, Sugiura M, Sakamoto K et al (1967) Rationale for transthoracic esophageal transection for bleeding varices. *Diseases of the Chest* **52**: 621–631.

Idezuki Y, Sanjo K, Bandai Y et al (1990) Current strategy for esophageal varices in Japan. *American Journal of Surgery* **160**: 98–104.

Inokuchi K (1985) Present status of surgical treatment of esophageal varices in Japan: a nationwide survey of 3588 patients. *World Journal of Surgery* **9**: 171–180.

Johnston GW (1977) Treatment of bleeding varices by esophageal transection with SPTU gun. *Annals of the Royal College of Surgeons of England* **59**: 404–408.

Kuzmak LI (1981) Use of EEA stapler in transection of esophagus in severe hemorrhage from esophageal varices. *American Journal of Surgery* **141**: 387–390.

Sugiura M & Futagawa S (1973) A new technique for treating esophageal varices. *Journal of Thoracic and Cardiovascular Surgery* **66**: 667–685.

Sugiura M & Futagawa S (1977) Further evaluation of Sugiura procedure in the treatment of esophageal varices. *Archives of Surgery* **112**: 1317–1321.

Walker RM (1960) Transection operation for portal hypertension. *Thorax* **15**: 218–224.

Wexler MJ (1980) Treatment of bleeding esophageal varices by transabdominal esophageal transection with the EEA stapling instrument. *Surgery* **88**: 406–416.

10
Prophylaxis of first variceal bleeding

GERHARD KLEBER
HASAN ANSARI
TILMAN SAUERBRUCH

In cirrhosis, the most common cause of portal hypertension, portal pressure is increased because the resistance to portal blood outflow inside the liver is elevated. The consequent development of portosystemic collaterals partly compensates for the increased portal pressure by diverting blood away from the portal vascular territory directly to the vena cava. Furthermore, systemic and splanchnic blood flows are increased in cirrhotic patients, tending to maintain portal hypertension despite the presence of portosystemic collaterals (Groszmann et al, 1988). The increased portal pressure and the existence of portosystemic collateral vessels are associated with typical endoscopic alterations such as varices and congestive gastropathy which indicate that the patient is at risk for bleeding.

NATURAL HISTORY AND ENDOSCOPIC FINDINGS

Oesophagogastric varices and congestive gastropathy are frequent findings in cirrhosis. Varices are seen in 50–60% (Calès and Pascal, 1988) and congestive gastropathy in approximately 60–90% (Papazian et al, 1986; D'Amico et al, 1990; Vigneri et al, 1991) of cirrhotic patients. About 30% of patients with oesophageal varices experience variceal bleeding (Calès and Pascal, 1988) and varices have been identified as the bleeding source in 65–80% of patients with liver cirrhosis and upper intestinal haemorrhage (Sauerbruch et al, 1988; Poynard et al, 1991). Even today, mortality following variceal haemorrhage is in the range 40–50% (Sauerbruch et al, 1988; Poynard et al, 1991).

Varices in the gastric fundus are less frequently the source of upper intestinal bleeding in cirrhotic patients. They are observed in approximately 12% of the patients and account for 6–12% of the upper intestinal bleeding episodes (Mathur et al, 1990; Kleber et al, 1991a).

Portal hypertensive gastropathy (congestive gastropathy) corresponds histologically to dilatation of the mucosal precapillaries and small venules as well as submucosal oedema (Hashizume et al, 1983; Pienkowski, 1989). Overt bleeding from gastropathy has been reported in 30–60% of cirrhotic patients and is associated with a mortality of less than 10% (D'Amico et al, 1990).

A further potential source of bleeding is the peptic ulcer. Its prevalence in portal hypertensive patients is increased about five-fold when compared to non-portal hypertensive patients (Rabinovitz et al, 1990). However, the propensity to bleed has not been investigated in patients with portal hypertension. Provided the natural history of peptic ulcers is similar in patients with and without portal hypertension, about 10% of cirrhotic patients with ulcers will eventually experience ulcer bleeding (Pulvertraft, 1968).

BLEEDING RISK SIGNS

Only one-third of all patients with liver cirrhosis and oesophageal varices eventually bleed (Calès and Pascal, 1988). Measures for the prevention of bleeding should be confined to these patients. Therefore, it is of paramount importance to select candidates with a high bleeding risk.

The likelihood of varix rupture depends on the wall tension of the vessels (Groszmann et al, 1988). According to Laplace's law the wall tension of a vessel is directly proportional to the blood pressure in the vessel, the diameter of the vessel and the properties of the wall (e.g. thickness). Accordingly, for a similar intravariceal blood pressure, large varices have a higher wall tension and thus rupture more easily than small varices. Follow-up studies showed that large varices bleed more than twice as often as small varices (Baker et al, 1959; Garcia-Tsao et al, 1985).

Further risk parameters are the so-called red colour signs—cherry-red or haematocystic spots, red weal markings (Japanese Research Society for Portal Hypertension, 1980)—which correspond to dilated blood-filled channels lying within or below the squamous epithelium of the variceal surface and communicating with the submucosal variceal network of the oesophagus (Spence et al, 1983). Patients with a positive red colour sign bleed two to four times more frequently than those without (North Italian Endoscopic Club for the Study and Treatment of Esophageal Varices, 1988; Kleber et al, 1991a).

Recently it has also been reported that patients with concomitant fundic varices and oesophageal varices bleed nearly three times as often from their oesophageal varices as patients without fundic varices (Kleber et al, 1991a).

A possible correlation between the bleeding risk and haemodynamic parameters has been assumed. The variceal blood pressure was slightly higher in patients who had bled than in those without previous bleeding (Rigau et al, 1989). This is in accordance with the finding that the presence of endoscopic risk indicators (variceal size, red colour sign, fundic varices) is associated with a significantly higher variceal pressure than their absence (Fischer et al, 1990; Kleber et al, 1989). Variceal pressure is related to portal pressure (Rigau et al, 1989). The relationship of portal pressure to the incidence of upper intestinal bleeding has been extensively studied. Bleeding episodes were considerably less likely when portal pressure (as assessed by measurement of hepatic venous pressure gradient) was less than

12 mmHg (Garcia-Tsao et al, 1985; Groszmann et al, 1990; Triger et al, 1991). The significance of elevated portal pressure for the development of variceal haemorrhage has recently been confirmed in a study of serial portal pressure measurements in patients with acute variceal haemorrhage (Ready et al, 1991): patients who experienced variceal rebleeding within 72 h of the initial bleeding episode had a significantly higher portal pressure (20 ± 1 mmHg) than patients without rebleeding (16 ± 1 mmHg). Therefore, serial portal pressure measurements during pharmacological treatment to reduce portal pressure may be useful to ensure an adequate pressure decrease (Groszmann et al, 1990).

In portal hypertensive gastropathy the following macroscopic changes have been described: a fine pink speckling also called the 'scarlatina-like' pattern or a 'mosaic-like' pattern (D'Amico et al, 1990). More severe stages are characterized by cherry-red spots on a finely granular mucosa showing confluent areas of diffuse bleeding (D'Amico et al, 1990). In severe portal hypertensive gastropathy, bleeding is much more frequent than in the mild form.

The liver function as assessed by the Child status or development of ascites also influences the probability of bleeding but to a lesser degree (Calès et al, 1990; Kleber et al, 1991a; Poynard et al, 1991). In one study over a period of 21 months, the bleeding risk in Child B/C patients was 1.5 times higher than that in Child A patients (Kleber et al, 1991a).

It is remarkable that in cirrhotic patients with varices, the majority of bleeding episodes occur within the first 12 months after diagnosis of varices. In one study comprising a mean follow-up of 3.3 years, more than two-thirds of all bleeding episodes were observed during the first year (Baker et al, 1959). In other words, patients with a longer history of varices have a lower bleeding risk than patients with newly diagnosed varices.

RATIONALE FOR PROPHYLAXIS OF A FIRST BLEEDING EPISODE AND TREATMENT OPTIONS

A prophylactic regimen should have two major aims: prolongation of survival and improvement of life quality. As outlined above, oesophagogastric varices develop in every other patient with cirrhosis. Given a 30% risk of bleeding from these varices and a 50% mortality associated with bleeding, complete prevention of bleeding theoretically improves life quality (no bleeding) in 15% and prolongs survival in 8% of all patients with cirrhosis. Therefore, in randomized, controlled trials prophylactic treatment regimens have been investigated only in high-risk patients, who present with at least one of the above-mentioned risk indicators. Only recently, another approach has been proposed: early clonidine treatment reduces the degree of portal hypertension and the development of portosystemic shunts in animal models (Lin et al, 1991). This may hinder the development of varices. Prevention of the development of varices may be expected to be more effective than prevention of bleeding from varices.

TREATMENT OPTIONS

There are surgical, endoscopic and pharmacological treatment options for prophylaxis of a first upper intestinal haemorrhage in portal hypertension.

Surgical procedures

There are two surgical principles used for prophylaxis or treatment of upper intestinal bleeding in portal hypertension: one diminishes portosystemic collateral flow by reducing portal pressure (portal decompressive surgery, e.g. portocaval shunt operation), and the other interrupts portosystemic collaterals without affecting portal pressure (portal non-decompressive surgery: oesophageal transection and devascularization operations). The perioperative mortality of these operations is relatively high, reaching 8–10% (Jackson et al, 1968; Conn and Lindenmuth, 1968; Resnick et al, 1969; Conn et al, 1972; Conn, 1990). Furthermore, encephalopathy may be exacerbated by portosystemic surgery.

Endoscopic approach (sclerotherapy)

Oesophageal variceal injection sclerotherapy leads to an intravariceal thrombosis together with inflammation and scarring of the perivenular tissue. The sclerosant and the injection technique vary. This, however, has no major impact on treatment results (Sauerbruch et al, 1991). In contrast to sclerotherapy for acute haemorrhage, prophylactic treatment seldom has an acute effect, since it is impossible to localize the potential bleeding site exactly. Therefore, the bleeding risk is not lowered until most of the varices have been obliterated, which requires on average 2–3 months (six to eight sessions). However, even after multiple sclerotherapy sessions for prophylaxis of rebleeding, about 30% of patients bleed from recurrent varices or varices that have not been sufficiently treated (Sauerbruch et al, 1987). This phenomenon has been observed primarily in patients with decompensated liver function (Sauerbruch et al, 1987). It may be caused by incomplete obliteration of the vascular feeders of the varices. In a recent study (Takase et al, 1990) recurrence of varices was found in 70% of the patients when obliteration was incomplete, but in only 7% after complete obliteration. Furthermore, sclerotherapy has no positive influence on potential extra-oesophageal bleeding sources (gastric varices and congestive gastropathy).

Prophylactic sclerotherapy carries an overall cumulative risk of major complications of 20–40% with a cumulative procedure-related mortality of 1–2% (Sauerbruch et al, 1991). It is obvious that complication rates are lower in the hands of an experienced operator. The main complications are sequelae of sclerotherapy-induced oesophageal ulcers such as bleeding, perforation or pleural effusion. A further relatively frequent complication is oesophageal stenosis. While histamine H_2 antagonists do not seem to reduce the risk of bleeding in otherwise untreated patients with varices (Idéo et al, 1988), omeprazole may play a role in reducing the rate of sclerotherapy-induced ulcers and thus ulcer-related bleeding events during sclerotherapy

(Gimson et al, 1990). Due to the associated complications, repeated sclerotherapy is only justified in those patients who have a high risk of bleeding from oesophageal varices.

β-blockers

Portal pressure is determined by the product of blood outflow resistance of the portal tributary vascular territory and its blood inflow. The outflow resistance of the portal tributary vascular territory is determined both by the intrahepatic vascular resistance to portal blood flow and the portocollateral vascular resistance (resistance to blood flow through portosystemic shunts).

Portal pressure may be lowered pharmacologically by reduction of the increased inflow to the portal venous tributary vascular territory (e.g. β-blockers, nitrates), reduction of the increased intrahepatic vascular resistance (e.g. calcium antagonists, serotonin antagonists), reduction of the portocollateral vascular resistance (e.g. nitrates, serotonin antagonists) or an increase in vascular capacitance of the portal and mesenteric veins (e.g. nitrates). These different pharmacological approaches show variable effects on portal pressure (Reichen and Le, 1986; Cummings et al, 1988; Hadengue et al, 1989; Iwao et al, 1991; Navasa et al, 1989; Vorobioff et al, 1989; Garcia-Pagán et al, 1990; Mastai et al, 1989; Vinel et al, 1990; Alvarez et al, 1991; Desmorat et al, 1991; Yang et al, 1991). Combination of drugs with different modes of action is a new investigational approach and seems to be promising (Hadengue et al, 1989; Roulot et al, 1989; Garcia-Pagán et al, 1990, 1991). Variceal pressure may also be independently influenced by pharmacological elevation of lower oesophageal sphincter tone, e.g. metoclopramide (Kleber et al, 1991b).

Catecholamine plasma concentrations are increased in cirrhotic patients and contribute to the systemic and splanchnic hyperdynamic state seen in cirrhosis (Gaudin et al, 1991). Therefore, the bulk of experimental studies has been performed with β-blockers. By reducing sympathetic nervous activity (e.g. by blockade of adrenergic β-receptors), it should be possible to improve haemodynamics in portal hypertension. Non-cardioselective ($β_1$/$β_2$-antagonists, e.g. propranolol, nadolol) or cardioselective ($β_1$-antagonists, e.g. atenolol) β-blockers have been studied. $β_1$-blockade reduces cardiac output and thereby splanchnic blood flow. $β_2$-blockade probably leads to unopposed α-adrenergic tone in the splanchnic vascular territory and thus to splanchnic arterial vasoconstriction. Reduction of splanchnic blood flow is, therefore, achieved by both mechanisms and leads to a reduction of portal pressure (Groszmann et al, 1990). Non-selective β-blockers are more effective than selective $β_1$-blockers, e.g. atenolol (Mills et al, 1984; Westaby et al, 1984).

β-blockers are not effective in all patients. The reason is that β-blockers produce only a slight reduction in portal pressure (13–26%) in cirrhotic patients (Rector, 1985; Garcia-Tsao et al, 1986; Vorobioff et al, 1987), only rarely lowering portal pressure to values less than 12 mmHg (Groszmann et al, 1990), the critical pressure threshold above which variceal bleeding occurs. According to haemodynamic studies (Garcia-Tsao et al, 1986;

Vorobioff et al, 1987), 30–50% of cirrhotic patients do not show a significant portal pressure reduction (non-responders), because β-blocker-induced portal pressure reduction is paralleled by an increase in portocollateral resistance. The latter is probably increased due to passive reduction of the lumen of the vessels when blood flow is reduced. This increased portocollateral resistance may partly antagonize the portal-pressure-lowering effect of β-blockers. Therefore, combining β-blockers with drugs which lower portosystemic collateral resistance, e.g. nitrates, serotonin antagonists (Hadengue et al, 1989; Garcia-Pagán et al, 1990), is beneficial. There are further explanations for treatment failures. Catecholamine concentrations are primarily elevated in patients with severely impaired liver function (Child C category). Thus, β-blockers should be particularly effective in this patient group. However, the natural history of these patients is probably determined by the impaired liver function rather than by variceal bleeding. Furthermore, catecholamine concentrations are increased in most cirrhotic patients, but the response to catecholamines may be reduced (Moreau et al, 1987; Bernardi et al, 1991; MacGilchrist et al, 1991). Catecholamine concentrations may also increase during propranolol treatment, leading to reduced efficacy of the drug in cirrhotic patients (Bendtsen et al, 1991). In addition, other vasoregulatory systems also contribute to the haemodynamic alterations in cirrhosis (Lebrec et al, 1990) and may compensate for the propranolol-induced haemodynamic effects.

CLINICAL, RANDOMIZED, CONTROLLED TRIALS

Two major end-points have been used in prophylactic trials for the prevention of upper gastrointestinal bleeding in cirrhotic patients with varices: prolongation of survival and reduction of first bleeding events. As mentioned, there are various reasons why prophylactic sclerotherapy or β-blocker treatment may fail. However, an effective bleeding prophylaxis may not necessarily prolong survival, since bleeding may be a terminal event in end-stage liver failure (Child B/C category). Prevention of bleeding would not necessarily change the fatal outcome. On the other hand, most patients in good condition (Child A category) will not succumb to bleeding. In these patients prevention of bleeding would only be justified if it led to an improvement in the quality of life. Thus, the aim of reducing mortality by prophylaxis of haemorrhage is rather ambitious and only achievable when the prophylactic measure has a high level of safety and efficacy. The same holds true for the improvement of life quality. The reduction of bleeding episodes probably only improves life quality if the treatment is safe, effective and minimally invasive.

To date the clinical value of some of the above-described surgical (portal decompressive and non-decompressive operations), endoscopic (sclerotherapy) and pharmacological (β-blockers) treatment options has been studied in randomized controlled trials.

Prophylactic portal decompressive surgery

Nearly 30 years ago, several randomized controlled trials studying the benefit of prophylactic portocaval anastomosis were published (Conn and Lindenmuth, 1968; Jackson et al, 1968; Resnick et al, 1969; Conn et al, 1972). These studies showed that the portocaval shunt operation is a very effective procedure in preventing initial haemorrhage from oesophagogastric varices or hypertensive gastropathy. However, the operation is probably not sufficiently safe to allow a significant reduction in mortality. Also, late hepatic failure may be more frequent after a shunt operation. Last but not least, portocaval anastomosis renders liver transplantation technically more difficult. For these reasons, resurrection of prophylactic shunt surgery appears to be unlikely.

Prophylactic portal non-decompressive surgery

A very recent, multicentre, randomized, controlled trial (Inokuchi and Cooperative Study Group of Portal Hypertension of Japan, 1990) showed the beneficial effect of non-decompressive surgery. Within a median follow-up of 49 months, 22% of the treated patients compared with 49% of the controls died. The cumulative bleeding rate at 5 years was reduced from 46% to 7%. The trial comprised only Child A and B patients with a high variceal bleeding risk (Japanese Research Society for Portal Hypertension, 1980). The devascularization procedures such as oesophageal transection, cardiotomy, gastric transection and Hassaab procedure were heterogeneous and varied from clinic to clinic. In rare instances (10 of 60 patients) selective shunt operation was used in the trial. The significant positive impact of these operations on survival and bleeding is impressive.

In a reflective editorial (Conn, 1990), some points of concern, however, have been raised despite the merits of the study: the low operative mortality of 3% (lower than published in earlier trials of the same investigators); the high mortality in the control group, even though only Child A/B patients were included the low rate of fatal liver failure in the operated group compared to the controls; the constant risk of bleeding in the controls, which normally decreases with time after randomization; and the heterogeneity of operative procedures, making it difficult to define the most appropriate approach. One lesson derived from this study may be that it is more realistic to allow each centre to perform the procedure in which the surgeon has the greatest experience than to attempt to establish a standard approach in all centres.

Prophylactic sclerotherapy

As seen in Table 1 and Figures 1 and 2, there are 13 fully published trials on prophylactic sclerotherapy. The bleeding incidence was significantly reduced in six trials (Figure 1). In five trials there was no beneficial effect and in two studies bleeding occurred more often in the sclerotherapy group.

Table 1. Endoscopic sclerotherapy (ST) in the prophylaxis of first variceal haemorrhage versus control patients (C).

Study	No. of patients ST	No. of patients C	Selection criteria	Child C (%) ST	Child C (%) C	Alcoholics (%) ST	Alcoholics (%) C	Mean follow-up (months)	Bleeding (%) Overall ST	Bleeding (%) Overall C	Bleeding (%) Oesophageal varices ST	Bleeding (%) Oesophageal varices C	Death (%) Overall ST	Death (%) Overall C	Death (%) Variceal bleeding related ST	Death (%) Variceal bleeding related C
Paquet (1982)	32	33	Cirrhosis, large varices, coagulation factors <30	?	?	?	?	24?	6	66	?	?	6	42	All deaths?	All deaths?
Witzel et al (1985)	56	53	Cirrhosis, small and large varices	21	17	80	81	25	?	?	9	57	21	55	4	36
Koch et al (1988)	30	30	Cirrhosis, large varices	3	17	53	73	36	30	33	13	30	37	33	0	20
Wördehoff and Spech (1987)	25	24	Cirrhosis, large varices	16	21	48	42	44	20	63	?	?	56	67	4	33
Santangelo et al (1988)	49	46	Chronic liver disease, large varices	?	?	88	91	13	35	15	?	?	24	24	18	4
Sauerbruch et al (1988)	68	65	Cirrhosis, large varices	18	22	63	69	22	32	43	28	37	35	46	15	17
Piai et al (1988)	71	69	Cirrhosis, large varices	24	32	34	33	13	?	?	14	42	23	38	7	28
Pötzi et al (1989)	45	42	Cirrhosis, large varices	28	33	60	45	up to 48?	?	?	29	34	22	45	12	22
Russo et al (1989)	21	20	Cirrhosis, large varices	14	15	0	0	17	?	?	0	15	0	15	0	10
Kobe et al (1990)	30	33	Large varices Red colour sign (RCS)	27	19	40	39	45	30	72	?	?	46	58	13	43
Andreani et al (1990)	42	41	Cirrhosis	23	24	81	81	?	21	32	14	24	43	44	5	10
Veterans Affairs Cooperative Variceal Sclerotherapy Group (1991)	143	138	Cirrhosis >3 varices	34	26	100	100	22.5†	22	17	?	?	32	17	7	4‡
Triger et al (1991)	33	35	Cirrhosis portal pressure: >12 mmHg	12	17	46	40	61*	70	74	39	40	61	60	18	11

* Median.
† Duration of study—treatment phase.
‡ Upper gastrointestinal bleeding.

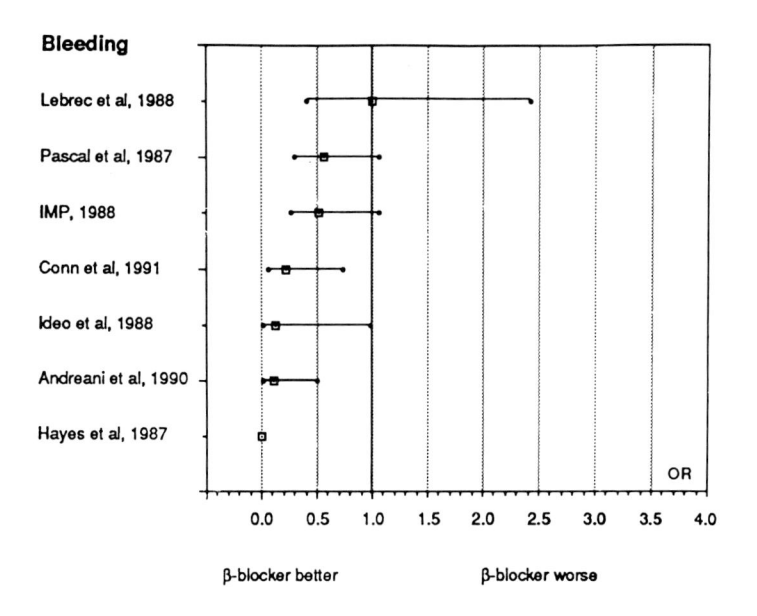

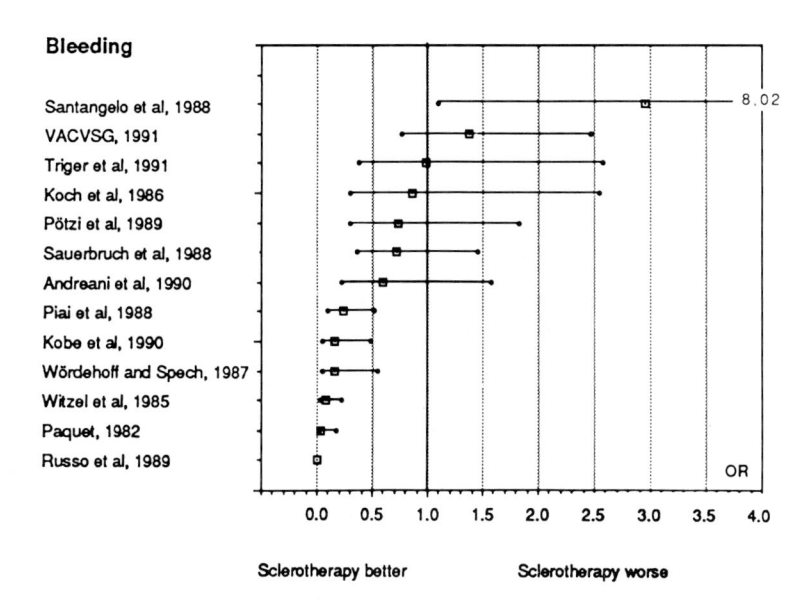

Figure 1. Randomized controlled trials for the prevention of first bleeding. Upper figure: β-blocker versus no treatment. Lower figure: sclerotherapy versus no treatment. Squares represent odds ratios (OR), horizontal bars represent 95% confidence intervals. The odds ratios were calculated as OR = ad/bc, where a and c are the numbers of bleeding patients and b and d the numbers of non-bleeding patients in the treatment and control groups, respectively.

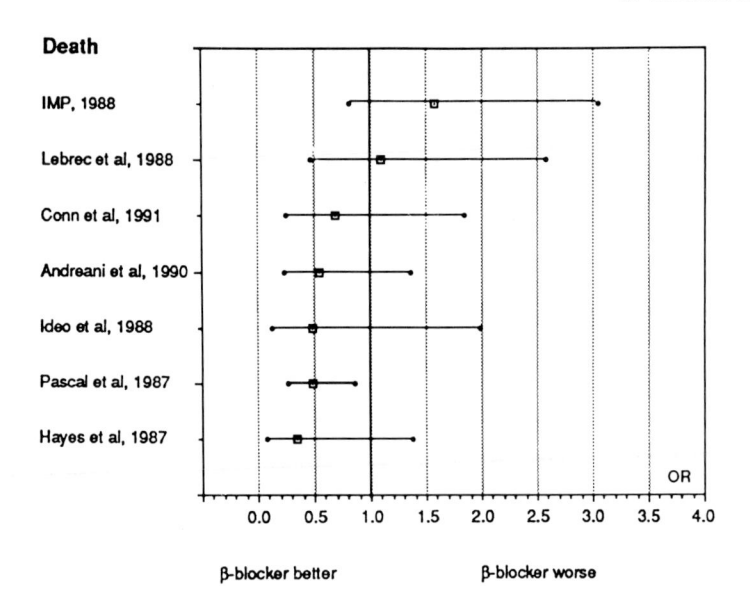

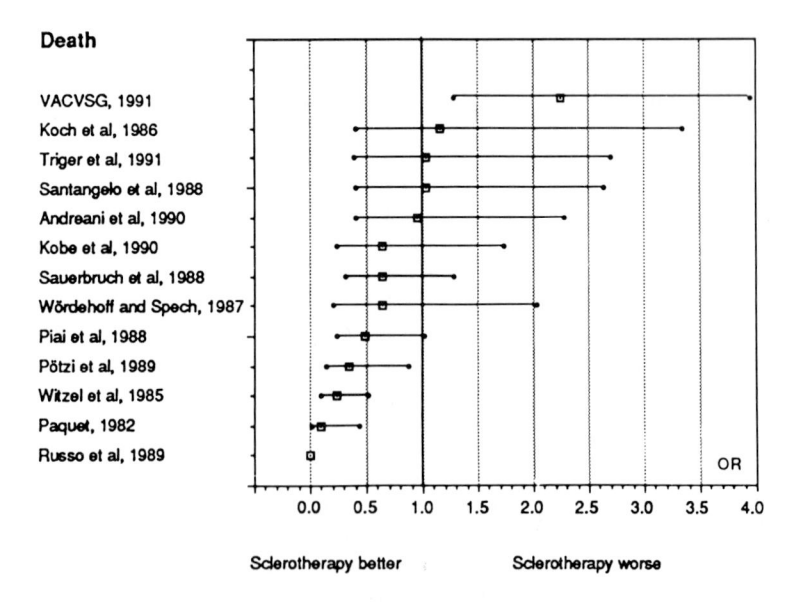

Figure 2. Randomized controlled trials for the prevention of first bleeding (influence on mortality). Upper figure: β-blocker versus no treatment. Lower figure: sclerotherapy versus no treatment. Squares represent odds ratios, horizontal bars represent 95% confidence intervals. The odds ratios were calculated as $OR = ad/bc$, where a and c are the numbers of dying patients and b and d the numbers of surviving patients in the treatment and control groups, respectively.

Both the latter trials were carried out in North America (Santangelo et al, 1988; Veterans Affairs Cooperative Variceal Sclerotherapy Group, 1991). The reduction in the number of bleeding events was associated with an improved survival rate in 4 of the 13 randomized, controlled trials (Figure 2). Four further studies showed a trend towards a lower mortality in the treated patients, especially in those with alcoholic cirrhosis (Sauerbruch et al, 1988; Pötzi et al, 1989; Triger et al, 1991), possibly due to a positive effect on drinking habits. In contrast, the most recent study found an increased mortality in the group randomized to sclerotherapy, although the bleeding incidence was not significantly different from the controls (Veterans Affairs Cooperative Variceal Sclerotherapy Group, 1991). The authors of this study have no conclusive explanation for this increased mortality. They believe that it was due to sclerotherapy. However, complete obliteration of varices was only achieved in 50 out of their 143 patients. Furthermore, there is no clear information about the treatment carried out in the case of acute haemorrhage in this study. Last, but not least, patients receiving sclerotherapy suffered significantly more often from other medical illnesses. On the other hand, the study had one advantage over all previous trials in that the control group received a sham treatment. The compliance to sclerotherapy was presumably lower than in other trials because only male alcoholics had been included. This may be one explanation for the high discontinuation rate. No figures are given concerning compliance in the control group. Sclerotherapy was thus insufficient in more than half of the patients of this trial. This may explain the discrepancies with most other studies.

In summary, analysis of the available controlled trials shows that the results of prophylactic sclerotherapy are heterogeneous (Table 1, Figures 1 and 2). However, there is a trend in favour of sclerotherapy concerning bleeding and survival, especially in patients with alcoholic cirrhosis (Sauerbruch et al, 1988; Pötzi et al, 1989; Triger et al, 1991) and moderately decompensated liver cirrhosis (Child B) (Sauerbruch et al, 1988). In those studies which did not include a sham-treated control group, these results may have been influenced by more intensive care of treated patients. Prophylactic sclerotherapy with its potential complications is probably only justified in patients with high-risk oesophageal varices and moderately decompensated alcoholic cirrhosis who are compliant.

Prophylactic β-blockers

Altogether, 912 cirrhotic patients have been studied in seven randomized, controlled trials so far (Table 2, Figures 1 and 2). They received either propranolol (Hayes et al, 1987; Pascal et al, 1987; Italian Multicenter Project for Propranolol in Prevention of Bleeding, 1988; Andreani et al, 1990; Conn et al, 1991) or nadolol (Idéo et al, 1988; Lebrec et al, 1988) or a control medication which consisted of a true placebo, vitamin K (Italian Multicenter Project for Propranolol in Prevention of Bleeding, 1988) or ranitidine (Idéo et al, 1988). In one study (Andreani et al, 1990) patients

Table 2. β-blocker (BB) in the prophylaxis of first variceal haemorrhage versus control patients (C).

Study	No. of patients BB	No. of patients C	Selection criteria	Child C (%) BB	Child C (%) C	Alcoholics (%) BB	Alcoholics (%) C	Mean follow-up (months)	Bleeding (%) Overall BB	Bleeding (%) Overall C	Bleeding (%) Oesophageal varices BB	Bleeding (%) Oesophageal varices C	Death (%) Overall BB	Death (%) Overall C	Death (%) Variceal bleeding related BB	Death (%) Variceal bleeding related C
Lebrec et al (1988)	53*	53	Cirrhosis, varix >4 mm bilirubin <100	—‡	—‡	74	74	16	24	25	11	15	28	26	8	15
Idéo et al (1988)	30*	49	Cirrhosis, large varices	27	22	47	55	18	3	22	3	16	10	18	0	8
Italian Multicenter Project for Propranolol in Prevention of Bleeding (1988)	85†	89	Cirrhosis, large varices	7	6	36	34	22	19	30	13	16	35	25	9	10
Pascal et al (1987)	118†	112	Cirrhosis, large varices	(8.7)	(8.4)§	91	88	14	17	27	?‖	?‖	21	36	9	16
Hayes et al (1987)	47†	48	?	(6.3)	(6.7)‡§	43	44	12¶	0	6	0	4	6	17	0	4
Conn et al (1991)	51†	51	Cirrhosis	10	6	76	80	16	8	28	4	22	16	22	4	6
Andreani et al (1990)	43†	41	Cirrhosis	31	24	77	81	?	5	32	5	24	30	44	2	10

* Nadolol.
† Propranolol.
‡ Only Child A and B.
§ Mean Pugh value.
‖ 29 of 50 patients with bleeding had an endoscopy at this time. 27 of 29 patients had variceal bleeding.
¶ Duration of the study.

were also randomized to a third group which received endoscopic sclerotherapy of the varices. The original data of four of the trials (Pascal et al, 1987; Idéo et al, 1988; Italian Multicenter Project for Propranolol in Prevention of Bleeding, 1988; Lebrec et al, 1988) were re-analysed (Poynard et al, 1991). Only two trials were double blind (Hayes et al, 1987; Conn et al, 1991); the other trials were single blind (Pascal et al, 1987; Idéo et al, 1988; Italian Multicenter Project for Propranolol in Prevention of Bleeding, 1988; Lebrec et al, 1988) or non-blind (Andreani et al, 1990). Thus, observer influence cannot be completely ruled out.

The dosage of the β-blockers used in the studies ranged from 40 to 160 mg for nadolol and from 40 to 320 mg for propranolol. In most of the studies the dose was titrated until a 25% reduction of the heart rate was achieved. In one trial (Conn et al, 1991) the dose of propranolol was titrated in each individual patient until the hepatic venous pressure gradient was reduced by 25% or to at least 12 mmHg or until the heart rate was reduced to at least 55 beats/min. This was achieved with doses comparable to those used in the other studies.

General exclusion criteria for β-blocker prophylaxis were hepatocellular carcinoma, anticipated non-compliance and severe non-hepatic diseases. The size of the varices and liver function were the main selection criteria and varied between the studies (Table 2). In one study only patients with a hepatic venous pressure gradient above 12 mmHg, the pressure threshold separating variceal bleeders from non-bleeders (Garcia-Tsao et al, 1985), were included.

Forty to seventy per cent of patients with varices and no previous bleeding were eligible and randomized to the studies. Treatment and control groups were comparable at the time of inclusion. The percentage of patients lost to follow-up was less than 10% in all trials and compliance was at least 80% in patients who had no drug-related side-effects. Cardiovascular (heart failure, conduction defects, bradycardia), pulmonary (asthma), neurological (hepatic encephalopathy, depression), haematological (thrombocytopenia) and gastrointestinal (diarrhoea) side-effects were reported in the trials. Side-effects which necessitated discontinuation of treatment occurred in 3–4% of patients treated with nadolol and in 11–14% of patients treated with propranolol. The lower incidence of side-effects in the nadolol trials was attributed to the fact that this drug is not metabolized in the liver, is not lipid soluble and does not reduce renal blood flow. Only two trials documented the side-effects in the control groups (Lebrec et al, 1988; Coun et al, 1991). From these trials it may be concluded that specific (treatment-related) side-effects occurred in only 5% of the patients treated with propranolol.

All trials were analysed on an intention-to-treat basis. The bleeding incidence in the control groups ranged from 6% to 39% during follow-up and was significantly higher in all seven trials than the bleeding incidence in the treated patients, which ranged from 0% to 16% (Table 2). Propranolol and nadolol were equally effective with respect to the reduction of the bleeding incidence. β-blocker treatment also reduced the incidence of bleeding from portal hypertensive gastropathy. Although the results of subgroup analysis are inconclusive, according to the available data the clinical efficacy of β-blockers and the haemodynamic response induced appear to be independent of liver function. Although alcohol consumption in treated and control patients was similar, the positive effect of β-blockers on the bleeding rate was more pronounced in alcoholics than in non-alcoholics.

β-blocker treatment reduced the total bleeding incidence and also the rate of fatal haemorrhages which accounted for about 50% of all bleeding events and between 4% and 29% of the observed deaths. Accordingly, a tendency towards increased survival was found in patients treated with β-blockers in all studies. In summary, 123 of the 443 control patients and 94 of the 427 patients receiving β-blockers died during follow-up. The overall difference, however, is not significant. Survival was significantly improved in only one of the seven trials (Pascal et al, 1987). The failure of β-blocker treatment to prolong life expectancy may be due to the rather low total incidence of fatal bleeding events in the studies or a rather high incidence of other causes of death.

β-blockers or sclerotherapy?

In one recent trial (Andreani et al, 1990) patients were randomized to three groups, receiving placebo, sclerotherapy or propranolol. β-blocker treatment was superior to sclerotherapy or placebo but did not increase survival (Tables 1 and 2).

SUMMARY

Surgical, endoscopic and pharmacological treatment options are available for prophylaxis of first upper intestinal haemorrhage in cirrhotic patients. Randomized controlled trials have revealed that a prophylactic portocaval shunt operation should not be performed because its beneficial effect on the bleeding rate is outweighed by a slightly increased mortality. Prophylactic portal non-decompressive surgery (mainly gastro-oesophageal vascular disconnection) has been shown to reduce the bleeding rate and mortality in Japanese cirrhotic patients. However, further trials in different populations must confirm this positive effect. β-blockers have fewer side-effects and are probably more effective for prophylaxis of the first bleed than sclerotherapy, but survival is only marginally influenced. Nadolol is preferable to propranolol. The effect of sclerotherapy is in part related to the technical experience of the physician. Although sclerotherapy has only minor effects on the bleeding rate, it is associated with a trend towards a prolonged survival. This may be caused by non-specific effects. On the basis of the published trials, only preliminary recommendations can be given. Prophylactic treatment may be useful in cirrhotic patients who are at high risk of bleeding. Life quality may be improved with continuous β-blocker treatment. Some studies suggest that alcoholics with large varices may also profit from regular prophylactic sclerotherapy performed by experienced physicians.

Acknowledgement

The expert secretarial help of M. Bäurer is gratefully acknowledged.

REFERENCES

Alvarez D, Mastai R, Lennie A et al (1991) Noninvasive measurement of portal venous blood flow in patients with cirrhosis: effects of physiological and pharmacological stimuli. *Digestive Diseases and Sciences* **36:** 82–86.

Andreani T, Poupon RE, Balkau BJ et al (1990) Preventive therapy propranolol of first gastrointestinal bleeding in patients with cirrhosis: results of a controlled trial comparing propranolol, endoscopic sclerotherapy and placebo. *Hepatology* **12:** 1413–1419.

Baker LA, Smith C & Liebermann G (1959) The natural history of esophageal varices. *American Journal of Medicine* **26:** 228–237.

Bendtsen F, Christensen NJ, Sorensen TIA & Henriksen JH (1991) Effect of oral propranolol administration on azygos, renal and hepatic uptake and output of catecholamines in cirrhosis. *Hepatology* **14:** 237–243.

Bernardi M, Rubboli A, Trevisani F et al (1991) Reduced cardiovascular responsiveness to exercise-induced sympathoadrenergic stimulation in patients with cirrhosis. *Journal of Hepatology* **12:** 207–216.

Calès P & Pascal JP (1988) Histoire naturelle des varices oesophagiennes au cours de la cirrhose (de la naissance à la rupture). *Gastroenterologie Clinique et Biologique* **12:** 245–254.

Calès P, Desmorat H, Vinel JP et al (1990) Incidence of large varices in patients with cirrhosis: application to prophylaxis of first bleeding. *Gut* **31:** 1298–1302.

Conn HO (1990) Why is prophylactic portal nondecompressive surgery effective in preventing hemorrhage from esophageal varices? *Hepatology* **12:** 166–169.

Conn HO & Lindenmuth WW (1968) Prophylactic portacaval anastomosis in cirrhotic patients with esophageal varices. Interim results, with suggestions for subsequent investigations. *New England Journal of Medicine* **279:** 725–732.

Conn HO, Lindenmuth WW, May CJ & Ramsby GR (1972) Prophylactic portal anastomosis. A tale of two studies. *Medicine* **51:** 27–40.

Conn HO, Grace ND, Bosch J et al (1991) Propranolol in the prevention of the first hemorrhage from esophagogastric varices: a multicenter, randomized clinical trial. *Hepatology* **13:** 902–912.

Cummings SA, Kaumann AJ & Groszmann RJ (1988) Comparison of the hemodynamic responses to ketanserin and prazosin in portal hypertensive rats. *Hepatology* **8:** 1112–1115.

Dagradi AE (1972) The natural history of esophageal varices in patients with alcoholic liver cirrhosis. An endoscopic and clinical study. *American Journal of Gastroenterology* **57:** 520–540.

D'Amico G, Montalbano L, Traina M et al (1990) Natural history of congestive gastropathy in cirrhosis. *Gastroenterology* **99:** 1558–1564.

Desmorat H, Vinel JP, Lahlou O et al (1991) Systemic and splanchnic hemodynamic effects of molsidomine in rats with carbon tetrachloride-induced cirrhosis. *Hepatology* **13:** 1181–1184.

Fischer G, Kleber G, Geigenberger G & Sauerbruch T (1990) Fundusvarizen und Wandektasien deuten bei Patienten mit portaler Hypertension auf einen hohen transmuralen Varizendruck. *Zeitschrift für Gastroenterologie* **24:** 475 (abstract).

Garcia-Pagán JC, Navasa M, Bosch J et al (1990) Enhancement of portal pressure reduction by the association of isosorbide-5-mononitrate to propranolol administration in patients with cirrhosis. *Hepatology* **11:** 230–238.

Garcia-Pagán JC, Feu F, Bosch J et al (1991) Propranolol compared with propranolol plus isosorbide-5-mononitrate for portal hypertension in cirrhosis. *Annals of Internal Medicine* **114:** 869–873.

Garcia-Tsao G, Groszmann RJ, Fisher RL et al (1985) Portal pressure, presence of gastroesophageal varices and variceal bleeding. *Hepatology* **5:** 419–424.

Garcia-Tsao G, Grade ND, Groszmann RJ et al (1986) Short-term effects of propranolol on portal venous pressure. *Hepatology* **6:** 101–106.

Gaudin C, Braillon A, Poo JL et al (1991) Plasma catecholamines in patients with presinusoidal portal hypertension: comparison with cirrhotic patients and nonportal hypertensive subjects. *Hepatology* **13:** 913–916.

Gimson A, Polson R, Westaby D & Williams R (1990) Omeprazole in the management of intractable esophageal ulceration following injection sclerotherapy. *Gastroenterology* **99:** 1829–1831.

Groszmann RJ, Blei AT & Atterbury CE (1988) Portal hypertension. In Arias IM, Jakoby WB, Popper H, Schachter D & Shafritz DA (eds) *The Liver: Biology and Pathobiology*, pp 1147–1159. New York: Raven Press.

Groszmann RJ, Bosch J, Grace ND et al (1990) Hemodynamic events in a prospective randomized trial of propranolol versus placebo in the prevention of a first variceal hemorrhage. *Gastroenterology* **99:** 1401–1407.

Hadengue A, Moreau R, Cerini R et al (1989) Combination of ketanserin and verapamil or propranolol in patients with alcoholic cirrhosis: search for an additive effect. *Hepatology* **9:** 83–87.

Hashizume M, Tanaka K & Inokuchi K (1983) Morphology of gastric microcirculation in cirrhosis. *Hepatology* **3:** 1008–1012.

Hayes PC, Crichton S, Shepherd AN & Bouchier IAD (1987) Propranolol in chronic liver disease: a controlled trial of its effect and safety over twelve months. *Quarterly Journal of Medicine* **65:** 823–834.

Idéo G, Bellati G, Fesce E & Grimoldi D (1988) Nadolol can prevent the first gastrointestinal bleeding in cirrhotics: a prospective, randomized study. *Hepatology* **8:** 6–9.

Inokuchi K & Cooperative Study Group of Portal Hypertension of Japan (1990) Improved survival after prophylactic portal nondecompression surgery for esophageal varices: a randomized clinical trial. *Hepatology* **12:** 1–6.

Italian Multicenter Project for Propranolol in Prevention of Bleeding (1988) Propranolol for prophylaxis of bleeding in cirrhotic patients with large varices: a multicenter, randomized clinical trial. *Hepatology* **8:** 1–5.

Iwao T, Toyonaga A, Sumino M et al (1991) Hemodynamic study during transdermal application of nitroglycerin tape in patients with cirrhosis. *Hepatology* **13:** 124–128.

Jackson FC, Perrin EB, Smith AG et al (1968) A clinical investigation of the portacaval shunt. II. Survival analysis of the prophylactic operation. *American Journal of Surgery* **115:** 22–42.

Japanese Research Society for Portal Hypertension (1980) The general rules for recording endoscopic findings on esophageal varices. *Japanese Journal of Surgery* **10:** 84–87.

Kleber G, Sauerbruch T, Fischer G & Paumgartner G (1989) Pressure of intraoesophageal varices assessed by fine needle puncture: its relation to endoscopic signs and severity of liver disease in patients with cirrhosis. *Gut* **30:** 228–232.

Kleber G, Sauerbruch T, Ansari H & Paumgartner G (1991a) Prediction of variceal hemorrhage in cirrhosis: a prospective follow-up study. *Gastroenterology* **100:** 1332–1337.

Kleber G, Sauerbruch T, Fischer G et al (1991b) Reduction of transmural oesophageal variceal pressure by metoclopramide. *Journal of Hepatology* **12:** 362–366.

Kobe E, Zipprich B, Schentke KU & Nilius R (1990) Prophylactic endoscopic sclerotherapy of esophageal varices—a prospective randomized trial. *Endoscopy* **22:** 245–248.

Koch H, Henning H, Grimm H & Soehendra N (1986) Prophylactic sclerosing of esophageal varices—results of a prospective controlled study. *Endoscopy* **18:** 40–43.

Lebrec D, Poynard T, Capron JP et al (1988) Nadolol for prophylaxis of gastrointestinal bleeding in patients with cirrhosis. A randomized trial. *Journal of Hepatology* **7:** 118–125.

Lebrec D, Braillon A, Abergel A et al (1990) Effect of pithing on hyperdynamic circulation of portal hypertensive rats. *FASEB Journal* **4:** A1191 (abstract).

Lin HC, Saubrane O & Lebrec D (1991) Prevention of portal hypertension and portosystemic shunts by early chronic administration of clonidine in conscious portal vein-stenosed rats. *Hepatology* **14:** 325–330.

MacGilchrist AJ, Sumner D & Reid JL (1991) Impaired pressor reactivity in cirrhosis: evidence for a peripheral vascular defect. *Hepatology* **13:** 689–694.

Mastai R, Rocheleau B & Huet PM (1989) Serotonin blockade in conscious, unrestrained cirrhotic dogs with portal hypertension. *Hepatology* **9:** 265–268.

Mathur SK, Dalvi AN, Someshwar V et al (1990) Endoscopic and radiological appraisal of gastric varices. *British Journal of Surgery* **77:** 432–435.

Mills PR, Rae AP, Farah DA et al (1984) Comparison of three adrenoreceptor blocking agents in patients with cirrhosis and portal hypertension. *Gut* **25:** 73–78.
Moreau R, Lee SS, Hadengue A et al (1987) Hemodynamic effects of a clonidine-induced decrease in sympathetic tone in patients with cirrhosis. *Hepatology* **7:** 149–154.
Navasa M, Chesta J, Bosch J & Rodés J (1989) Reduction of portal pressure by isosorbide-5-mononitrate in patients with cirrhosis. Effects on splanchnic and systemic hemodynamics and liver function. *Gastroenterology* **96:** 1110–1118.
North Italian Endoscopic Club for the Study and Treatment of Esophageal Varices (1988) Prediction of the first variceal hemorrhage in patients with cirrhosis of the liver and esophageal varices. *The New England Journal of Medicine* **319:** 933.
Papazian A, Braillon A, Dupas JL et al (1986) Portal hypertensive gastric mucosa: an endoscopic study. *Gut* **27:** 1199–1203.
Paquet KJ (1982) Prophylactic endoscopic sclerosing treatment of the esophageal wall in varices—a prospective controlled randomized trial. *Endoscopy* **14:** 4–5.
Pascal JP, Calès P & Multicenter Study Group (1987) Propranolol in the prevention of first upper gastrointestinal tract hemorrhage in patients with cirrhosis of the liver and esophageal varices. *New England Journal of Medicine* **317:** 856–861.
Piai G, Cipolletta L, Claar M et al (1988) Prophylactic sclerotherapy of high-risk esophageal varices: results of a multicentric prospective controlled trial. *Hepatology* **8:** 1495–1500.
Pienkowski P (1989) Étüde fonctionelle, chez l'homme, de la gastropathie congestive au cours de la cirrhose par la mesure de la différence de potentiel. *Gastroentérologie Clinique et Biologique* **13:** 763–788.
Pötzi R, Bauer P, Reichel W et al (1989) Prophylactic endoscopic sclerotherapy of oesophageal varices in liver cirrhosis. A multicentre prospective controlled randomised trial in Vienna. *Gut* **30:** 873–879.
Poynard T, Calès P, Pasta L et al (1991) Beta-adrenergic-antagonist drugs in the prevention of gastrointestinal bleeding in patients with cirrhosis and esophageal varices. An analysis of data and prognostic factors in 589 patients from four randomized clinical trials. *New England Journal of Medicine* **324:** 1532–1538.
Pulvertraft C (1968) Comments on the incidence and natural history of gastric and duodenal ulcer. *Postgraduate Medical Journal* **44:** 597–602.
Rabinovitz M, Schade RR, Dindzans V et al (1990) Prevalence of duodenal ulcer in cirrhotic males referred for liver transplantation: does the etiology of cirrhosis make a difference? *Digestive Diseases and Sciences* **35:** 321–326.
Ready JB, Robertson AD, Goff JS & Rector WG Jr (1991) Assessment of the risk of bleeding from esophageal varices by continuous monitoring of portal pressure. *Gastroenterology* **100:** 1403–1410.
Rector WG (1985) Propranolol for portal hypertension. *Archives of Internal Medicine* **145:** 648–650.
Reichen J & Le M (1986) Verapamil favorably influences hepatic microvascular exchange and function in rats with cirrhosis of the liver. *Journal of Clinical Investigation* **78:** 448–455.
Resnick RH, Chalmers TC, Ishihara AM et al (1969) A controlled study of the prophylactic portacaval shunt. A final report. *Annals of Internal Medicine* **70:** 675–688.
Rigau J, Bosch J, Bordas JM et al (1989) Endoscopic measurement of variceal pressure in cirrhosis: correlation with portal pressure and variceal haemorrhage. *Gastroenterology* **96:** 873–880.
Roulot D, Gaudin C, Braillon A et al (1989) Hemodynamic effects of a combination of clonidine and propranolol in conscious cirrhotic rats. *Canadian Journal of Physiology and Pharmacology* **67:** 1369–1372.
Russo A, Giannone G, Magnano A et al (1989) Prophylactic sclerotherapy in nonalcoholic liver cirrhosis: preliminary results of a prospective controlled randomized trial. *World Journal of Surgery* **13:** 149–153.
Santangelo CW, Dueno MI, Estes BL & Krejs GJ (1988) Prophylactic sclerotherapy of large esophageal varices. *New England Journal of Medicine* **318:** 814–818.
Sauerbruch T, Weinzierl M, Ansari H & Paumgartner G (1987) Injection sclerotherapy of oesophageal variceal haemorrhage. A prospective long-term follow-up study. *Endoscopy* **19:** 181–184.
Sauerbruch T, Wotzka R, Köpcke W et al (1988) Prophylactic sclerotherapy before the first

episode of variceal hemorrhage in patients with cirrhosis. *New England Journal of Medicine* **319:** 8–15.

Sauerbruch T, Fischer G & Ansari H (1991) Variceal injection sclerotherapy. *Baillière's Clinical Gastroenterology* **5:** 131–153.

Spence RAJ, Sloan JM, Johnston GW & Greenfield A (1983) Oesophageal mucosal changes in patients with varices. *Gut* **24:** 1024–1029.

Takase Y, Shibuya S, Chikamori F et al (1990) Recurrence factors studied by percutaneous transhepatic portography before and after endoscopic sclerotherapy for esophageal varices. *Hepatology* **11:** 348–352.

Triger DR, Smart HL, Hosking SW & Johnson AG (1991) Prophylactic sclerotherapy for esophageal varices: long-term results of a single-center trial. *Hepatology* **13:** 117–123.

Veterans Affairs Cooperative Variceal Sclerotherapy Group (1991) Prophylactic sclerotherapy for esophageal varices in men with alcoholic liver disease. A randomized, single-blind, multicenter clinical trial. *New England Journal of Medicine* **324:** 1779–1784.

Vigneri S, Termini R, Piraino A et al (1991) The stomach in liver cirrhosis. Endoscopic, morphological, and clinical correlations. *Gastroenterology* **101:** 472–478.

Vinel J-P, Monnin J-L, Combis J-M, Calès P, Desmorat H & Pascal J-P (1990) Hemodynamic evaluation of molsidomine: A vasodilator with antianginal properties in patients with alcoholic cirrhosis. *Hepatology* **11:** 239–242.

Vorobioff J, Picabea E, Villavicencio R et al (1987) Acute and chronic hemodynamic effects of propranolol in unselected cirrhotic patients. *Hepatology* **7:** 648–653.

Vorobioff J, Garcia-Tsao G, Groszmann R et al (1989) Long-term hemodynamic effects of ketanserin, a 5-hydroxytryptamine blocker, in portal hypertensive patients. *Hepatology* **9:** 88–91.

Westaby D, Bihari DJ, Gimson AES et al (1984) Selective and non-selective beta receptor blockade in the reduction of portal pressure in patients with cirrhosis and portal hypertension. *Gut* **25:** 121–124.

Witzel L, Wolbergs E & Merkl H (1985) Prophylactic endoscopic sclerotherapy of oesophageal varices. A prospective controlled study. *Lancet* **i:** 773–775.

Wördehoff D & Spech HJ (1987) Prophylaktische Ösophagusvarizensklerosierung. Ergebnisse einer prospektiven, randomisierten Langzeitstudie über 7 Jahre. *Deutsche Medizinische Wochenschrift* **112:** 947–951.

Yang SS, Ralls PW & Korula J (1991) The effect of oral nitroglycerin on portal blood velocity as measured by ultrasonic doppler. A double blind, placebo controlled study. *Journal of Clinical Gastroenterology* **13:** 173–177.

# 11

Pathophysiology and treatment of ascites and the hepatorenal syndrome

PAOLO GENTILINI
GIACOMO LAFFI

The term 'ascites' is used to describe the accumulation of free fluid inside the abdominal cavity. This condition was first described as early as the fifth century BC by Hippocrates, who used the word 'askites', which means 'fluid-filled bag'. Ascites may be related to disease processes that do not directly involve peritoneum, such as portal hypertension or hypoalbuminaemia, or to diseases in which peritoneum itself is involved (Table 1). Cirrhosis, malignant diseases, heart failure and tuberculosis account for 90% or more of patients with ascites. In this chapter we are mainly concerned with ascites complicating cirrhosis.

NATURAL HISTORY OF SODIUM AND WATER RETENTION IN CIRRHOSIS

Cirrhosis is usually associated with several abnormalities of renal function, which become more severe as the disease progresses. The most frequent of these alterations is an impairment in renal handling of sodium. In the pre-ascitic stage of the disease, patients may have a reduced ability to excrete an acute sodium load (Naccarato et al, 1981). Patients who develop ascites always have progressive sodium retention. The degree of this abnormality, however, varies considerably from one patient to another and, in the same patient, during the course of the disease. Therefore, some patients have a relatively high excretion of sodium, and the onset of ascites in these cases may be triggered by a high-sodium diet, or the administration of saline, mineralocorticoids or sodium-containing drugs, while a reduction of sodium intake may lead to the disappearance of ascites. Other patients show avid sodium retention and rapidly accumulate ascites and, subsequently, undergo spontaneous diuresis. The formation of ascites and peripheral oedema in cirrhosis is related to an imbalance in sodium metabolism, rather than to a disturbance in water handling, so that patients with decompensated cirrhosis can excrete urine at low osmolality when

Table 1. Causes of ascites.

Portal hypertension

Severe alcoholic hepatitis
Fulminant viral hepatitis
Liver cirrhosis
Chronic active hepatitis
Liver neoplasms:
   Primary (hepatoma, cholangiocarcinoma)
   Secondary
Circulatory changes:
   Prehepatic—portal vein obstruction
   Intrahepatic—veno-occlusive disease
   Posthepatic—right-side heart failure, constrictive pericarditis, tricuspid
      valve insufficiency, inferior vena cava obstruction, Budd–Chiari syndrome

Severe blood dyscrasia (hypoalbuminaemia)

Nephrotic syndrome
Protein-losing enteropathy
Malnutrition

Peritoneal diseases

During infection or infestation:
   Non-specific bacteria
   Tuberculosis
   Candidiasis
   Filariasis
Primary or secondary neoplasms
Granulomatous diseases:
   Crohn's disease
   Sarcoidosis
Vasculitis:
   Systemic lupus erythematosus
   Schonlein–Henoch syndrome

Miscellaneous

Trauma
Hypothyroidism (myxoedema)
Ovarian disease:
   Stromal tumours
   Meigs syndrome
Pancreatic diseases:
   Neoplasms
   Acute or chronic pancreatitis: pancreatic ascites
   Pseudocysts
Bile ascites
Chylous ascites:
   Infection or infestation
   Neoplasms, lymphomas, leukaemia
   Congenital dysplasia of the lymphatic system
Haemodialysis or peritoneal dialysis

given a water load. On the other hand, when a sodium load is administered to these patients, it is retained, favouring further accumulation of ascites (Epstein, 1988).

The second alteration of renal function is the reduced capacity for water excretion, leading to water retention and hyponatraemia. This disturbance usually occurs in patients with more advanced disease, who invariably have ascites. However, there are cirrhotic patients with ascites in whom free water clearance continues to be normal during the entire course of the disease, and there are others who develop an absolute failure to eliminate the water load, so that dilutional hyponatraemia becomes a major clinical problem. Hyponatraemia is especially frequent in patients who have a free water clearance during an oral water load, equal to or less than 1 ml/min (Arroyo et al, 1988).

The hepatorenal syndrome (HRS), also called functional renal failure (FRF) of cirrhosis, is the final and most severe disturbance of renal function in patients with cirrhosis. HRS is a syndrome characterized by a marked reduction in renal blood flow (RBF) and glomerular filtration rate (GFR), a progressive increase in blood urea nitrogen (BUN) and serum creatinine concentration, azotaemia and oliguria in the setting of advanced cirrhosis, with a marked reduction of liver function and ascites, often refractory to medical treatment (Epstein, 1988b; Gentilini and Laffi, 1989). Patients with HRS usually have a very low urinary sodium concentration (<10 mmol/l) and normal urine sediment (Table 2). Light and electron microscopic studies have revealed only modest or negligible pathological changes in the kidney, indicating the functional nature of this disorder. This is further confirmed by the observations that the kidneys from cirrhotic patients with HRS completely recover their function when transplanted to another subject or when the cirrhotic patients undergo liver transplantation (Epstein, 1988b). The immediate cause of HRS is an active vasoconstriction of the renal arteries, leading to a decrease in renal perfusion and GFR. In these patients,

Table 2. Renal dysfunction in cirrhosis.

Renal functional impairment (subclinical HRS)	Hepatorenal syndrome (acute renal failure of unexplained origin)
Clinical findings	
Plasma creatinine <1.5 mg/dl	Plasma creatinine >1.5 mg/dl
Significant reduction of RBF and GFR	Azotaemia
Sodium retention often present	Oliguria
	No signs of tubular dysfunction
	Urinary Na <10 mmol/l;
	U/Posm >1;
	U/P creat >30
	No improvement after volume expansion
Intrarenal haemodynamic alterations	
* arterial vasoconstriction	* arterial vasoconstriction
* cortical hypoperfusion	* cortical hypoperfusion
* arterio-venous shunts	* arterio-venous shunts

U/P, urinary versus plasma; osm, osmolality; creat, creatinine.

selective renal arteriography and kidney scan show that arterial vasoconstriction is associated with a marked vasomotor instability, redistribution of blood flow from the cortex to the medulla and the presence of intrarenal arteriovenous shunts (Epstein, 1988b). Despite extensive studies, the relationship between sodium retention and the altered renal haemodynamics in cirrhosis with ascites is still incompletely defined. In the earlier stages of the disease, the two phenomena can run a separate course even if there is some reciprocal dependence. Thus, sodium retention usually occurs in the setting of a normal, or higher than normal, GFR. On the other hand, some degree of renal impairment may be observed even in patients without sodium retention and ascites. In fact, a reduction of RBF and GFR, as indicated by low para-aminohippurate and inulin clearances, was observed in some patients with both compensated cirrhosis and chronic hepatitis, in the absence of clinical signs of renal failure, i.e. an increase in BUN and plasma creatinine concentration (Gentilini et al, 1980). As the disease progresses, the association between these two phenomena becomes more frequent, so that patients with advanced disease and untreatable ascites usually have a marked reduction of renal function, often with clinically evident HRS.

In addition to the above alterations of renal function, patients with cirrhosis and ascites usually have several changes in splanchnic and systemic haemodynamics, vasoactive and neurohormonal factors, all of which usually

Table 3. Clinical and functional parameters during progressive phases of liver cirrhosis.

	Early cirrhosis	Compensated cirrhosis	Decompensated cirrhosis	Terminal cirrhosis
Portal pressure	=+	+	++	+++
Splanchnic blood flow	=+	+	++	+++
Peripheral resistance	=	−	−−	−−−
Cardiac output	=+	+	++	++
Total plasma volume	=	+	+	=+
Effective arterial plasma volume	=	−	−−	−−−
Mean arterial pressure	=	=	−	−−
Urinary sodium excretion	=	=	−−	−−−
Free water clearance	=	=	=−	−−
GFR	=−	−	−−	−−−
RBF	=−	−	−−	−−−
Ascites			+	++
Renal arteriovenous shunts	=+	+	++	++
Catecholamines	=	=	+	++
RAA system	=	=	++	+++
Antidiuretic hormone	=	=	=+	++
Atrial natriuretic peptide	=	=	+	++
Natriuretic hormone		=	+	+
Renal prostaglandins	=	=+	++	−−
Kinin–kallikrein system	=	=	+	−−

= normal values.
+ increased values.
− decreased values.

become progressively severe as the disease progresses (Table 3) (Gentilini and Laffi, 1989).

PATHOGENESIS OF SODIUM AND WATER RETENTION IN CIRRHOSIS

Pathogenic mechanisms involved in sodium and water retention in cirrhotic patients have been debated for many years and different theories have been proposed.

Before the theory of **peripheral vasodilatation** was conceived, two other hypotheses were formulated to explain the abnormal sodium and water retention in cirrhotic patients. The first was the *underfilling theory*. According to this, the primary element in sodium and water retention is the formation of ascites. Increased transcapillary hydrostatic pressure in the hepatic and splanchnic microcirculation leads to abnormal lymph formation in the liver. When lymphatic drainage is not sufficient to remove all fluid formed, it accumulates in the peritoneal cavity as ascites. Consequently, there is a decrease in plasma volume and arterial pressure and the stimulation of high-pressure baroreceptors of the carotid sinus and aortic arch. This in turn activates efferent mechanisms such as the renin angiotensin aldosterone (RAA) system, sympathetic nervous system (SNS) and release of vasopressin (ADH), which are responsible for sodium and water retention. This latter would not be sufficient to restore plasma volume because, due to the presence of increased hydrostatic forces at the sinusoidal level, the retained fluid translocates in the abdominal cavity as ascites (Schrier et al, 1988; Witte et al, 1971).

The underfilling theory, however, does not explain why plasma volume expansion by head-out water immersion to the neck, a manoeuvre that redistributes blood volume causing central hypervolaemia, is not able to elicit a natriuretic response in all patients (Epstein, 1988a). Moreover, total plasma volume is usually increased in cirrhotic patients accumulating ascites (Lieberman et al, 1970). On the other hand, in dogs with nitrosamine-induced cirrhosis, renal retention of sodium precedes the accumulation of ascites (Levy, 1988).

These observations led Lieberman and Reynolds to propose the *overflow theory* (Lieberman et al, 1970). According to this theory, the primary element in the formation of ascites is an early, volume-independent retention of sodium. The precise mechanism(s) of this primary abnormality, although not clearly outlined by these authors, was ascribed to a defective hepatic synthesis of an unknown natriuretic factor or to a decreased hepatic inactivation of an antidiuretic factor (Levy, 1988).

This theory, however, implies that at the onset of ascites, there is an inhibition of vasoactive and sodium-retaining systems, which, on the contrary, are usually stimulated in these patients (Schrier et al, 1988; Gentilini and Laffi, 1989). Moreover, plasma volume expansion by head-out water immersion is able to normalize renal sodium handling in a large group of patients, a finding not compatible with the overflow theory (Epstein et al, 1988a).

According to the most recent theory of *peripheral arterial vasodilatation* (Schrier et al, 1988), the initiating event in sodium retention and the formation of ascites is a peripheral arterial vasodilatation, which leads to intravascular underfilling, not because the intravascular blood volume is decreased, but because the intravascular compartment is enlarged. In compensated cirrhosis, the initial peripheral arterial vasodilatation, and thus the consequent underfilling, causes a transient sodium and water retention (probably due to baroreceptor-mediated transient activation of the RAA system and SNS). A new equilibrium is thus reached, in which the increased vascular capacity is compensated by an increase in circulating plasma volume and cardiac output. Subsequently, the increased plasma volume, related to the transient sodium retention, is no longer sufficient to maintain circulatory homeostasis, due to a further increase in peripheral arterial vasodilatation and to the extravasation of fluid from the sinusoidal and splanchnic capillaries into the peritoneal cavity. The arterial baroreceptors, sensing the vascular underfilling, activate the RAA system and SNS, and in turn sodium retention is promoted. The fluid retained by the kidney, however, is no longer effective in restoring the effective arterial blood volume (EABV), since it is now sequestered in the peritoneal cavity as ascites. The activation of the main vasoconstrictor systems contributes to counteract peripheral vasodilatation and thus maintains arterial pressure. According to this theory, HRS is the extreme manifestation of intravascular underfilling. In fact, patients with HRS have a greater reduction of arterial pressure than those with ascites and unimpaired renal function, together with very high levels of plasma renin activity (PRA), plasma noradrenaline and ADH (Schrier et al, 1988).

MECHANISMS INVOLVED IN SODIUM AND WATER RETENTION AND IN THE PATHOGENESIS OF THE HEPATORENAL SYNDROME

The mechanisms involved in sodium and water retention and the pathogenesis of HRS in liver diseases are considered in Figure 1 and can be listed as follows:

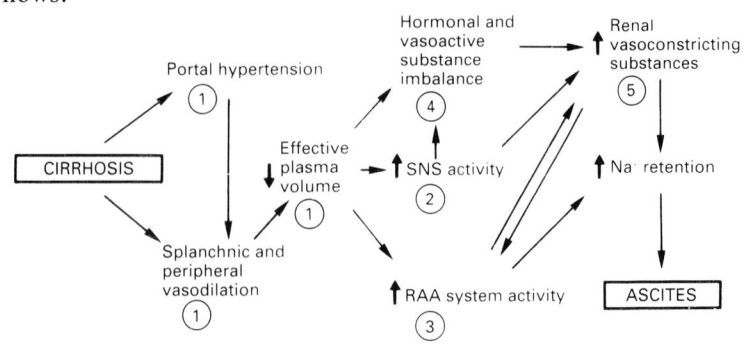

Figure 1. Principal mechanisms involved in the pathogenesis of ascites in liver cirrhosis. From Gentilini et al (1991).

1. Portal hypertension.
2. Activation of sympathetic nervous system.
3. Activation of the renin angiotensin aldosterone system.
4. Antidiuretic hormone.
5. Natriuretic factors.
6. Endotoxins.
7. Imbalance of intrarenal vasoactive substances.

Portal hypertension

Any liver disease that ultimately causes a block to intrahepatic flow eventually provokes an increased pressure in the corresponding venous district, i.e. the portal vein and its branches. Portal hypertension is the *sine qua non* for the formation of ascites.

There is a large body of evidence from clinical and experimental studies that the liver is the main site for ascites formation. Flux of fluid across the hepatic sinusoid (which is highly permeable to albumin) is determined solely by changes in the hydrostatic pressure. The increased sinusoidal pressure causes transudation of plasma into the space of Disse and then to lymphatic vessels (Levy, 1988). As soon as the production of hepatic lymph exceeds the drainage capacity, lymph produced by the liver passes into the peritoneal cavity with the subsequent formation of ascites. The splanchnic capillaries, on the other hand, have mechanisms of autoregulation and respond to an increase in portal pressure with modifications in pre-capillary and post-capillary sphincter tone so that only 60% of the increase in portal pressure is transmitted to the capillaries. The capillaries in the splanchnic area are barely permeable to proteins and the increased hydrostatic pressure is rapidly compensated by an increase in intracapillary oncotic pressure which opposes excessive filtration (Levy, 1988).

In the subsequent stages of the disease, there are numerous alterations in the hepatic and splanchnic microcirculation, such as the capillarization of the sinusoids, that is, the appearance inside the liver of unfenestrated capillaries with basal membranes which are impermeable to albumin. This leads to the establishment of an effective gradient of oncotic pressure. In such an advanced stage of the disease, gastrointestinal capillaries are also altered, with a partial loss of their ability to autoregulate hydrostatic pressure and flow, as demonstrated by the constant presence of an increased splanchnic inflow (Levy, 1988).

In decompensated cirrhosis, in fact, resistance in the splanchnic area is greatly reduced and splanchnic blood flow is increased, as indicated by the finding that hepatic blood flow is normal or near normal despite the development of a wide system of portosystemic collaterals which divert up to 80% of portal flow outside the liver (Schrier et al, 1988).

Activation of the sympathetic nervous system

Cirrhotic patients with ascites usually have an activation of the SNS, as indicated by an increase in plasma noradrenaline levels, which has been shown to be due to an increased release and not to an impaired degradation, since noradrenaline clearance is not significantly altered in cirrhosis (Zambraski and DiBona, 1988). In cirrhotic patients with ascites and high plasma noradrenaline levels, intravenous clonidine administration causes a reduction of arterial pressure, together with an inhibition of sympathetic activity, indicating that the activation of the SNS in cirrhosis is part of the homeostatic mechanism aimed at maintaining arterial pressure (Willett et al, 1986).

The activation of the SNS also takes place within the kidney, as evidenced by an increased noradrenaline concentration in the renal vein, with a positive venous-arterial gradient, which is usually negative in healthy subjects (Zambraski and DiBona, 1988). The activation of the SNS in cirrhosis is thought to play a major role in sodium and water retention and the decrease in renal function in these patients. In fact, a significant negative correlation between plasma noradrenaline concentration and urinary sodium excretion, GFR, RBF and free water clearance, is usually observed in this setting (Zambraski and DiBona, 1988).

However, the importance of SNS activation in impairing renal function is contradicted by some evidence. The infusion of alpha-blockers, such as phentolamine, directly into the renal artery did not produce any increase in RBF (Zambraski and DiBona, 1988). This negative result, however, might be secondary to the transitory systemic hypotension, induced by phentolamine, which could have resulted in a reduction in renal perfusion. Moreover, cirrhotic patients with ascites, submitted to head-out water immersion, usually show a significant increase in creatinine clearance, diuresis and natriuresis, not always accompanied by a reduction of circulating noradrenaline levels (Zambraski and DiBona, 1988). Nevertheless, it cannot be excluded that in the terminal stages of cirrhosis, the persistent and intense activation of the SNS, together with other vasoconstrictive factors, could determine an irreversible vasoconstriction (Gentilini and Laffi, 1989).

Activation of the renin angiotensin aldosterone system

Several studies have established that the RAA system is activated in cirrhotic patients with ascites and avid sodium retention. Activation of the RAA system, as measured by PRA, is more marked in patients with ascites and HRS, whereas patients without ascites have normal values of PRA (Epstein and Norsk, 1988). Even if a diminished hepatic extraction of renin may contribute to the elevated PRA in liver disease, the major determinant of the high PRA is an augmented renal release of renin. Different explanations have been proposed for the activation of the RAA system in cirrhosis. Renal hypoperfusion, which can follow activation of the SNS, may represent the primary event. Another cause can be the decreased EABV, as suggested by experiments with head-out water immersion (Epstein and Norsk, 1988).

Several lines of evidence indicate that aldosterone plays a major role in the pathogenesis of sodium retention in cirrhosis (Arroyo et al, 1988). A significant, inverse correlation between plasma aldosterone concentration

(PAC) and urinary sodium excretion has been shown in cirrhotics (Wilkinson et al, 1979). The existence of patients with avid sodium retention and normal PAC has been explained by the existence of an increased tubular sensitivity to aldosterone, since spironolactone, an aldosterone antagonist, is able to reverse sodium retention in these patients (Wilkinson et al, 1979; Arroyo et al, 1988). According to some authors, aldosterone plays only a permissive role, the major component of the abnormal sodium retention being a reduced distal delivery of filtrate (Epstein, 1988a). However, activation of the RAA system is a determinant in maintaining arterial pressure in cirrhotic patients. Administration of saralasin, an angiotension II (AII) antagonist, or ACE-inhibitors, significantly reduced arterial pressure in cirrhotic patients with ascites (Schroeder et al, 1976; Pariente et al, 1985). The integrity of the RAA system is also a determinant for the maintenance of GFR in cirrhotic patients with ascites; in fact, administration of low-dose captopril (12.5 mg) to patients with cirrhosis and ascites caused a reduction in GFR and sodium excretion without affecting arterial pressure to any appreciable extent (Gentilini et al, 1991b).

Antidiuretic hormone (ADH)

Plasma levels of ADH are usually elevated in cirrhotic patients with ascites who exhibit a reduced capacity to excrete a water load (Arroyo et al, 1988). Administration of demeclocycline, which interferes with the tubular action of ADH, increases urinary flow with a concomitant decrease in urinary osmolality in decompensated cirrhotic patients (Arroyo et al, 1988). Administration of a specific antagonist of the hydro-osmotic effect of ADH normalizes the impaired water excretion in an experimental model of cirrhosis (Claria et al, 1989). The increased ADH activity in patients with liver disease seems to be related to an increased non-osmotic release of ADH. In fact, the administration of a water load was not able to suppress ADH in a group of patients with an evident reduction of EABV and low plasma osmolality (Bichet et al, 1982). Plasma volume expansion, obtained by the insertion of the LeVeen shunt, led to the normalization of circulating ADH levels (Reznick et al, 1983). Finally, the administration of a specific antagonist of the vascular effects of ADH to rats with experimental cirrhosis, ascites and ADH hypersecretion induced a marked reduction in arterial pressure, suggesting that ADH hypersecretion contributes to the maintenance of arterial pressure in cirrhosis (Claria et al, 1991).

Natriuretic factors

Atrial natriuretic peptide (ANP)

At least two hormones with natriuretic activity have been identified: ANP and the natriuretic hormone (NH) (Ballermann et al, 1991). Recently, other peptides similar to ANP have also been described, such as the brain natriuretic peptide (BNP) (Sudoh et al, 1988).

Atrial natriuretic peptide is a cardiac hormone with several biological activities including natriuresis, diuresis, inhibition of renin and aldosterone secretion, and vasodilatation (Ballermann et al, 1991). Available evidence indicates that cirrhotics with ascites usually have higher plasma ANP levels than healthy subjects (Gines et al, 1988a; Laffi et al, 1989). The increase in plasma levels of ANP seems to be due to its greater production by the myocardium and not to a reduced hepatic inactivation (Gines et al, 1988a). Cirrhotic patients with ascites retain sodium despite high plasma levels of ANP, suggesting that these patients are resistant to the renal effects of this natriuretic hormone. This argument is strengthened by studies in which pharmacological doses of ANP were infused to cirrhotic patients (Laffi et al, 1989). Studies on ANP levels during head-out water immersion contributed to the clarification of causes of the renal resistance. In fact, in these studies, despite the rise in ANP level following immersion, a rather heterogeneous diuretic and natriuretic response was observed. The rise in ANP level in these studies was accompanied by a comparable increase in urine cyclic guanosine monophosphate (cGMP) excretion, indicating intact agonist-receptor interaction and guanylate cyclase activation. Patients who exhibited a barely discernible or absent natriuretic response showed a clear reduction of EABV, as indicated by the higher PRA and PAC. The natriuretic and diuretic capacity of the hormone may be overwhelmed by the striking activation of vasoconstrictor and sodium-retaining systems such as the RAA systems, SNS and ADH (Skorecki et al, 1988).

Natriuretic hormone (NH)

This is a still unknown substance, presumably produced in the hypothalamus. NH has a marked natriuretic activity, which occurs in the absence of any change in RBF and GFR and is probably related to its ability to inhibit Na-K-ATPase present on the basolateral membrane of the renal tubular cells. Unlike ANP, NH is a vasoconstrictor and may cause a rise in arterial pressure. These actions are comparable to those of drugs with digitalis-like action, and led to the suggestion that NH is the endogenous agonist of receptors for digitalis and to its description as the 'endogenous digitalis-like substance' (De Wardener and Clarkson, 1985). The activity of NH is usually assessed by measuring the main biological activities associated with the presence of this hormone in plasma or urinary extracts. All these activities have recently been found to be increased in urinary extracts from cirrhotic patients with ascites (Figure 2), providing indirect evidence of NH hypersecretion in cirrhosis (La Villa et al, 1990). The more recent identification by Hamlyn et al (1991) of NH with ouabain, if confirmed, will allow direct measurements of this hormone in physiological and pathological conditions, including cirrhosis of the liver.

Brain natriuretic peptide (BNP)

First isolated in the brain of pigs (Sudoh et al, 1988), BNP is a 32 amino acid peptide analogous to ANP, but different in amino acid composition. It is secreted by the hearts of mammals and induces an increase in cGMP

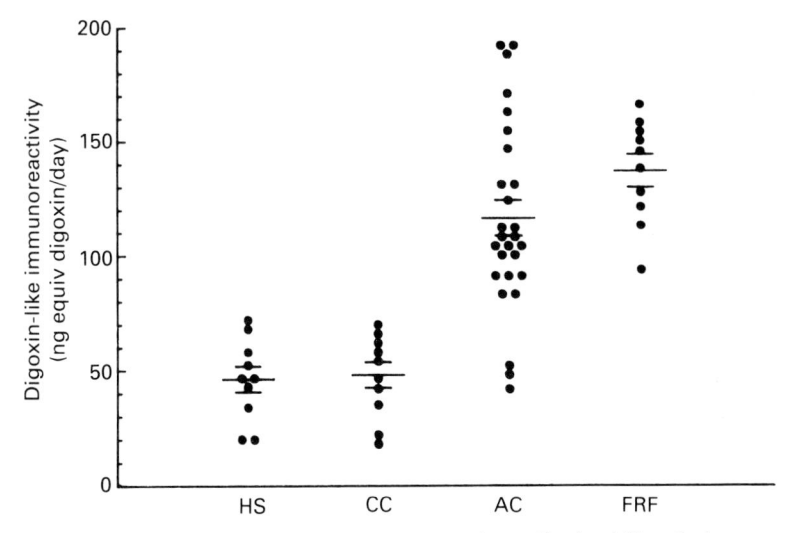

Figure 2. Individual values of natriuretic hormone as estimated by the ability of urinary extracts to cross-react with anti-digoxin antibodies, in healthy subjects (HS), and in patients with compensated cirrhosis (CC), ascitic cirrhosis (AC), and functional renal failure (FRF). AC and FRF patients had significantly higher levels of natriuretic hormone than HS and CC ($p<0.01$). From La Villa G. et al (1990) Natriuretic hormone activity in the urine of cirrhotic patients. *Hepatology* 12: 467–475.

concentration and an increase in natriuresis, together with vasodilatation and inhibition of renin and aldosterone secretion. Recent data obtained in our laboratory suggest that plasma BNP levels are increased in cirrhotic patients with ascites, with and without FRF (La Villa et al, 1992).

From all these data it is evident that water and sodium retention in cirrhosis is not due to a deficit of endogenous natriuretic factors in general, but rather to an increase in these hormones. The mechanisms responsible for the increased ANP, BNP and NH production in these patients are still unknown; possibly the increased synthesis of these factors may compensate for the activation of the RAA system and the SNS, which have a powerful sodium retaining activity. An alternative hypothesis is that the increased release of natriuretic factors is a consequence of the systemic haemodynamic alterations found in liver cirrhosis, consisting of an increase in circulating plasma blood volume, cardiac output and venous return, in the presence of a marked reduction in total peripheral resistances and EABV (Schrier et al, 1988). The simultaneous presence of arterial hypovolaemia, sensed by high pressure baroreceptors in the aortic arc and carotid sinus, and central venous hypervolaemia sensed by low-pressure receptors in the atria and intrathoracic large veins, could explain the paradoxical situation of activation of both natriuretic and sodium-retaining factors.

Endotoxins

Lipopolysaccharides contained in the wall of Gram-negative bacteria normally present in the human gut are generally found in low quantities in intestinal venous blood and are taken up and completely inactivated by Kupffer cells. In liver cirrhosis, when there is a proliferation of intestinal saprophytes, a diminished phagocytic capacity of hepatic mesenchymal cells and extensive portosystemic collaterals, endotoxins can be found in the systemic circulation (Bourgoignie and Valle, 1988). Recent studies using a chromogenic assay, which has improved sensitivity and allows quantitation, have confirmed the presence of high endotoxin levels in most patients with alcoholic cirrhosis (Triger, 1991). Their presence has been thought to be linked to the renal damage often found in cirrhosis, on the basis that experimental investigations in animals have demonstrated that endogenous administration of endotoxins causes renal vasoconstriction, as well as fibrin deposition inside periglomerular and peritubular capillaries (Bourgoignie and Valle, 1988).

Wang et al (1988) showed that endotoxins also induce the release of significant amounts of platelet-activating factor (PAF, 1-O-alkyl-2-acetyl-sn-glyceryl-3-phosphorylcholine) by rat glomerular mesangial cells. Intravenous infusion of PAF to animals decreases peripheral vascular resistance, mean blood pressure, RBF, GFR, urinary flow rate and urinary sodium excretion (Snyder, 1990). Plasma levels of PAF are elevated in patients with compensated cirrhosis, and even higher in those with ascites (Caramelo et al, 1987). Administration of BN-52021, a PAF receptor antagonist, to cirrhotic rats, has been shown to correct deranged systemic haemodynamics which characterize this disease (Villamediana et al, 1986).

Imbalance in intrarenal vasoactive substances

A large body of data provides compelling evidence that the *renal prostaglandin system* has an important role in regulating renal haemodynamics in cirrhotic patients. Several studies (Laffi et al, 1986; Zipser and Lifschitz, 1988) clearly showed that in patients with cirrhosis, ascites and maintained renal haemodynamics, urinary excretion of vasodilating prostaglandins PGE_2 and 6-keto-$PGF_{1\alpha}$, the non-enzymatic metabolite of prostaglandin PGI_2, are increased, together with Thromboxane TxB_2, the non-enzymatic metabolite of vasoconstrictor TxA_2, suggesting an overall activation of the system (Figure 3). This event may be due to the reduction of EABV, which activates vasoconstricting factors such as AII and noradrenaline, which are potent activators of renal prostaglandin synthesis. The increased renal synthesis of vasodilator prostaglandins is thought to contribute to the maintenance of RBF and GFR, despite the activation of vasoconstricting and sodium-retaining systems (Laffi et al, 1986). This contention is strongly supported by studies with non-steroidal anti-inflammatory drugs (NSAIDs), which reduce prostaglandin synthesis by inhibiting cyclo-oxygenase activity. In fact, while NSAIDs have no effect upon renal function in healthy subjects, they dramatically reduce RBF, GFR and sodium excretion in cirrhotic patients with ascites (Boyer et al, 1979). NSAID-induced renal failure in cirrhosis can be prevented by the infusion of PGA_1 (Boyer et al, 1979). The determinant role of vasodilating prostaglandins in the maintenance of renal haemodynamics in cirrhotic patients with ascites is further confirmed by the observation that HRS is associated with a marked reduction of the excretion of these compounds (Figure 3), suggesting an exhaustion of the renal prostaglandin system (Laffi et al, 1986; Zipser and Lifschitz, 1988). In this latter condition, the renal production of vasoconstrictor TxA_2 seems to be less affected, as indicated by studies showing that in patients with HRS, urinary excretion of TxB_2 is higher than in normal subjects, or similar to normal subjects, while the urinary excretion of PGE_2

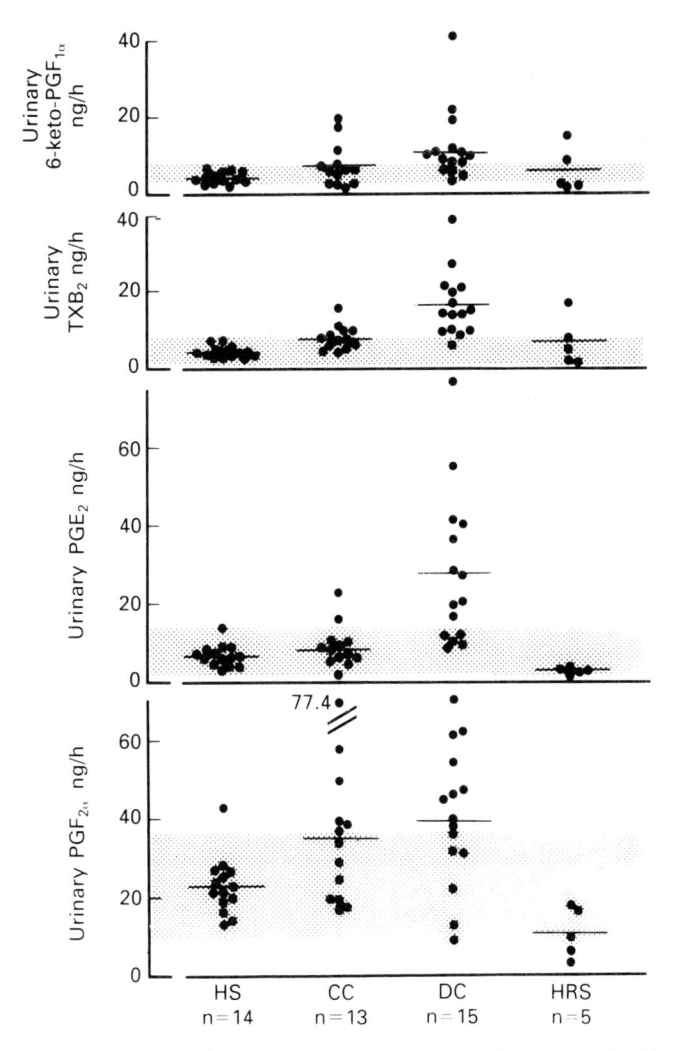

Figure 3. Urinary 6-keto-$PGF_{1\alpha}$, TxB_2, PGE_2, and $PGF_{2\alpha}$ excretion rates in healthy subjects (HS) as compared with patients with compensated cirrhosis (CC), decompensated cirrhosis (DC), or hepatorenal syndrome (HRS). Stippled areas indicate the normal range (mean ± 2SD). From Laffi et al (1986).

is markedly reduced. The pattern of excretion of urinary 6-keto-PGF$_{1\alpha}$ in these patients is very variable (Zipser and Lifschitz, 1988). These data suggest that an imbalance between vasodilator and vasoconstrictor metabolites of arachidonic acid and the relative prevalence of the latter compounds, together with other endogenous vasoconstrictors, such as AII, noradrenaline and ADH, can contribute to the pathogenesis of the irreversible vasoconstriction which characterizes the HRS (Laffi et al, 1986; Zipser and Lifschitz, 1988).

The renal prostaglandin system correlates with other renal systems such as the *kallikrein–kinin* and RAA system, as well as the SNS (Zipser and Lifschitz, 1988). Low circulating values of pre-kallikrein and bradykinin have been observed in patients with alcoholic cirrhosis and are thought to be responsible for the decreased availability of kinins (Wong et al, 1977). However, direct measurement of urinary kallikrein, which may be considered an expression of intrarenal kinin activity, has produced some conflicting results, with values sometimes raised (Perez-Ayuso et al, 1984), sometimes normal (Gentilini et al, 1983), and sometimes lower than normal (Zipser et al, 1981). In general, it seems that urinary kallikrein excretion is reduced in more advanced stages, with the lowest values during HRS (Perez-Ayuso et al, 1984).

Leukotrienes (LTC4, LTD4, and LTE4) are potent vasoconstrictors and may play a role in renal disorders (Zipser and Lifschitz, 1988). Urinary excretion of LTE4 is markedly increased in cirrhotic patients with HRS as compared to normal controls, suggesting that LTE4 may participate in the pathogenesis of this syndrome (Moore et al, 1990).

TREATMENT OF ASCITES

General considerations

Ascites due to chronic liver disease does not, except in extreme cases, require immediate therapeutic manoeuvres, but should be considered an important complication of liver cirrhosis, since it worsens prognosis (Gines et al, 1987b). Ascites, by raising intra-abdominal pressure, favours gastro-oesophageal reflux, which may precipitate variceal bleeding; it may predispose to pulmonary atelectasis and pneumonia by elevation of the diaphragm and induce anorexia by compressing the upper gastrointestinal tract. The increased intra-abdominal pressure facilitates the development of umbilical, inguinal and hiatal hernias. The presence of ascites also provokes oedema of splanchnic tissues, thus reducing the filter effect physiologically exerted by the lymphatic system and mesothelial walls on intestinal bacteria. In about 10% of cases, ascites is complicated by spontaneous bacterial peritonitis (SBP), with abdominal pain, increase in wall tension, intermittent or remittent fever, frequent neutrophil leukocytosis and bacteraemia (Conn and Atterbury, 1987). Finally, HRS only develops in patients with ascites. All these considerations justify treatment aimed at relieving ascites.

Side-effects of diuretic therapy

In cirrhotic patients with ascites, effective diuretic therapy should lead to a loss of body weight between 300 and 900 g/day, given the limited possibility of fluid reabsorption from the peritoneal cavity, which does not exceed 900 ml/day (Shear et al, 1970).

While it is relatively easy to monitor diuretic therapy in the hospital, it is much more difficult when the patient has been discharged, so certain parameters must be repeatedly checked:

1. Serum and urinary electrolytes.
2. Haematocrit.
3. BUN, serum creatinine and creatinine clearance.

BUN and serum creatinine do not accurately reflect renal function, which can be better assessed by measuring creatinine clearance and calculating the creatinine index (daily creatinine excretion/body weight) (Papadakis and Arieff, 1987). In fact, serum creatinine is also affected by reduced production due to the loss of muscular mass.

One of the most important and frequent complications of diuretic therapy is *prerenal azotaemia*, observed in 20–55% of patients, who show an increase in BUN and serum creatinine (Gines et al, 1989). This complication seems to be a direct consequence of the rapid decrease in plasma volume which follows aggressive diuretic therapy; it is less frequent in patients who also have peripheral oedema, as fluid from the interstitial space is reabsorbed more easily than ascites, protecting the patients from volume contraction (Pockros and Reynolds, 1986). Reduction of plasma volume leads to a decrease of renal perfusion, GFR and oliguria. Due to very high sodium and water reabsorption which takes place mainly in the proximal tubule, urine is hyperconcentrated and virtually free of sodium. Prerenal azotaemia usually improves after diuretic withdrawal and the administration of plasma expanders, in contrast to HRS, which is unaffected by plasma expansion (Galambos, 1979).

Another complication of aggressive diuretic therapy is *dilutional hyponatraemia*, which is related to the inability of the kidney to excrete free water, because loop diuretics, blocking the reabsorption of chloride and sodium in the thick ascending limb of the loop of Henle, impair the mechanism of dilution (Frommer et al, 1986). Diuretics also lead to a reduction of plasma volume, with further non-osmotic stimulation of ADH hypersecretion; at the same time, proximal sodium reabsorption markedly increases, decreasing sodium delivery to the diluting segment of the nephron (Frommer et al, 1986). In these conditions, diuretics should be withdrawn and patients should be given albumin or other plasma expanders (Gentilini and Laffi, 1989; McCormick et al, 1990).

Patients receiving aldosterone antagonists may develop *hyperkalaemia* and *metabolic acidosis*, due to the inhibition of aldosterone-mediated potassium and hydrogen secretion in the collecting duct (Frommer et al, 1986). Addition of frusemide to aldosterone antagonists protects against hyperkalaemia and metabolic acidosis (Arroyo et al, 1989). *Gynaecomastia* is another long-term side-effect of antialdosterone antagonists, especially spironolactone, while it is less frequent in patients given potassium canrenoate (Gentilini, 1991). In contrast, loop diuretics frequently induce *hypokalaemia* and *metabolic alkalosis* (Frommer et al, 1986). In these cases, sodium not reabsorbed in the loop of Henle is exchanged with hydrogen ions in the distal tubule with consequent loss of positive charges. At the same time, there is an increase in plasma bicarbonate concentration, due to hypovolaemia. Hypovolaemia also stimulates the RAA system, so that the large quantities of aldosterone increases sodium/potassium exchange in the distal tubules leading to alkalosis.

Another complication of diuretic therapy is the onset of *portosystemic encephalopathy*. In these patients, loop diuretics and thiazides provoke excessive loss of potassium with subsequent hypokalaemic alkalosis. This is responsible for an increased production of ammonia in the kidney, with increased ammonia transport to the central nervous system (Gines et al, 1989).

Renal prostaglandins are involved in the renal response to diuretics, as demonstrated by the reduction of the diuretic and natriuretic effects of frusemide following the administration of NSAIDs (Daskalopoulos et al, 1985). These latter drugs must therefore be avoided in cirrhotic patients with ascites.

Sequential treatment of sodium and water retention

In well-conducted sequential therapy, serious side-effects are uncommon (Gentilini et al, 1986b). In contrast, aggressive diuretic therapy trying to obtain the disappearance of ascites in a short time could be very harmful.

In patients with tense ascites, especially if there is respiratory distress or other consequences of increased abdominal pressure, therapeutic paracentesis must be performed, with infusion of human albumin or other plasma expanders (Gines et al, 1987a). This procedure also allows analysis of the ascitic fluid, for a correct diagnosis.

When the diagnosis has already been made and ascites is not tense, it is possible to start a *sequential diuretic therapy*. This is a stepwise therapy aimed at obtaining a satisfactory result with the lowest doses of diuretics; in the absence of adequate therapeutic response, patients are progressively moved from one step to the next. The response to diuretic treatment is assessed by monitoring body weight, whereas measurement of urinary sodium excretion allows evaluation of sodium balance and the compliance of the patients to the diet. The various stages of sequential therapy can be easily standardized as follows (Figure 4).

Bed rest and low sodium diet

Bed rest, by increasing central volume, reduces the activity of the RAA system and SNS, favours spontaneous mobilization of ascites and improves the response to diuretics (Ring-Larsen et al, 1986). The diet should be restricted in sodium; about 40 mmol of sodium (corresponding to 2.3 g of

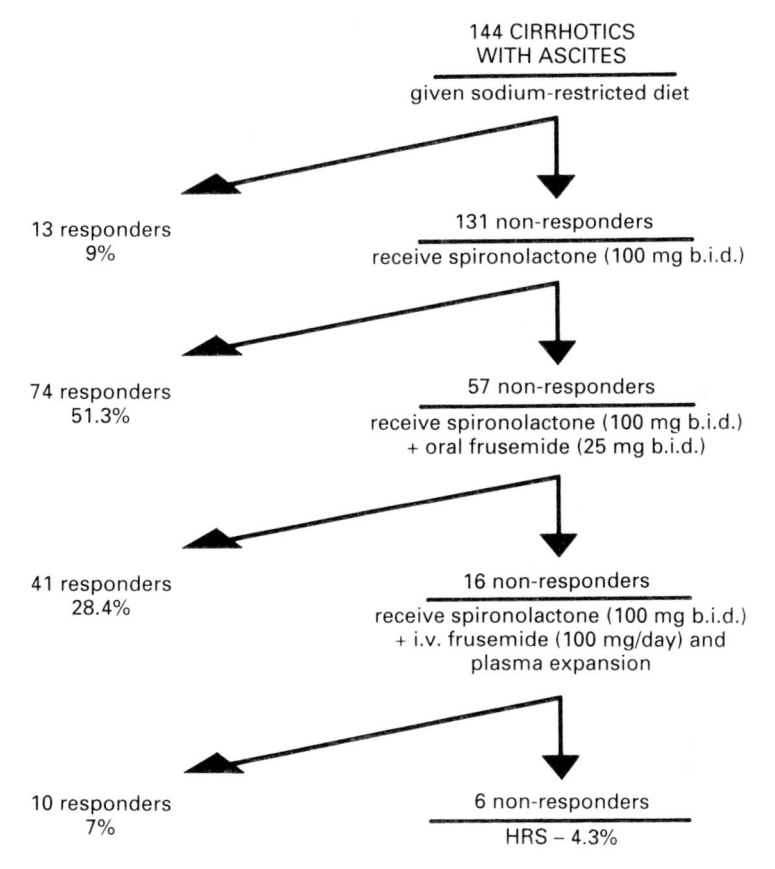

```
                    144 CIRRHOTICS
                     WITH ASCITES
                given sodium-restricted diet
                             ↓
13 responders        131 non-responders
    9%         receive spironolactone (100 mg b.i.d.)
                             ↓
74 responders         57 non-responders
   51.3%       receive spironolactone (100 mg b.i.d.)
                   + oral frusemide (25 mg b.i.d.)
                             ↓
41 responders         16 non-responders
   28.4%       receive spironolactone (100 mg b.i.d.)
                 + i.v. frusemide (100 mg/day) and
                          plasma expansion
                             ↓
10 responders         6 non-responders
    7%                   HRS – 4.3%
```

Figure 4. Sequential treatment of cirrhotic patients with ascites. From Gentilini et al (1986b).

sodium chloride) per day is sufficient for a palatable diet with adequate caloric content. Excessive sodium restriction (below 20 mmol/day) makes the diet unappetizing and can predispose to the onset of a dilutional hyponatraemia and prerenal hyperazotaemia (Galambos, 1979). The lack of compliance to a low-sodium diet can cause resistance to diuretic therapy and further ascites accumulation (Arroyo et al, 1989).

Bed rest and a low-sodium diet induce the disappearance of ascites in 10–20% of patients, according to the various reports in the literature (Figure 4). A favourable response to this regimen is more likely to occur in patients who have not had ascites previously, who excrete more than 10 mmol of sodium into urine per day, and who have normal renal function and free water clearance (Rocco and Ware, 1986).

Treatment with aldosterone antagonists

Patients not responding to a low-sodium diet and bed rest must be given an aldosterone-antagonist such as spironolactone or potassium canrenoate

(Gentilini et al, 1986b; Arroyo et al, 1989). The bioavailability of these drugs is high, with an intestinal absorption around 70% of the dose taken, which can also be improved by food intake. Binding to plasma proteins is extensive. Canrenone is a major metabolite of spironolactone and can be interconverted enzymatically with its hydrolytic product canrenoate (Weiner, 1990). The diuretic response to these drugs is slow, so their effectiveness can be assessed after a 3–5 day observation period. Treatment can be started with spironolactone, or better with potassium canrenoate, which has less anti-androgenic activity (Gentilini, 1991). Despite their low natriuretic potency (aldosterone antagonists bring about a 2% increase in elimination of filtered sodium, compared with 30% of frusemide), these drugs are the first choice in the treatment of cirrhotic patients with ascites. In fact, the administration of a loop diuretic alone gives a good natriuretic response in only 50% of non-azotaemic patients with ascites, whereas spironolactone is effective in most patients (Perez-Ayuso et al, 1983). The administration of 200 mg/day of an aldosterone antagonist allows an adequate response (a body weight loss of 300 g/day) in about 50% of patients (Figure 4). Higher doses may be required in patients with marked hyper-aldosteronism (Arroyo et al, 1989). In our experience, however, these high doses result in a significant increase in side-effects such as hyperkalaemia and metabolic acidosis. Therefore, in patients not responding to bed rest, a low-sodium diet and the administration of 200 mg/day of an aldosterone antagonist, it is preferable to add low doses of a loop diuretic (Gentilini et al, 1986b).

Addition of loop diuretics

Frusemide is the most widely used loop diuretic, and is also active in patients with renal failure (Weiner, 1990). This drug is rapidly absorbed from the gastrointestinal tract and its bioavailability is about 60%. Frusemide is extensively bound to plasma proteins and rapidly secreted by the organic acid transport system in the proximal tubule. When in the lumen, it is carried to the ascending limb of the loop of Henle where it inhibits a specific co-transport system, the Na^+–$2Cl^-$–K^+ carrier, thus blocking sodium reabsorption. Frusemide has a short half-life and the duration of its action is in the range of 3–6 hours (Weiner, 1990). The usual dose is 50 mg/day, but after the first few days of treatment, it is already possible to adjust the dosage to induce an adequate response. A further 25–30% of patients respond to the addition of a loop diuretic (Figure 4).

Other loop diuretics, such as bumetanide, piretanide and ethacrynic acid have been used with similar effect (Gines et al, 1989). Recently, a new loop diuretic, torasemide, has been proposed for the treatment of ascites in cirrhotic patients. This drug, a sulphonyl urea derivative, when administered in equipotent doses as frusemide, exerts a two-fold greater diuretic and natriuretic activity, whereas it has a similar effect on kaliuresis (Figure 5) (Laffi et al, 1991).

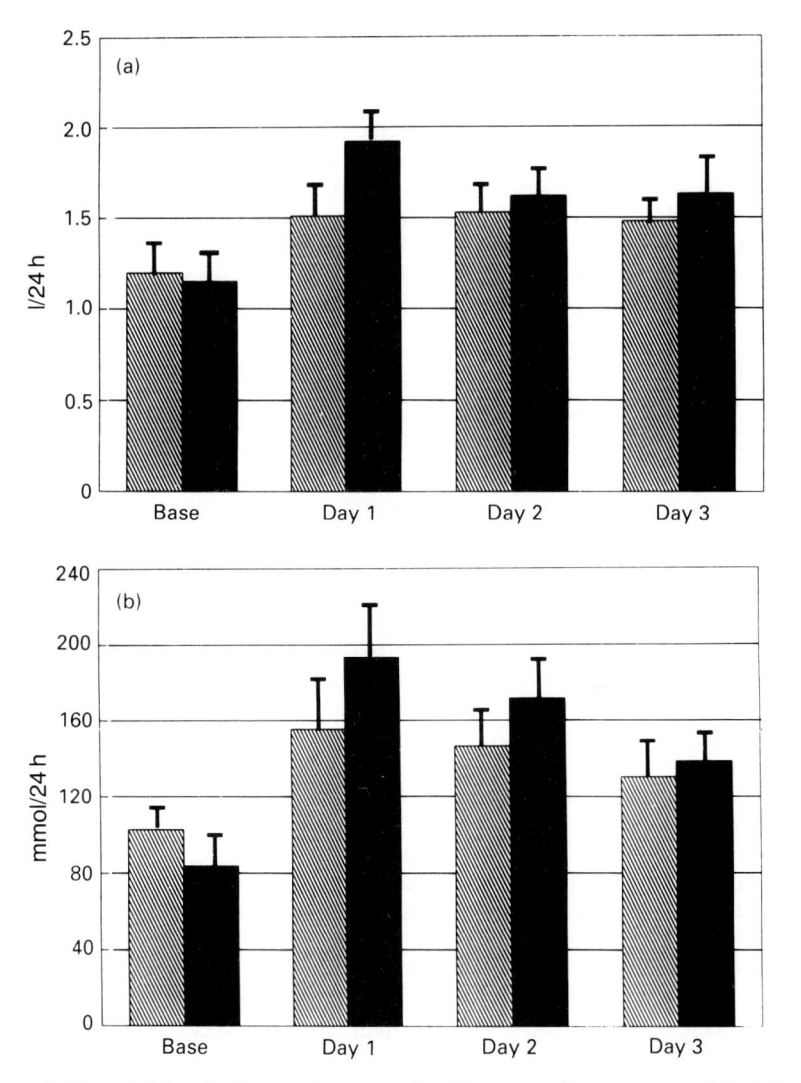

Figure 5. Diuresis (a) and urinary sodium excretion (b) measured in two groups of 12 cirrhotic patients with ascites after five days of 200 mg/day potassium canrenoate administration (BASE) and addition of 25 mg frusemide (hatched columns) or 10 mg torasemide (black columns) (mean ± SEM). (b), torasemide versus frusemide, $p < 0.02$. From Laffi et al (1991).

Addition of plasma expanders and high-dose diuretics

When the three steps mentioned above fail to induce an adequate natriuresis and the disappearance of ascites, patients should be given higher doses of a loop diuretic, possibly intravenously, with the addition of human albumin (up to 160–200 mg of frusemide and 100 ml of 25% human albumin) (Gentilini et al, 1986b). Albumin has the advantage of having a half-life of about 20 days and is well tolerated, whereas dextran and haemaccel® have much shorter half-lives and can cause idiosyncratic reactions. Plasma expansion compensates, at least partially, for the decrease in plasma volume and improves systemic and renal haemodynamics, thus inducing a better response to diuretic administration. With these procedures, a further 8% of cases show an adequate response (Figure 4). Patients who do not respond to 160–200 mg/day of frusemide (or equivalent doses of other loop diuretics) are usually insensitive to higher doses. In our experience, prolonged plasma expansion with human albumin (50 ml/day) improves the response to diuretics in any stage of therapy.

Refractory ascites

Patients who do not respond to high-dose diuretics (up to 400 mg spironolactone and 160 mg frusemide/day) and/or do not tolerate an effective diuretic regimen due to the appearance of serious side-effects (electrolyte imbalance, renal failure, hepatic encephalopathy) and are said to have refractory (diuretic-resistant) ascites (Arroyo et al, 1989; Gentilini et al, 1991a). In our experience, this occurs in about 4% of all cases (Figure 4).

The mechanism by which these patients do not respond to high doses of diuretics is unclear. A major factor may be the decrease in GFR often occurring in these patients, with a consequent decrease in filtered sodium load, and enhanced sodium reabsorption in the proximal tubule (Arroyo et al, 1989). It is well known that the natriuretic effects of loop diuretics strictly depend on the amount of drug reaching the lumen of the loop of Henle (Weiner, 1990). Thus, an additional mechanism of diuretic resistance may be related to an impaired secretion of loop diuretics into the tubular lumen (Pinzani et al, 1987). Another factor explaining the resistance seems to be related to ageing. In fact, we observed that the mean age of patients responding to the various stages of the diuretic treatment rose progressively from 44 to 63 years, whereas the mean age of those who did not respond at all was 66 years (Gentilini et al, 1986a).

The presence of refractory ascites carries a poor prognosis and patients generally do not survive more than two to three months. Refractory ascites usually occurs in patients with serious liver impairment complicated by renal insufficiency, hepatic encephalopathy and possible haemorrhage. HRS is a fairly frequent association, the presence of which is often worsened by diuretic administration.

TREATMENT OF REFRACTORY ASCITES AND THE HEPATORENAL SYNDROME

Prolonged administration of high-dose diuretics has been reported to be of some use, even in patients with refractory ascites (Stanley et al, 1989). However, these drugs must be used cautiously because EABV is usually markedly reduced in these patients (Schrier et al, 1988) and renal function is often reduced even in the presence of normal BUN and serum creatinine

levels (Papadakis and Arieff, 1987). In these patients, therefore, more invasive manoeuvres are often required (Gentilini et al, 1991a), including:
1. Repeated aspiration paracentesis.
2. Insertion of LeVeen shunt.
3. Experimental medical treatment.
4. Portosystemic shunts.
5. Orthotopic liver transplantation.

Repeated therapeutic paracentesis

Paracentesis has always been considered an effective procedure for the treatment of ascites in cirrhosis. However, the introduction of diuretic agents and some reports describing severe side-effects following paracentesis led to a decline of this procedure at the end of the 1950s. More recently, a large series of controlled trials have compared large volume paracentesis plus intravenous albumin infusion (6–8 g/L of ascitic fluid removed) with standard diuretic therapy in cirrhotic patients with tense ascites (Gines et al, 1987a). Therapeutic paracentesis plus intravenous albumin infusion was associated with a shorter duration of hospital stay and a lower rate of complications such as hyponatraemia, renal impairment and hepatic encephalopathy than conventional diuretic therapy. This procedure did not induce any significant change in standard liver function tests, systemic and renal haemodynamics, plasma volume, serum electrolytes and hormonal parameters (Gines et al, 1987a). On the other hand, paracentesis without albumin infusion was associated with a marked increase in PRA and a higher incidence of side-effects such as hyponatraemia and renal impairment, indicating that an expansion in intravascular volume is essential in order to avoid a contraction of EABV after paracentesis (Gines et al, 1988b). Albumin, which is expensive and not easily available, can be replaced by less expensive plasma expanders, such as dextran-70, dextran-40 and 5% haemaccel® (Planas et al, 1990; Salerno et al, 1991).

Paracentesis does not correct sodium retention in cirrhotic patients with ascites. Therefore, patients treated with paracentesis should also be given diuretics and a low-sodium diet to prevent reaccumulation of ascites. Recently, a controlled trial was performed comparing therapeutic paracentesis plus intravenous albumin infusion with a LeVeen shunt in patients with refractory ascites: both procedures were found to be equally effective in relieving ascites (Gines et al, 1991).

Insertion of LeVeen shunt

The shunt is made of a silicone tube with a unidirectional valve which is inserted into the peritoneal cavity, and, by a subcutaneous route, reaches the internal jugular vein and superior vena cava. When the pressure in the abdominal cavity rises to more than 3 cm H_2O above that of the vena cava, the valve opens, allowing ascitic fluid to flow directly into the systemic venous circulation. Due to the unidirectional valve, blood cannot flow back into the peritoneal cavity (LeVeen et al, 1974). Other forms of drainage similar to the LeVeen shunt have been introduced, such as the Denver and Hakim–Cordis shunts, but without any clear advantages over the LeVeen shunt (Arroyo et al, 1989).

Insertion of a peritoneovenous LeVeen shunt can lead to the disappearance or net reduction of ascitic fluid, particularly in patients on a low-sodium diet receiving low doses of diuretics.

Reabsorption of fluid from the peritoneal cavity allows the correction of the majority of haemodynamic and neuroendocrine changes found in cirrhosis, with increased plasma volume and cardiac output and normalization of plasma levels of ADH, noradrenaline, renin and aldosterone. There is a contemporaneous improvement in renal function and generally a reduction in portal pressure (Arroyo et al, 1989). However, insertion of the LeVeen shunt is not devoid of complications, which can be fairly frequent. These include disseminated intravascular coagulation, acute pulmonary oedema, haemorrhage from ruptured gastro-oesophageal varices, local and systemic bacterial infections (Arroyo et al, 1989). Prophylactic measures may consist of the administration of antibiotics active on *Staphylococcus aureus*, the mobilization of ascitic fluid before surgical insertion and the application of a titanum tip to the catheter in order to reduce the possibility of thrombosis (Arroyo et al, 1989).

Insertion of the LeVeen shunt is now performed in a restricted number of patients, so that it is difficult to compare its efficacy with other suggested procedures for conservative treatment of refractory ascites. The survival rate of patients undergoing LeVeen shunting does not appear to be greater than that obtained with other therapies and the prognosis of these patients is more dependent on the degree of hepatic impairment than on the presence of ascites or its response to treatment (Stanley et al, 1989; Gines et al, 1991).

Experimental medical treatment

Vasoconstrictor agents have been used to counteract peripheral vasodilatation and sustain arterial pressure in patients with refractory ascites and/or HRS, but the results have been disappointing (Epstein, 1988b). The use of ornithine-vasopressin has also been proposed more recently; in patients with decompensated cirrhosis and deteriorating renal function, Lenz et al (1991) demonstrated that this drug is able to correct the hyperdynamic state of these patients and to improve renal function, increasing renal sodium and water excretion.

Recently, there has been some interest in the potential therapeutic application of ANP in patients with refractory ascites. Besides its well-known diuretic and natriuretic activities, ANP markedly influences renal haemodynamics, increasing RBF and GFR; furthermore, it inhibits the release of renin and the synthesis and release of aldosterone (Ballermann et al, 1991).

However, the administration of synthetic human ANP to patients with cirrhosis and ascites induced a heterogeneous response, ranging from an appropriate natriuresis to no appreciable change in urinary sodium excretion. Patients resistant to the natriuretic effect of ANP had a greater reduction of EABV and during ANP infusion exhibited a further increase in PRA and PAC, together with an increase in heart rate, suggesting an activation of SNS, triggered by the concomitant ANP-induced hypotension (Laffi et al, 1989).

In patients with HRS, the renal production of vasodilating prostaglandin is markedly reduced, whereas urinary excretion of TxA_2 tends to be relatively elevated or maintained (Zipser and Lifschitz, 1988; Laffi et al, 1986). The administration of PGE_1 directly into the renal artery failed to reverse HRS (Zusman et al, 1977). More recently, oral administration of the prostaglandin analogue misoprostol, together with albumin infusion, to four patients with ascites and HRS, was able to improve GFR, diuresis and natriuresis (Fevery et al, 1990).

Administration of thromboxane-synthase inhibitors was tried in order to reduce renal synthesis of the potent vasoconstrictor TxA_2. Administration of dazoxiben to a small group of patients with HRS did not induce any favourable results (Zipser and Lifschitz, 1988). On the other hand, inhibition of renal TxA_2 synthesis by OKY 046 significantly improved the diuretic and natriuretic effect of frusemide in decompensated cirrhotics (Pinzani et al, 1988). More recently, we administered the thromboxane antagonist ONO 3708 to patients with cirrhosis and ascites, and observed a significant improvement in free water clearance and urine output. These studies suggest a role for renal TxA_2 as a modulator of water handling in these patients (Gentilini et al, 1989).

Portosystemic shunts

Other treatments, such as more invasive portosystemic surgery in well-selected patients can produce a relatively long survival without reformation of ascites or haemorrhage even in the absence of specific treatment (Franco, 1983).

However, there is a risk of perioperative mortality varying from 10% to 40% of cases, and surgery is followed by a high rate of encephalopathy. The majority of patients with refractory ascites have hepatic and renal impairment which does not permit high-risk surgery, even in conditions of relative water and electrolyte compensation.

Orthotopic liver transplantation

Refractory ascites or HRS may be considered indications for liver transplantation. In a recent study by Gonwa et al (1991), 31 patients with advanced liver disease and HRS underwent liver transplantation. In the immediate post-transplant period, these patients received exclusively azathioprine and prednisone until diuresis was established. Patients with HRS exhibited a striking improvement in GFR at one and two years after transplantation. Perioperative mortality and long-term survival were comparable with those observed in transplanted patients without HRS.

SUMMARY

Ascites indicates the accumulation of fluid in the peritoneal cavity, due to a wide range of causes. These causes can be classified according to the presence of portal hypertension, severe blood dyscrasia and peritoneal disease. Cirrhosis is the most frequent cause of ascites. The occurrence of ascites in cirrhosis is due to portal hypertension, which is responsible for the increase in hydrostatic pressure at the sinusoidal level and the alterations of splanchnic and systemic haemodynamics. These latter include increased splanchnic inflow, reduced systemic resistance and increased plasma volume and cardiac output. Portal hypertension also plays a major role in determining sodium retention, which occurs in the setting of increased RAA system and SNS activity. The mechanisms by which portal hypertension leads to the activation of antinatriuretic factors and sodium retention are not completely understood; three main hypotheses have been proposed to explain this relationship, namely the underfilling, the overflow and the peripheral arterial vasodilatation theories.

In patients with cirrhosis and ascites, there is an overall activation of the renal prostaglandin system, which probably acts to maintain renal haemodynamics and GFR by counteracting the vasoconstricting effects of AII and noradrenaline on renal circulation. In advanced stages, ascites may become refractory to medical treatment and renal function shows a progressive impairment and eventually acute renal failure, the so-called HRS, due to a marked vasoconstriction of the renal arteries and the opening of the intrarenal-arteriovenous (A-V) shunts. In this condition, the reduced renal synthesis of vasodilating prostaglandins is probably of pathogenic importance. Treatment of ascites is usually based on bed rest, low-sodium diet and administration of aldosterone antagonists and loop diuretics. A sequential treatment of ascites based on the progressive addition of more potent drugs is the best way to relieve ascites while avoiding potentially dangerous side-effects. Patients who fail to respond to the above manoeuvres are said to have refractory ascites. Current treatment of this latter condition is mainly based on therapeutic paracentesis and the application of the LeVeen shunt, but long-term results are unsatisfactory.

REFERENCES

Arroyo V, Bernardi M, Epstein M et al (1988) Pathophysiology of ascites and functional renal failure in cirrhosis. *Journal of Hepatology* **6:** 239–257.

Arroyo V, Epstein M, Gallus G et al (1989) Refractory ascites in cirrhosis: mechanism and treatment. *Gastroenterology International* **2:** 195–207.

Ballermann BJ, Zeidel ML, Gunning ME et al (1991) Vasoactive peptides and the kidney. In Brenner BM & Rector FC (eds) *The Kidney*, 4th edn, vol. 1, pp 510–583. Philadelphia: WB Saunders.

Bichet D, Szatalowicz V, Chaimovitz C et al (1982) Role of vasopressin in abnormal water excretion in cirrhotic patients. *Annals of Internal Medicine* **96:** 413–417.

Bourgoignie JJ & Valle GA (1988) Endotoxin and renal dysfunction in liver disease. In Epstein M (ed.) *The Kidney in Liver Disease*, 3rd edn, pp 486–507. Baltimore: Williams & Wilkins.

Boyer TD, Zia P & Reynolds TB (1979) Effect of indomethacin and prostaglandin A1 on renal function and plasma renin activity in alcoholic liver disease. *Gastroenterology* **77**: 215–222.

Caramelo C, Fernandez-Gallardo S, Santos JC et al (1987) Increased levels of platelet-activating factor in blood from patients with cirrhosis of the liver. *European Journal of Clinical Investigation* **17**: 7–11.

Claria J, Jimenez W, Arroyo V et al (1989) Blockade of the hydroosmotic effect of vasopressin normalizes water excretion in cirrhotic rats. *Gastroenterology* **97**: 1294–1299.

Claria J, Jimenez W, Arroyo V et al (1991) Effect of V1-vasopressin receptor blockade on arterial pressure in conscious rats with cirrhosis and ascites. *Gastroenterology* **100**: 494–501.

Conn HO & Atterbury CE (1987) Cirrhosis. In Schiff L & Schiff ER (eds) *Diseases of the Liver*, 6th edn, pp 725–864. Philadelphia: Lippincott.

Daskalopoulos G, Kronborg J, Katkov W et al (1985) Sulindac and indomethacin suppress the diuretic action of furosemide in patients with cirrhosis and ascites. Evidence that sulindac affects renal prostaglandins. *American Journal of Kidney Diseases* **6**: 217–221.

De Wardener HE & Clarkson EM (1985) Natriuretic hormone. In Seldin DW & Giebisch G (eds) *The Kidney: Physiology and Pathophysiology*, pp 1013–1031. New York: Raven Press.

Epstein M (1988a) Renal sodium handling in liver disease. In Epstein M (ed.) *The Kidney in Liver Disease*, 3rd edn, pp 3–30. Baltimore: Williams & Wilkins.

Epstein M (1988b) Hepatorenal syndrome. In Epstein M (ed.) *The Kidney in Liver Disease*, 3rd edn, pp 89–118. Baltimore: Williams & Wilkins.

Epstein M & Norsk P (1988) Renin-angiotensin system in liver disease. In Epstein M (ed.) *The Kidney in Liver Disease*, 3rd edn, pp 331–355. Baltimore: Williams & Wilkins.

Fevery J, Van Cutsem E, Nevens F et al (1990) Reversal of hepatorenal syndrome in four patients by peroral misoprostol (prostaglandin E_1 analogue) and albumin administration. *Journal of Hepatology* **11**: 153–158.

Franco D (1983) Traitement de l'ascite irreductible du cirrhotique par la derivation portal. *Gastroenterologie Clinique Biologique* **7**: 533–539.

Frommer JP, Wesson DE & Eknoyan E (1986) Side effects and complications of diuretic therapy. In Eknoyan G & Martinez-Maldonado M (eds) *The Physiological Basis of Diuretic Therapy in Clinical Medicine*, pp 293–309. Orlando: Grune & Stratton.

Galambos JT (1979) *Cirrhosis*. Philadelphia: WB Saunders.

Gentilini P (1991) Spironolactone and canrenoate: different antialdosteronic diuretic agents. Hepatology elsewhere. *Hepatology* **13**: 999–1000.

Gentilini P & Laffi G (1989) Renal functional impairment and sodium retention in liver cirrhosis. *Digestion* **43**: 1–32.

Gentilini P, Laffi G, Buzzelli G et al (1980) Functional renal alterations in chronic liver disease. *Digestion* **20**: 73–78.

Gentilini P, Sicuteri F, Laffi G et al (1983) The kinin system and other vasoactive substances in chronic liver disease. In Fritz H, Back N, Dietze G & Haberland GL (eds) *Kinins-III*, Part B, pp 1161–1166. New York: Plenum Publishing.

Gentilini P, Laffi G, La Villa G et al (1986a) Aging and liver cirrhosis. Reduced response to diuretic treatment of ascites. In Courtois Y, Faucheux B, Forette B et al (eds) *Modern Trends in Aging Research*, Colloque INSERM, vol. 147, pp 185–191. London: John Libbey Eurotext.

Gentilini P, La Villa G, Laffi G et al (1986b) Sodium retention in cirrhosis: aspects of pathophysiology and treatment. *Frontiers in Gastrointestinal Research* **9**: 203–218.

Gentilini P, Laffi G, Marra F et al (1989) Selective thromboxane A2 receptor antagonism increases free-water clearance in cirrhotic patients with ascites. *Hepatology* **10**: 717(A).

Gentilini P, Laffi G, La Villa G & Romanelli RG (1991a) Experimental therapy of refractory ascites. *Gastroenterology International* **4**: 114–119.

Gentilini P, Maggiore Q, Romanelli RG et al (1991b) Angiotensin II maintains renal hemodynamics in patients with cirrhosis. *Gastroenterology* **100**: A746.

Gines P, Arroyo V, Quintero E et al (1987a) Comparison of paracentesis and diuretics in the treatment of cirrhotics with tense ascites. Results of a randomized study. *Gastroenterology* **93**: 234–241.

Gines P, Quintero E, Arroyo V et al (1987b) Compensated cirrhosis: natural history and prognostic factors. *Hepatology* **7**: 122–128.

Gines P, Jimenez W, Arroyo V et al (1988a) Atrial natriuretic factor in cirrhosis with ascites. Plasma levels, cardiac release and splanchnic extraction. *Hepatology* **8**: 636–642.

Gines P, Tito L, Arroyo V et al (1988b) Randomized comparative study of therapeutic paracentesis with and without intravenous albumin in cirrhosis. *Gastroenterology* **94**: 1493–1502.

Gines P, Arroyo V & Rodes J (1989) Treatment of ascites and renal failure in cirrhosis. *Baillière's Clinical Gastroenterology* **3**: 165–186.

Gines P, Arroyo V, Vargas V et al (1991) Paracentesis with intravenous infusion of albumin as compared with peritoneovenous shunting in cirrhosis with refractory ascites. *New England Journal of Medicine* **325**: 829–835.

Gonwa TA, Morris C, Goldstein RM et al (1991) Long-term survival and renal function following liver transplantation in patients with and without hepatorenal syndrome—experience in 300 patients. *Transplantation* **51**: 428–430.

Hamlyn JM, Blaustein MP, Bova S et al (1991) Identification and characterization of a ouabain-like compound from human plasma. *Proceedings of the National Academy of Science USA* **88**: 6259–6263.

Laffi G, La Villa G, Pinzani M et al (1986) Altered renal and platelet arachidonic acid metabolism in cirrhosis. *Gastroenterology* **90**: 274–282.

Laffi G, Pinzani M, Meacci E et al (1989) Renal hemodynamic and natriuretic effects of human atrial natriuretic factor infusion in cirrhosis with ascites. *Gastroenterology* **96**: 167–177.

Laffi G, Marra F, Buzzelli G et al (1991) Comparison of the effects of torasemide and furosemide in nonazotemic cirrhotic patients with ascites: a randomized, double-blind study. *Hepatology* **13**: 1101–1105.

La Villa G, Asbert M, Jimenez W et al (1990) Natriuretic hormone activity in the urine of cirrhotic patients. *Hepatology* **12**: 467–475.

La Villa G, Romanelli RG, Casini Raggi V et al (1992) Plasma levels of brain natriuretic peptide in patients with cirrhosis of the liver. *Hepatology* (in press).

Lenz K, Hortnagl H, Druml W et al (1991) Ornipressin in the treatment of Functional Renal Failure in decompensated liver cirrhosis. *Gastroenterology* **101**: 1060–1067.

LeVeen H, Christoudias G, Moon JP et al (1974) Peritoneo-venous shunting for ascites. *Annals of Surgery* **180**: 580–591.

Levy M (1988) Pathophysiology of ascites formation. In Epstein M (ed.) *The Kidney in Liver Disease*, 3rd edn, pp 209–243. Baltimore: Williams & Wilkins.

Lieberman FL, Denison EK & Reynolds RB (1970) The relationship of plasma volume, portal hypertension, ascites, and renal sodium retention in liver cirrhosis: the overflow theory of ascites formation. *Annals of the New York Academy of Sciences* **170**: 202–212.

McCormick PA, Mistry P, Kaye G et al (1990) Intravenous albumin infusion is effective therapy for hyponatraemia in cirrhotic patients with ascites. *Gut* **31**: 204–207.

Moore KP, Taylor GW, Maltby NH et al (1990) Increased production of cysteinyl leukotrienes in hepatorenal syndrome. *Journal of Hepatology* **11**: 263–271.

Naccarato R, Messa P, D'Angelo A et al (1981) Renal handling of sodium and water in early chronic liver disease. *Gastroenterology* **81**: 205–210.

Papadakis MA & Arieff AI (1987) Unpredictability of clinical evaluation of renal function in cirrhosis. *American Journal of Medicine* **82**: 945–952.

Pariente EA, Bataille C, Bercoff E & Lebrec D (1985) Acute effects of captopril on systemic and renal hemodynamics and on renal function in cirrhotic patients with ascites. *Gastroenterology* **88**: 1255–1259.

Perez-Ayuso RM, Arroyo V, Planas R et al (1983) Randomized comparative study of efficacy of furosemide versus spironolactone in non-azotemic cirrhosis with ascites. *Gastroenterology* **84**: 961–968.

Perez-Ayuso RM, Arroyo V, Camps J et al (1984) Renal kallikrein excretion in cirrhotics with ascites: relationship to renal hemodynamics. *Hepatology* **4**: 247–252.

Pinzani M, Daskalopoulos G, Laffi G et al (1987) Altered furosemide pharmacokinetics in chronic alcoholic liver disease with ascites contributes to diuretic resistance. *Gastroenterology* **92**: 294–298.

Pinzani M, Laffi G, Meacci E et al (1988) Intrarenal thromboxane A2 generation reduces the furosemide-induced sodium and water diuresis in cirrhosis with ascites. *Gastroenterology* **95**: 1081–1087.

Planas R, Gines P, Arroyo V et al (1990) Dextran-70 versus albumin as plasma expanders in cirrhotic patients with tense ascites treated with total paracentesis. Results of a randomized study. *Gastroenterology* **99**: 1736–1744.

Pockros PJ & Reynolds TB (1986) Rapid diuresis in patients with ascites from chronic liver disease: the importance of peripheral edema. *Gastroenterology* **90:** 1827–1833.

Reznick RK, Langer B, Taylor BR et al (1983) Hyponatremia and arginine vasopressin secretion in patients with refractory hepatic ascites undergoing peritoneovenous shunting. *Gastroenterology* **84:** 713–718.

Ring-Larsen H, Henriksen JH, Wilken C et al (1986) Diuretic treatment in decompensated cirrhosis and congestive heart failure: effect of posture. *British Medical Journal* **292:** 1351–1353.

Rocco VK & Ware AJ (1986) Cirrhotic ascites. Pathophysiology, diagnosis, and management. *Annals of International Medicine* **105:** 573–585.

Salerno F, Badalamenti S, Lorenzano E et al (1991) Randomized comparative study of hemaccel vs. albumin infusion after total paracentesis in cirrhotic patients with refractory ascites. *Hepatology* **13:** 707–713.

Schrier RW, Arroyo V, Bernardi M et al (1988) Peripheral arterial vasodilation hypothesis: a proposal for the initiation of renal sodium and water retention in cirrhosis. *Hepatology* **8:** 1151–1157.

Schroeder ET, Anderson GH, Goldman SH & Streeten DHP (1976) Effects of blockade of angiotensin II on blood pressure, renin and aldosterone in cirrhosis. *Kidney International* **9:** 511–519.

Shear L, Ching S & Gabuzda GJ (1970) Compartmentalization of ascites and edema in patients with hepatic cirrhosis. *Gastroenterology* **282:** 1391–1396.

Skorecki KL, Leung WM, Campbell P et al (1988) Role of atrial natriuretic peptide in the natriuretic response to central volume expansion induced by head-out water immersion in sodium-retaining cirrhotic subjects. *American Journal of Medicine* **85:** 375–382.

Snyder F (1990) Platelet-activating factor and related acetylated lipids as potent biologically active cellular mediators. *American Journal of Physiology* **259:** C697–C708.

Stanley MM, Ochi S, Lee KK et al (1989) Peritoneovenous shunting as compared with medical treatment in patients with alcoholic cirrhosis and massive ascites. *New England Journal of Medicine* **321:** 1632–1638.

Sudoh T, Kangawa K, Minamino N & Matsuo H (1988) A new natriuretic peptide in porcine brain. *Nature* **332:** 78–81.

Triger DR (1991) Endotoxemia in liver disease-time for re-appraisal? *Journal of Hepatology* **12:** 136–138.

Villamediana LM, Sanz E, Fernandez-Gallardo S et al (1986) Effects of platelet-activating factor antagonist BN 52021 on the hemodynamics of rats with experimental cirrhosis of the liver. *Life Sciences* **39:** 201–205.

Wang J, Kester M & Dunn MJ (1988) The effect of endotoxin on platelet-activating factor synthesis in cultured rat glomerular mesangial cells. *Biochimica Biophysica Acta* **969:** 217–224.

Weiner IM (1990) Diuretics and other agents employed in the mobilization of edema fluid. In Gilman AG, Rall TW, Nies AS & Taylor P (eds) *Goodman & Gilman's Pharmacological Basis of Therapeutics*, 8th edn, pp 713–731. New York: Pergamon Press.

Wilkinson SP, Jowett JDH, Slater JDH et al (1979) Renal sodium retention in cirrhosis: relationship to aldosterone and nephron site. *Clinical Science* **56:** 169–177.

Willett JR, Jennings G, Esler M & Dudley FJ (1986) Sympathetic tone modulates portal venous pressure in alcoholic cirrhosis. *Lancet* **2:** 939–943.

Witte MH, Witte CL & Dumond AE (1971) Progress in liver disease: physiological factors involved in the causation of cirrhotic ascites. *Gastroenterology* **61:** 742–750.

Wong P, Talamo RC & Williams GH (1977) Kallikrein-kinin and renin-angiotensin systems in functional renal failure of cirrhosis of the liver. *Gastroenterology* **73:** 1114–1118.

Zambraski EJ & DiBona GF (1988) Sympathetic nervous system in hepatic cirrhosis. In Epstein M (ed.) *The Kidney in Liver Disease*, 3rd edn, pp 469–485. Baltimore: Williams & Wilkins.

Zipser RD, Kerlin P, Hoefs JC et al (1981) Renal kallikrein excretion in alcoholic cirrhosis. *American Journal of Gastroenterology* **75:** 183–187.

Zipser RD & Lifschitz MD (1988) Prostaglandins and related compounds. In Epstein M (ed.) *The Kidney in Liver Disease*, 3rd edn, pp 393–416. Baltimore: Williams & Wilkins.

Zusman RM, Axelrod L & Tolkoff-Rubin N (1977) The treatment of the hepatorenal syndrome (HRS) with intrarenal administration of prostaglandin E1. *Prostaglandins* **13:** 819–830.

12
Recent developments in the pathophysiology and treatment of hepatic encephalopathy

KARIN WEISSENBORN

PATHOPHYSIOLOGY

In spite of decades of intensive research, the pathogenesis of hepatic encephalopathy (HE) has still not been clarified. The reasons for this are, on the one hand, the lack of adequate animal models for studying HE—especially in its chronic form—and, on the other, the impossibility of simulating in a model the interaction of several possible causation factors.

Three mechanisms in the pathogenesis of HE are discussed: a disturbance of cerebral energy metabolism, alterations in the composition and function of neuronal membranes and, finally, a change in the neurotransmitter status with predominance of the inhibitory neurotransmission. The basis for these changes are, according to current understanding, the synergism of neurotoxically effective substances such as ammonia, mercaptans, short- and medium-chain fatty acids and phenols, changes in neurotransmission because of an altered amino acid metabolism, an altered permeability of the blood–brain barrier, and changes in the density and affinity of neuronal receptors.

This chapter attempts to present the current state of the discussion concerning the significance of the individual factors in the development of HE.

Ammonia

At the beginning of the century clinical and experimental observations led to the conclusion that there was a connection between raised ammonia levels in the blood and the occurrence of HE. In 1922, for example, Matthews surmised that ammonia is a causal factor in meat poisoning in Eck fistula dogs, and Kirk showed, in 1936, that precoma occurred in cirrhotic patients given ammonium citrate. In 1952 Phillips and co-workers established a regular relationship between raised ammonia levels and the development of HE (Zieve, 1991). From that time ammonia has been a constant element in the discussions on HE.

Ammonia is generated from the catabolism of proteins, amino acids, purines and pyrimidines as well as biogenic amines. For a long time it was assumed that the intestinal bacterial metabolism of nitrogenous substances—especially from food proteins and from urea diffused in the lumen of the intestines—was the main source of ammonia. Meanwhile it has been established that the bacteria only account for 40% of the synthesis of ammonia in the gastrointestinal tract. The remaining 60% originates from the digestion of dietary protein and the metabolism of circulating glutamine in the small intestine. Besides the intestines, the liver, kidneys, brain and muscle are also involved in the synthesis of ammonia. Participation of the kidneys and brain is only slight (Crossley et al, 1983; Gerok, 1985).

Ammonia detoxication is effected essentially in the liver, where it is converted into urea and glutamine. Urea synthesis is the most important detoxication process. It occurs in the urea cycle, specific to the liver, by which urea is formed from ammonia, carbon dioxide and the amino group of aspartate using four high-energy phosphates. Urea is an ideal detoxication product because it is biologically inert and can be eliminated via the kidneys with a high clearance rate. Glutamine synthesis is not specific to the liver. In addition, the muscle and brain contain the enzyme glutamine synthetase which catalyses, in a ATP-dependent reaction, the production of glutamine from ammonia and glutamate. Glutamine essentially aids the transport of ammonia in non-toxic form from various organs to the liver where, with the help of glutaminase, glutamine is split into ammonia and glutamate again. As Häussinger (1983) showed, glutamine splitting and urea synthesis or glutamine production are localized in different parts of the liver. While glutamine production takes place in the hepatocytes around the central vein of a liver acinus, glutamine splitting and urea synthesis occur in the periportal area. The metabolic heterogeneity of hepatocytes increases the effectiveness of ammonia detoxication. Urea synthesis requires high ammonia concentrations for entry into the cycle. This concentration is to be found periportally. The efficacy of periportal urea synthesis is enhanced by the addition of substrate supplied by periportal glutamine degradation. Glutamine synthesis takes place in the presence of even lower concentrations of ammonia. Small amounts of ammonia which elude urea synthesis can therefore still be detoxicated via glutamine synthesis. Ammonia levels in healthy people are regulated within a narrow range by these mechanisms. In cases of hepatic diseases, on the other hand, hyperammonaemia occurs as a result of a disturbance in urea and glutamine synthesis. Additionally, because of increased catabolism, ammonia production often increases (James et al, 1979). However, this contributes to hyperammonaemia only in cases of disturbed detoxication.

Reduction in ammonia detoxication can be caused either metabolically or haemodynamically. A combination of the two is more usual, when the haemodynamic component is considered the more important. Ammonia metabolism is presumably disturbed as a result of a decreased activity of the two rate-limiting enzymes of the urea cycle, carbamylphosphate synthetase and arginosuccinate synthetase (Maier et al, 1979). It is not absolutely certain, however, that the reduced ammonia metabolism in the liver is of decisive importance for hyperammonaemia, as the activity of the participating enzymes can be considerably raised by a gradual increase in oral protein intake even in severe liver disease (Maier and Gerok, 1985). Ammonia detoxication is possibly more significantly affected by the ammonia-rich portal blood bypassing the liver via portocaval anastomoses. Arguably, ammonia detoxication could take place in the muscle in this situation, but the importance of this metabolic route is restricted because of the extreme loss of muscle mass in many cirrhotic patients.

About 47% of ammonia present in arterial blood is extracted in one passage through the brain (Crossley et al, 1983). In cases of hyperammonaemia, therefore, ammonia levels in the brain are inevitably raised. Ammonia in the brain is detoxicated predominantly in the cytosol of astrocytes via the amination of glutamate to glutamine (Norenberg, 1987). This metabolic pathway is of pathological significance. Glutamine levels are increased two to five times in the brains of cirrhotic patients, as they are in the brains of rats following portocaval shunt (PCS) (Butterworth, 1991). When glutamine synthesis is inhibited by methionine-sulphoximine, animals survive a lethal dose of ammonium salts (Gerok, 1985).

Originally it was assumed that the toxic effect of ammonia was partly due to the reductive amination of α-ketoglutarate by ammonia, thus depleting the brain of this intermediary in the citrate cycle and inhibiting the formation of ATP. This supposition has not been proven. As Hindfelt et al (1977) showed, depletion of high-energy phosphates does not occur in the *early* stages of HE, induced in PCS rats by an additional ammonia load. Only when ammonia intoxication produced coma did the animals develop an abnormal cerebral energy state, with a reduction of ATP and a decrease in the ATP/ADP ratio in all brain regions. This long-term depletion of ATP is possibly due to a block in citrate formation. Hindfelt's study showed increased glycolysis and correspondingly raised pyruvate levels in PCS rats after ammonia loading. On the other hand, citrate levels dropped, which leads to the conclusion that the linkage between glycolysis and the citrate cycle was disturbed. In contrast to citrate, malate and α-ketoglutarate levels were raised.

As a result of increased supplies of pyruvate, greater production of alanine and oxaloacetate occurred with the expenditure of aspartate. The lowered aspartate levels, in combination with reduced concentrations of glutamate, due to increased glutamine production, lead to inhibition of the malate–aspartate shuttle and thereby, delayed, to reduced oxidative phosphorylation. This could possibly be of importance in the causation of coma.

Another ammonia-dependent mechanism under discussion in the pathogenesis of HE is the depletion of glutamate, an essential excitatory neurotransmitter, as a result of increased glutamine production in hyperammonaemia. However, it has been shown that, while a reduction of the glutamate contents occur in the brains of patients with HE as well as animals following PCS (Holmin et al, 1983; Lavoie et al, 1987), this reduction did not affect the neurotransmitter pool (Moroni et al, 1983). According to more recent findings, hyperammonaemia affects the glutamatergic neurotransmission in other ways (Szerb and Butterworth, 1991): astrocytes and neurones are closely connected in the glutamatergic synaptic regulation.

Glutamate released in the synaptic cleft either stimulates the postsynaptic receptor or is taken up again into the perineural astrocytes. There, by the action of glutamine synthetase, it is converted into glutamine which is partly transported back to the presynaptic part of the neurone and thereby into the surplus within the neurotransmitter pool. In cases of chronic hyperammonaemia, straining of the astrocytes occurs due to increased energy-consuming glutamine synthesis. Other functions such as the uptake of glutamate from the synaptic cleft or extrusion of sodium cations from the cell interior are impeded. In these ways functional, morphological and biochemical changes take place in the astrocytes. Finally the activity of glutamine synthetase is also reduced so that cerebral mechanisms which could deal with an acute increase in ammonia are affected. The reduced reuptake of glutamate should also lead to a down-regulation of the glutamatergic N-methyl-D-aspartate (NMDA) receptors and thereby to an inhibition of the excitatory neurotransmission (Peterson et al, 1990).

Further points concerning the glutamatergic neurotransmission are a lowering of glutaminase activity by ammonia and a hitherto unexplained postsynaptic effect. As a result, ammonia reduces the firing rate of hippocampal pyramidal cells which has been induced by glutamate applied iontophoretically, and disrupts the glutamatergic neurotransmission of Schaffer collaterals to CA1 pyramidal cells in hippocampal slices (Fan et al, 1990).

Serotoninergic and catecholaminergic neurotransmissions are also believed to be affected by hyperammonaemia because of an increase in the transport of their precursor amino acids over the blood–brain barrier. Details of these changes can be found elsewhere in this chapter.

Further pathogenetic mechanisms of the effect of ammonia in HE are inhibition of the Na^+/K^+-dependent ATPase as a result of competition of ammonia with potassium with a consequent toxic effect upon the neuronal cell membrane and an impairment of the postsynaptic inhibition in the brain-stem and cortex by inactivation of chloride extrusion from the neurones (Butterworth, 1991).

It cannot be proved that the above-mentioned mechanisms are, in fact, important in the development of HE. However, if one compares HE with a pure ammonia intoxication, there are a number of facts which illustrate the significance of hyperammonaemia in the development of HE:

1. The administration of ammonia-producing substances can induce encephalopathy in patients with hepatic cirrhosis (Zieve, 1984a).
2. Reduction of bacterial ammonia synthesis, through administration of, for example, neomycin or lactulose, or a decrease in protein intake, leads to amelioration of HE (Conn and Lieberthal, 1978).
3. Congenital defects of the urea cycle, which induce hyperammonaemia, lead to neuropsychiatric symptoms similar to those observed with HE (Gerok, 1985).
4. Changes in astrocytes, induced by raised ammonia levels, in both animal experiments and astrocyte cultures, are similar to those found in cases of HE (Norenberg, 1987).

5. There is a close correlation between the degree of HE and concentrations of glutamine and α-ketoglutarate in the cerebrospinal fluid (CSF). Both substances reflect the ammonia content of the brain (Zieve, 1991).
6. Ammonia concentrations in the blood correlate well with the clinical picture in individual cases (Zieve, 1984a).

The following arguments are put forward against the pathogenetic significance of hyperammonaemia in HE:

1. Ammonia intoxication leads to hyperkinetic, preconvulsive or convulsive states and not to clouding of consciousness and a hypokinetic syndrome which are seen in HE.
2. Plasma levels of ammonia correlate poorly with HE. About 10% of HE patients have normal ammonia levels, and many patients with hyperammonaemia do not have HE. Of course, it must be remembered that the ammonia concentrations in the brain, and not in the blood, are critical in the development of HE and that concentrations in the blood are essentially influenced by muscle metabolism (Zieve, 1984a). Nevertheless, these findings support the view that ammonia is not the only important factor in the development of HE (Zieve, 1984a, 1991).

Mercaptans, phenols and short- and medium-chain fatty acids

Besides ammonia, mercaptans, phenols and short- and medium-chain fatty acids accumulate in hepatic failure. All three substances are basically able to induce coma, although the toxic levels necessary for this are far above those observed in either animal experiments or patients with HE. Zieve et al, however, showed that these toxins could each exert their own individual effect at lower doses when they were present simultaneously than when acting singly. Under the former conditions, the necessary toxic levels lay within the pathophysiological range. On the basis of these results, Zieve put forward the hypothesis that the above-mentioned substances act synergistically with ammonia in the pathophysiology of HE (Zieve, 1984b).

Among the mercaptans, until recently methanethiol was considered to be of the greatest pathophysiological importance. However, as recent studies by Tangerman et al have shown (Tangerman, 1991), there is no correlation between methanethiol levels (measured as methanethiol mixed disulphides) and the degree of HE compared to controls. Plasma levels were only raised in patients in stages III and IV of HE. Comparable findings were seen in rats with PCS or following hepatic ischaemia, and in dogs with HE. In their opinion, the fact that a patient with a deficiency in hepatic methionine adenosyltransferase and massively raised dimethylsulphide levels in the expired air or methanethiol mixed disulphide levels in serum and urine showed no signs of HE rules out the pathogenetic significance of methanethiol. They think that hydrogen sulphide is more likely to be pathogenetically important because its levels were increased in both animal experiments and preliminary examinations in HE patients. These findings still have to be confirmed.

The significance of phenols in the development of HE is even less clear than that of mercaptans. Phenols are produced in the intestines and the liver from the amino acids phenylalanine and tyrosine. They are detoxified primarily in the liver by conjugation with glucuronic or sulphuric acid. In cases of hepatic insufficiency, there is an increase of phenols in the blood, CSF and urine. As phenols *per se* can induce coma, they are considered to be significant in the development of HE. This supposition is supported by the results of Zieve et al, which showed that the administration of phenols in doses which alone were not sufficient to induce a coma nevertheless reduced by 25% the amount of ammonia necessary to trigger a coma in animal experiments (Zieve, 1984b). The mechanism of the effect of phenols is not clear.

A synergistic action of short- and medium-chain fatty acids together with other neurotoxins has also been proved (Zieve, 1984b). Here, too, the mechanism is not clear. However, it is postulated that the fatty acids inhibit urea synthesis (Zieve, 1984b). Furthermore, it could be significant that they displace tryptophan in plasma protein binding so that increased amounts of free tryptophan can pass into the brain and be converted into serotonin (Curzon and Knott, 1977).

Neurotransmitters

In the recent past, changes of neurotransmission have been discussed frequently as pathophysiological factors in HE. It is postulated that an imbalance between excitation and inhibition with predominance of the latter exists in cases of HE. Potential causes for this imbalance include changes in catecholamine and indole metabolism, alterations in glutamatergic and GABAergic neurotransmission, which will be discussed.

Dopamine, noradrenaline and false neurotransmitters

Characteristically, an imbalance between aromatic amino acids (AAA) and branched-chain amino acids (BCAA) is found in the plasma of cirrhotic patients, but the cause is not clear. It is assumed that stimulation of glucagon secretion and the subsequent rise in gluconeogenesis from amino acids occur as a result of hyperammonaemia. This, in turn, leads to a further increase in ammonia production and a rise in insulin secretion. The glucose level in serum is kept within the normal range by these means, but the uptake and metabolism of BCAAs are simultaneously stimulated in the musculature. While the plasma levels of BCAAs decrease, at the same time a rise in the levels of AAAs, such as tryptophan, tyrosine, phenylalanine and methionine, takes place because their metabolism in the liver is reduced (James et al, 1979).

Taking these changes in the amino acid pattern with HE into account, Fischer and Baldessarini (1971) developed their hypothesis of 'false neurotransmitters'. This is essentially based on the following train of thought: in consequence of the plasma amino acid imbalance, the concentration of AAAs increases and that of BCAAs decreases in the brain because the amino acids compete for the same carrier system at the blood–brain barrier and the transport is dependent on concentrations. The raised concentration of tryptophan in the brain then leads to an increase in the synthesis of the inhibitory neurotransmitter serotonin. The raised phenylalanine levels inhibit tyrosine-3-mono-oxygenase and thereby the hydroxylation of tyrosine to dopa. In that way the biosynthesis of dopamine and noradrenaline is inhibited and phenylalanine and tyrosine are metabolized via an alternative route, namely to phenylethanolamine or octopamine. Both these substances bind to catecholamine receptors, but have only a fraction of the effectiveness of true transmitters. For example, the sympathomimetic effect of octopamine is only 2% of that of noradrenaline.

According to this theory, HE can be seen as the consequence of a reduction in catecholaminergic neurotransmission with simultaneous increase of serotoninergic neurotransmission.

The hypothesis was first supported by a series of observations. Raised levels of tryptophan, tyrosine and phenylalanine were found in the plasma and brains of patients with fulminant hepatic failure (FHF) as well as a reduction in the levels of noradrenaline and dopamine in the brains of patients who had died of FHF (Fischer and Baldessarini, 1971; Bloch et al, 1978). In dogs with HE from a PCS, Smith et al (1978) found raised tryptophan, tyrosine and phenylalanine levels in the CSF. After the animals had been treated with a solution of amino acids enriched with BCAAs, their general state became normal, as did the plasma amino acid pattern and the levels of phenylalanine, tyrosine, tryptophan, phenylethanolamine, octopamine and 5-hydroxyindoleacetic acid in the CSF.

The hypothesis is also supported by the fact that the octopamine plasma levels in patients with liver cirrhosis are raised and that they correlate with the stage of HE (Nespoli et al, 1981).

James et al (1979) proposed a modification of the hypothesis in that they tried to amalgamate the ammonia hypothesis with that of false neurotransmitters. They saw the possibility of uniting the two hypotheses in the following way.

1. Raised ammonia levels, through increased glucagon secretion, directly influence the composition of the plasma amino acid spectrum.
2. As a result of the raised cerebral ammonia levels, increased conversion of glutamate to glutamine takes place which results in a rapid exchange of brain glutamine for plasma neutral amino acids. By these means increased quantities of AAAs reach the brain and provide the basis for the production of false neurotransmitters.

The 'hypothesis of false neurotransmitters' has been questioned in the meantime. Zieve and Olsen (1977), in animal experiments, reassessed the importance of octopamine in the development of coma in HE. Following intraventricular administration of octopamine in a concentration up to 20 000 times greater than normal and simultaneous reduction of dopamine and noradrenaline levels by 90%, they found no changes in the vigilance or motor activity of the animals. Later it could be shown in a series of experiments that the production of catecholamines in the brain is not affected in HE. When examining the brains of patients with HE and liver cirrhosis, Cuilleret et al

(1980) found no essential changes in dopamine or noradrenaline levels compared to controls. The octopamine levels were significantly higher in the controls than in the cirrhotic patients. Comparable findings were published by Bergeron et al (1989a,b). On autopsy examination of brain sections from cirrhotic patients with HE, they found, in comparison to controls, that although the phenylalanine and tyrosine levels were raised in HE patients (as was to be expected according to the hypothesis of false neurotransmitters), there was no difference in the respective levels of BCAAs (valine, leucine and isoleucine). Additionally, they showed that there was no reduction in the levels of dopamine and noradrenaline in the brains of HE patients but that regionally, with stable dopamine levels, raised levels of the dopamine metabolites homovanillinic acid and 3-methoxytyramine were present (which indicates increased dopamine metabolism) and also that the noradrenaline level was simultaneously raised.

As early as 1982, Borg et al (1982) found raised noradrenaline, adrenaline and dopamine levels in the CSF of patients with HE. At the same time they also found raised levels of the false neurotransmitters octopamine and tyramine. Compared to controls, the dopa levels were unchanged. Borg et al interpreted the raised catecholamine levels in the CSF to be the result of an increased availability of tyrosine and increased release of noradrenaline from storage.

Recently, Moos Knudsen et al (1991) queried, with good reason, the hypothesis that an increase of the amino acid transport over the blood–brain barrier has an influence on neurotransmitter metabolism. In a study of the function of the carrier system for neutral amino acids across the blood–brain barrier in patients with cirrhosis and HE, they established that the permeability of the blood–brain barrier for neutral amino acids is unchanged. Consequently, the rise in the amino acid levels in the brain is not the sequel of altered carrier function but reflects only the altered plasma amino acid levels. In this connection, Moos Knudsen et al maintain that it is questionable to infer changes in the synaptic cleft from increased transport of transmitter precursors in the brain, especially since the permeability of the barrier for amino acids passing from the brain into the blood is 10–20 times as high as in the other direction and only one-sixth of the neutral amino acids which are transported into the brain are actually metabolized. The rest are promptly passed back into the blood.

Tryptophan and indole metabolism

In the hypothesis of false neurotransmitters, besides catecholamines, tryptophan metabolism is also regarded as important. Tryptophan is the precursor of the inhibitory neurotransmitter serotonin. It is present in the blood mostly bound to albumin. In cirrhotic patients, as a result of disturbed tryptophan metabolism (Rössle et al, 1986) and a displacement of tryptophan by free fatty acids or even bilirubin from plasma protein binding (Curzon and Knott, 1977), a rise in the free tryptophan plasma level occurs. Cirrhotic patients with HE show a significantly higher free tryptophan level, on average, than those without HE (Ono et al, 1978).

As Curzon and Knott (1977) showed, the synthesis of serotonin (5-hydroxytryptamine) is determined by the tryptophan concentration in the brain. Serotonin cannot pass the blood–brain barrier, and therefore all brain serotonin is produced inside the serotonergic neurones. The first step in serotonin synthesis is the hydroxylation of tryptophan. This is the rate-limiting process. The corresponding enzyme, tryptophan hydroxylase, is not usually saturated with tryptophan. Increased substrate, therefore, leads to augmented serotonin synthesis. The serotonin synthesis takes place in the cytoplasm. Part of the serotonin is then stored in vesicles and the rest is metabolized directly in the cytoplasm: into 5-hydroxyindoleacetic acid (5-HIAA) or, in negligible amounts, into the neurotoxic metabolite 5-hydroxytryptophol. The 5-HIAA levels are considered a measure of serotonin metabolism. In humans, serotonin synthesis only plays a small role in the total tryptophan metabolism. Tryptophan is mainly metabolized into kynurenines by means of a pyrrolase in the liver, kidney, intestines and brain. Both metabolites, serotonin as well as the kynurenines, are supposed to be of significance in the pathophysiology of HE.

An indication of the involvement of the serotonergic system in HE is the rise in the levels of serotonin, tryptamine, 5-hydroxytryptophan (5-HTP), the direct precursor of serotonin, and 5-HIAA in the CSF of patients in stages II and III of HE. In stage IV the levels of serotonin and tryptamine fall although they still lie above those of the control group.

5-HTP levels sink below the control levels and the 5-HIAA levels continue to rise (Borg et al, 1982). These findings suggest increased serotonin metabolism, but it is not clear whether this is significant for serotonergic neurotransmission.

Serotonin is usually to be found in high concentrations in the medulla oblongata and substantia nigra, and in medium concentrations in the putamen, pallidum, thalamus and hypothalamus (Hardy et al, 1987). Changes in serotonin metabolism should therefore be studied in these areas of the brain, where possible. Bergeron et al (1989b) studied the levels of serotonin, 5-HTP and 5-HIAA in homogenates of the caudatum, and frontal and prefrontal cortex of cirrhotic patients who had died in hepatic coma. There were no changes found in the concentrations of serotonin or 5-HTP. On the other hand, 5-HIAA levels were markedly raised compared to the controls in both the caudatum and prefrontal cortex. These findings support the assumption of increased serotonin turnover, already postulated in several experiments, mostly in animals (Cummings et al, 1976; Borg et al, 1982; Bengtsson et al, 1985; Mans et al, 1987; Bugge et al, 1988).

In a subsequent study, Bergeron et al (1990) determined the 5-HTP, serotonin and 5-HIAA levels in various areas of the cortex and brain-stem and in the striatum of rats with PCS and compared them to sham-operated animals before and after ammonia loading. There was a slight elevation in the levels of serotonin in the cortex and an increase in 5-HTP and 5-HIAA levels in all the areas studied in the shunt-operated animals, when compared to the controls. The serotonin turnover was, therefore, raised in the PCS rats. Following ammonia administration, there was no significant change in the serotonin and 5-HTP levels in the PCS rats. By contrast, 5-HIAA levels rose in all brain regions studied, in precoma (10–15 min after injection) as well as in coma (about 20 min after injection). There were no differences in the two coma stages in terms of these changes. The changes in serotonin turnover, therefore, do not seem to be responsible for the coma in the animals. They seem, rather, to be important for the early signs of HE—such as disturbances in the sleep patterns and diurnal rhythms or a decrease in spontaneous voluntary movement. This is supported by the findings of Warbritton et al (1978), in which a reduction in the spontaneous and stimulated locomotor activity of rats was observed after intraventricular infusion of serotonin, and by the results of Wojcik et al (1980), which showed a rise in the levels of serotonin and 5-HIAA accompanied by changes in the sleep pattern of rats following intraperitoneal administration of tryptophan. The findings of Bergeron et al (1990) and of Bengtsson et al (1986, 1987), who could not establish a correlation between serotonin turnover and the degree of HE, refute the role of serotonin metabolism in the later HE stage.

Bengtsson (1991), on the grounds of his own very varied results in relation to serotonin turnover in different animal models of HE, questioned whether serotonin turnover had any part to play in the development of HE. He pointed out that, on the basis of the available data on both serotonin and catecholamine metabolism, it cannot be decided whether the neurotransmitter pool is involved. He recommends that, instead of further studies on metabolism, more attention should be paid to the modulation of monoamine receptors—as is already the case in biologically oriented psychiatric research.

As already mentioned, increased tryptophan levels in the plasma and brain lead to a rise of both serotonin and kynurenine synthesis, whereby the same doses of tryptophan in experiments increased kynurenine synthesis by many times more than that of serotonin (Freese et al, 1990). The most relevant kynurenine is quinolinic acid (QUIN). It is synthesized in astrocytes and is extremely neurotoxic. In animal experiments axon-sparing lesions were found after injection of QUIN directly into the brain (Schwarcz et al, 1983). QUIN is considered to be instrumental in the development of various neurological diseases—Huntington's chorea, for example, and temporal lobe epilepsy. It could also play a role in the development of HE, for QUIN levels were raised in both the CSF of patients with hepatic failure (Moroni et al, 1986a) and the brains of PCS rats (Moroni et al, 1986b). The QUIN levels, like those of 5-HIAA, could be further raised in the brains of PCS rats after administration of ammonia. In this connection, the findings of Bucci et al (1982) are interesting: they found histological changes in the brains of PCS rats, in contrast to healthy controls, after long-term administration of tryptophan—an increased number of enlarged astrocytes and neuronal lesions. Whether these changes, too, are partly due to the effect of QUIN is open to discussion.

Another mechanism involving QUIN which should be discussed is the reduced binding of glutamate to its NMDA receptor, because QUIN acts as an NMDA receptor agonist (Peterson et al, 1990).

Glutamate

Glutamate and aspartate appear to be the most important excitatory neurotransmitters in the mammalian brain. They act through three different receptor systems which are differentiated via various synthetic agonists: NMDA, quisqualate and kainate. The levels of aspartate and glutamate are decreased in the brains of cirrhotic patients, especially in the caudatum as well as prefrontally and in the brain-stem (Butterworth et al, 1987; Lavoie et al, 1987). In hepatectomized rats, PCS rats and those injected intraperitoneally with ammonium salts, total glutamate levels were lowered in the brain whereas the neurotransmitter pool portion of the glutamate rose (Hindfelt et al, 1977; Moroni et al, 1983). Peterson et al (1990) showed that the binding of L-glutamate to the NMDA receptor around the corpus striatum, in various cortical areas and in the hippocampus, was lowered by almost 40% in rats following portocaval anastomosis. Binding to the quisqualate and kainate receptors was unchanged. The cause of reduced glutamate binding to the NMDA receptor is not known. Besides the already mentioned possible QUIN effect, a down-regulation of the receptor as a result of an increased glutamate availability in the synaptic cleft is discussed. This is the consequence of reduced reuptake from the synaptic cleft, the cause of which has also not yet been explained. The supposition that ammonia inhibits the reuptake of glutamate and aspartate has been investigated in a study by Grüngreiff et al (1991a). Following the incubation of hippocampal slices of rats in the CSF or serum of patients with HE, the high-affinity uptake of glutamate and aspartate was significantly lower than that in control serum or control body fluid; the inhibition of the uptake correlated with the degree of HE and with the ammonia levels. In a series of experiments in which the serum was progressively diluted and the ammonia concentration was kept constant, it could be shown that still other factors must play a role in the inhibition of the reuptake because, despite constant ammonia content, the least diluted samples of serum displayed the strongest inhibition.

The inhibition of glutamate and aspartate reuptake and the subsequent protracted stay of the transmitter in the synaptic cleft may be an explanation for the psychogenic changes in patients with HE, such as euphoria or anxiety. The lowered reuptake eventually leads to a depletion of the pool which could finally lead to lethargy and coma.

Gamma-aminobutyric acid (GABA)

GABA is the most important inhibitory neurotransmitter in the mammalian brain. Catalysed by glutamate dehydrogenase in the presynaptic neurones, it is synthesized from glutamate and stored in intracellular vesicles. When released from these storage sites, GABA binds to the specific GABA receptor in the postsynaptic membrane. The receptor is part of a so-called 'supramolecular complex' composed of several subunits surrounding chloride ionophore, which is the active component of the receptor. The width of the ionophore is regulated by the GABA receptor. Activation of the GABA receptor leads to the opening of the ionophore and chloride inflow with subsequent hyperpolarization of the postsynaptic membrane. The effect of GABA on the chloride channel can be modulated in various ways, for example by the benzodiazepine, (Bz) receptor, which is a further part of the 'supramolecular complex'. The frequency of the GABA-regulated chloride inflow at the ionophore rises in the presence of Bz receptor agonists. Barbiturates, on the other hand, modulate the effect of GABA in that they bind in the chloride channel and bring about an extension of the GABA-induced opening period of the ionophore.

Schafer and Jones (1982) put forward the hypothesis of an involvement of GABA in HE on the following grounds:

1. Similar visual evoked potentials (VEP) changes occurred in rabbits with galactosamine-induced FHF and those with barbiturate- or Bz-induced coma.
2. A 12-fold raised level of 'GABA-like' activity was measured in the plasma of rabbits with FHF employing a radio-receptor assay.
3. Intestinal flora synthesize GABA. In cases of limited hepatic functioning or marked PCS it is not catabolized by the liver in the usual way and, therefore, contributes to raised GABA plasma levels.
4. In cases of acute hepatic failure, there is increased permeability of the blood–brain barrier to aminoisobutyric acid, a GABA isomer.
5. In studies of receptor binding of [^{3}H]GABA and [^{3}H]flunitrazepam to postsynaptic membranes of rabbits with FHF, an increase of both GABA and Bz receptors could be shown.

On the basis of these experiments, Schafer and Jones formulated the following hypothesis. In cases of hepatic failure, GABA, produced by the intestinal flora, and present in the plasma in increased quantities because of reduced metabolization in the liver, passes through the blood–brain barrier and induces its own receptors at the postsynaptic neuronal membranes. In this manner GABA formed in the intestine participates in the development of HE. The increased numbers of GABA and Bz receptors are the cause of the raised sensitivity to barbiturates and benzodiazepines observed in patients with hepatic failure.

This hypothesis is questionable on various counts. It is doubtful, for example, whether the cause of a coma can be concluded from the form of VEP, as evoked potentials, like EEG, react to the most varied noxa in the same way. It is also controversial whether an increase in GABA plasma levels really occurs in HE. It is true that an increase in these levels has been described by various workers in animal experiments (Maddison et al, 1987) and in patients with FHF or portosystemic encephalopathy (PSE) (Ferenci et al, 1983; Minuk et al, 1985; Levy and Losowsky, 1989). However, radio-receptor binding, the method used frequently in these studies to determine the GABA in plasma, is not specific. When other methods were used, such as gas chromatography and mass spectrometry, no changes in the GABA plasma levels were established (Moroni et al, 1987). A further point against the GABA hypothesis is that the GABA level in plasma represents only a tenth of that in the brain, so that excessive amounts of GABA would have to pass the blood–brain barrier in order to show an effect (Mans, 1991). In fact, no changes in the GABA contents of the brain were identified in various animal experiments or in patients with HE (Record et al, 1976; Butterworth et al, 1987; Roy et al, 1988).

Contradictory findings are also documented concerning the transport of GABA over the blood–brain barrier. In rabbits with FHF, the passage of α-aminobutyric acid, a GABA isomer, as well as GABA itself has been demonstrated (van Berlo et al, 1987; Bassett et al, 1990), whereas no increased uptake of GABA was shown in the brains of rats with FHF (Knudsen et al, 1988). In experimental animals with PCS there was, likewise, no change in the cerebral uptake of GABA (Huet et al, 1984; Roy et al, 1988).

The known mechanisms of receptor regulation contradict the assumption of Schafer and Jones (1982) that raised cerebral GABA levels induce an increase in the density of GABA receptors. An excess of GABA should lead to a down-regulation of the receptors. Baraldi and Zeneroli (1982) support this view: although they, too, found an increased density of GABA receptors in rats with FHF, they did not attribute this to increased provision of GABA but to a reduction in the activity of glutamate dehydrogenase in the presynaptic neurone and, thereby, reduced GABA synthesis. The density and affinity of GABA receptors, as well as Bz receptors, in the various stages of HE have been examined in many different experimental animals and in post mortem studies, but no corresponding findings could be reported. This is attributed to the different methods used in the studies. If the results of studies to date are viewed in the light of known sources of methodical error, it seems more likely that there are no changes in the GABA receptors, or even the Bz receptors, in HE (Mans, 1991).

In general, the original hypothesis on the involvement of GABA in HE does not hold up. Nevertheless there are a number of findings which make increased GABA tonus in HE probable. Bassett et al (1987) reported the same findings in rabbits with FHF induced by galactosamine and HE stages II–III, in terms of behavioural changes and VEP, as in rabbits injected with diazepam or γ-vinyl-GABA, which inhibits the catabolism of GABA. Significant improvement in HE, with increased frequency of movement of the animals, increased awareness and return of the reaction to painful stimuli as well as normalization of muscle tone, was temporarily achieved by the administration of bicuculline, a GABA antagonist, or flumazenil, a Bz antagonist. The animals' VEP also became normal with these substances. Moreover, it was noticeable that the animals with HE demonstrated cerebral convulsions only after higher doses of bicuculline than the control animals. Isopropylbicyclophosphate, an antagonist of the GABA–Bz–Cl$^-$ ionophore, led to similar effects to those of bicuculline or flumazenil. The behavioural and VEP changes induced by γ-vinyl-GABA or diazepam could be eliminated, in the same way, by bicuculline or flumazenil.

The following conclusions may be drawn from these results:

1. In cases of FHF, HE coincides with increased GABA activity.
2. HE can be positively influenced by blockage of the GABA or Bz receptors.

3. Bz receptor antagonists could be valuable in the treatment of HE (GABA antagonists carry the risk of triggering convulsions).
4. A substance similar to a Bz receptor agonist could be present in HE.

These findings were confirmed in principle by Gammal et al (1990) in investigations on rats with FHF and HE induced by thioacetamide. Further confirmation of participation of the GABAergic system in HE came from the comprehensive studies by Basile et al (1991), who analysed the spontaneous activity from cerebellar Purkinje cells in rabbits with HE in stages II–III and controls. The spontaneous firing rate of the Purkinje cells dropped in both groups after administration of muscimol, a GABA agonist, whereby these cells in the HE group were four- to five-fold more sensitive. They were also hypertensive to flunitrazepam. Flumazenil induced a slight reduction of the firing rate in the controls, due to its limited intrinsic agonist activity; however, it caused an activation in the HE animals. Ro 14-7437, a pure Bz receptor antagonist, had no effect on the controls but produced a dose-dependent increase in the firing rate in the HE animals. When Ro 14-7437 was added to the incubation medium before the administration of muscimol, the HE neurones were no longer hypersensitive. These results suggest that Bz receptor agonists are present in HE, and increase the potency of the available GABA.

In order to demonstrate such Bz receptor ligands, Basile et al (1990) carried out autoradiographic studies on microsections of rabbit brains. They showed that in rabbits with HE the binding of [^{3}H]flumazenil was significantly decreased compared to controls. If the microsecretions were washed before incubation, there was no difference in the [^{3}H]flumazenil binding. The same results were achieved with [^{3}H]flunitrazepam. In a further experiment the binding of [^{3}H]flumazenil to Bz receptors on washed membranes of the cortex of healthy rats could be inhibited by brain extract from rats with HE. The extracts showed the characteristics of a typical Bz receptor agonist.

The group finally succeeded in extracting the Bz receptor agonist-like substances out of brain homogenate. Some of these substances had similar retention times to known benzodiazepines in the HPLC. The total amount of Bz receptor ligands was about four times as high in the HE rats as in the controls. In qualitative analyses diazepam and *N*-desmethyldiazepam could be demonstrated (Basile et al, 1991).

Meanwhile Olasmaa et al (1991) and Mullen et al (1990) have been able to show the presence of Bz-like substances in the CSF, plasma, urine and saliva of patients with HE. The Bz-like activity in the plasma correlated with the degree of HE (Mullen et al, 1990). The Bz-like substances showed the following characteristics: they are heat-stable, non-polar, resistant to proteolytic enzymes and have a molecular weight of less than 1000. In the blood they are mostly bound to proteins. They prove to be competitive inhibitors of the Bz binding. They bind specifically to the Bz receptors, whereby their receptor binding is strengthened, as is that of all Bz receptor agonists, by GABA.

The evidence for these Bz receptor ligands in animal models of HE as well as in patients with HE, and also reports on the successful application of Bz receptor antagonists in both animal models and patients with HE, allow the assumption that the BAGA-Bz receptor complex plays a part in the development of HE (Grimm et al, 1988; Bansky et al, 1989). To what extent this is so remains to be clarified.

THERAPY

Established means

In the treatment of HE most attention is still directed towards achieving a reduction in ammonia production or resorption, emphasizing the importance of ammonia in the pathogenesis of HE. Although the principles of HE therapy were introduced long ago and are well known, they will be briefly outlined here for the sake of completeness.

Factors precipitating an acute HE episode in cirrhotic patients include gastrointestinal bleeding, alkalosis and hypokalaemia with subsequent hyperammonaemia on administration of diuretics, infection, sedative overdosage or constipation. The elimination of these causes often leads to improvement without any further measures. If no such trigger can be identified, a 'spontaneous HE episode' must be assumed. As these are frequently the result of limited protein tolerance, it is sensible to prescribe a protein-free diet for several days and then slowly increase the protein intake again: from approximately 20 g/day, increasing by 10 g/day weekly up to at least 40 g/day, or better 60–60 g/day. If this amount is not tolerated, the protein can be partly replaced by a mixture of BCAAs which can produce a positive nitrogen balance to approximately the same order of magnitude as a corresponding amount of food protein, without precipitating HE (Horst et al, 1984). The fact that vegetable protein is better tolerated than animal protein is also of importance in this connection. The reasons for this are acceleration of gastrointestinal transit and increased ingestion and elimination of nitrogenous substances by the intestinal bacteria in a vegetarian diet (Maier, 1987). In fact, a wholly vegetarian diet is not usually accepted by patients because of gastrointestinal discomfort.

In addition to the above measures, the use of lactulose and neomycin in the treatment of HE is undisputed. Both substances significantly reduce ammonia synthesis in the intestine and, thereby, lead to a drop in the plasma ammonia level. Neomycin acts by reducing the intestinal flora and inhibiting glutamine splitting in the mucosa. The latter action is also attributed to lactulose. Further mechanisms of lactulose action discussed are: (1) acidification of the intestinal contents, which causes ammonia to be present in increased amounts as ammonium ion, which does not diffuse through the intestinal wall; (2) accelerated passage through the intestines; (3) stimulation of the incorporation of ammonia into bacterial protein; and (4) reduction of the metabolization of proteins and amino acids into short-chain fatty acids (Mortensen et al, 1990). Lactulose is preferred to neomycin because of its fewer side-effects. If a satisfactory result is not obtained, both substances can be administered in combination, whereby an additive effect is achieved. The lactulose should be given in doses which produce two to three soft stools a day. Administration of about 60–150 ml is usually required (Maier, 1987).

Recent developments

More recent treatment methods include giving lactitol instead of lactulose, administration of BCAAs parenterally or orally, administration of zinc sulphate, zinc acetate, sodium benzoate, sodium phenylacetate or ornithine-aspartate, and, finally, the use of Bz receptor antagonists.

Lactitol

Lactitol is a lactulose-analogous disaccharide which is neither metabolized nor resorbed in the small intestine but is excessively metabolized by the colonic bacteria. It can be manufactured in crystalline form and has the advantage over lactulose of not being very sweet. It is usually better tolerated by the patients. In controlled studies it was as effective as lactulose in the treatment of both acute HE episodes in cirrhotics and latent HE (Morgan and Hawley, 1987; Morgan et al, 1989). In cases of HE episodes the symptoms improved more rapidly with lactitol than with lactulose. Acceptance by the patients was comparable for the two substances.

BCAAs

BCAAs are introduced into the treatment of HE for two reasons: firstly, because of the amino acid imbalance observed in cases of HE which is considered to be one of its causes, and, secondly, because of the severe muscle catabolism which the provision of BCAAs should counteract. The effectiveness of BCAAs, both intravenously administered in cases of HE episodes and orally in patients with subclinical encephalopathy, has been investigated in a number of controlled studies (Maier, 1987; Marchesini et al, 1991). So far, however, no confirmatory results have been achieved. Even on meta-analyses of the above-mentioned studies, there are contradictory results. Eriksson and Conn (1989) found that BCAAs had no significant effect; Naylor et al (1989) came to the conclusion that BCAAs cause a decrease in the mortality rate for patients with HE episodes. The various authors agree that a positive nitrogen balance can be achieved with BCAA treatment and that, if necessary, BCAAs can be administered in patients with decompensating cirrhosis and protein intolerance in order to counteract catabolism (Horst et al, 1984).

Zinc

It has been known for decades that cirrhotic patients suffer from a lack of zinc. The plasma levels in patients with HE are even lower when compared to those without. Recently a closer connection between zinc and ammonia levels as well as the importance of zinc in normal brain functioning have been confirmed. A lack of zinc leads to deterioration of urea synthesis and hyperammonaemia. Furthermore, zinc is attributed with a role in regulating the activity of the key enzymes of GABA metabolism. Zinc is also thought to be important in the synthesis of nucleic acids and membrane stability (Grüngreiff et al, 1991b; Riggio et al, 1991). In the light of these facts, various investigations on the effect of zinc in HE have been carried out recently. Reding et al (1984), in a study involving 22 patients with chronic HE, reported a positive effect on both the synthesis of urea and the test results in Number Correction test (NCT). In case reports, too, a positive effect of zinc sulphate or zinc acetate was described (Riggio et al, 1991; van der Rijt et al, 1991). Riggio et al (1991), however, could find no significant effect of zinc treatment on the various parameters of the PSE index (mental state, flapping tremor, EEG, NCT and blood ammonia) in 14 cirrhotic patients with slight HE in a recent randomized cross-over study. The importance of this new therapy, therefore, cannot yet be assessed.

Sodium benzoate and sodium phenylacetate

To date, there are very few data available on the effectiveness of sodium benzoate or sodium phenylacetate. These substances increase the elimination of conjugated nitrogen in the urine and have been successfully used in the treatment of children with congenital hyperammonaemia. This was the reason for Mendenhall et al (1986) testing their effect on patients with chronic HE. In seven out of eight patients treated with sodium benzoate there was a decrease in the ammonia levels and a reduction in the PSE index of nearly 50%. The effect of sodium phenylacetate was not significant.

Amino acids involved in the urea cycle

Ammonia levels can also be lowered, giving ornithine- or arginine-containing substances. The first reports on this treatment appeared more than 30 years ago; however, there are very few controlled studies available. Leweling et al (1991) showed, in a study involving 16 patients with cirrhosis and HE 0–II, that ornithine-aspartate in a dose of 20 g or 40 g decreased the postprandial elevation of blood ammonia levels, compared to placebo. The practical importance of this is being investigated clinically at present.

Benzodiazepine receptor antagonists

In contrast to the many measures to bring about a reduction in the plasma ammonia levels, the use of Bz receptor antagonists such as flumazenil represents a new therapeutic principle. It is based on the evidence of raised GABA tonus in HE, as has been described in detail above. According to Meier and Bansky (1990), positive results of uncontrolled studies were obtained in two-thirds of 43 patients with cirrhosis or FHF and HE. The largest groups have been examined by Grimm et al (1988) and Bansky et al (1989). Grimm et al administered flumazenil, in the form of a brief infusion, in 11 patients with FHF and nine episodes of HE in cirrhotic patients. The dosage was varied according to effect and ranged from 2 mg over 5 min to 15 mg over 3 h. The therapy was obviously successful in six out of eleven HE episodes in cases of FHF and six out of nine episodes in cirrhotic patients. The improvement was evident within 3–60 min and led to a change in the degree of HE of about one stage. Complete recovery from the symptoms was not achieved. Four patients had no regression; in the others the improvement lasted 30–240 min. Bansky et al achieved improvement in 9 out of 14 cirrhotic patients with HE. The non-responders in both groups demonstrated additional complications such as cerebral oedema or renal failure, or showed only slight HE. In spite of these encouraging reports, the effectiveness of Bz antagonists in cases of HE cannot be regarded as having been confirmed. Unfortunately, 'spontaneous' improvement is often observed in cases of HE and it cannot be ruled out with certainty in all investigations that benzodiazepines still present in the blood were antagonized. In order to prove the effectiveness of Bz antagonists, therefore, larger, and, if possible, multi-centre, controlled studies are necessary.

SUMMARY

The pathophysiology of HE has not yet been clarified. At present the main mechanisms under discussion are the combined effects of different toxins, such as ammonia, mercaptans, phenols and short- and medium-chain fatty acids, as well as a change particularly in GABAergic and glutamatergic neurotransmission. In this chapter the current views on the importance of these individual factors in the pathophysiology of HE are discussed; possible connections between changes in neurotransmission and the effect of different neurotoxins are presented. In addition, possible therapies resulting from recent knowledge of the pathophysiology of this disease are discussed, such as the use of Bz receptor antagonists.

REFERENCES

Bansky G, Meier PJ, Riederer E et al (1989) Effects of the benzodiazepine receptor antagonist flumazenil in hepatic encephalopathy in humans. *Gastroenterology* **97:** 744–750.

Baraldi M & Zenerolli ML (1982) Experimental hepatic encephalopathy: changes in the binding of gamma-aminobutyric acid. *Science* **216:** 427–429.

Basile AS, Ostrowski NL, Gammal SH et al (1990) The $GABA_A$ receptor complex in hepatic encephalopathy: autoradiographic evidence for the presence of elevated levels of a benzodiazepine receptor ligand. *Neuropsychopharmacology* **3:** 61–71.

Basile AS, Skolnick P & Jones EA (1991) Benzodiazepine receptor ligands and hepatic encephalopathy: electrophysiological and neurochemical studies. In Bengtsson F, Jeppsson B, Almdal T & Vilstrup H (eds) *Progress in Hepatic Encephalopathy and Metabolic Nitrogen Exchange*, pp 131–136. Boca Raton: CRC Press.

Bassett ML, Mullen KD, Skolnick P et al (1987) Amelioration of hepatic encephalopathy by pharmacologic antagonism of the $GABA_A$–benzodiazepine receptor complex in a rabbit model of fulminant hepatic failure. *Gastroenterology* **93:** 1069–1077.

Bassett ML, Mullen KD, Scholz B et al (1990) Increased brain uptake of γ-aminobutyric acid in a rabbit model of hepatic encephalopathy. *Gastroenterology* **98:** 747–757.

Bengtsson F (1991) Round table discussion on brain monoamines: some personal reflections. In Bengtsson F, Jeppsson B, Almdal T & Vilstrup H (eds) *Progress in Hepatic Encephalopathy and Metabolic Nitrogen Exchange*, pp 233–239. Boca Raton: CRC Press.

Bengtsson F, Gage FH, Jeppsson B et al (1985) Brain monoamine metabolism and behaviour in portocaval shunted rats. *Experimental Neurology* **90:** 21–35.

Bengtsson F, Nobin A, Falck B et al (1986) Portocaval shunt in the rat: selective alterations in the behavior and brain serotonin. *Pharmacology, Biochemistry and Behaviour* **24:** 1611–1616.

Bengtsson F, Bugge M, Vagianos C et al (1987) Brain serotonin metabolism and behavior in rats with carbon-tetrachloride induced liver cirrhosis. *Research in Experimental Medicine* **187:** 429–438.

Bergeron M, Pomier Layrargues G & Butterworth RF (1989a) Aromatic and branched-chain amino acids in autopsied brain tissue from cirrhotic patients with hepatic encephalopathy. *Metabolic Brain Diseases* **4(3):** 169–176.

Bergeron M, Reader TA, Pomier Layrargues G & Butterworth RF (1989b) Monoamines and metabolites in autopsied brain tissue from cirrhotic patients with hepatic encephalopathy. *Neurochemical Research* **14(9):** 853–859.

Bergeron M, Swain MS, Reader TA et al (1990) Effect of ammonia on brain serotonin metabolism in relation to function in the portocaval shunted rat. *Journal of Neurochemistry* **55:** 222–229.

Bloch P, Delorme ML & Rapin JR (1978) Reversible modifications of neurotransmitters of the brain in experimental acute hepatic coma. *Surgery, Gynecology and Obstetrics* **146:** 551.

Borg J, Warter JM, Schlienger JL et al (1982) Neurotransmitter modifications in human cerebrospinal fluid and serum during hepatic encephalopathy. *Journal of the Neurological Sciences* **57:** 343–356.

Bucci L, Ioppolo A, Chiavarelli R & Biogotti A (1982) The central nervous system toxicity of long-term oral administration of L-tryptophan to portocaval shunted rats. *British Journal of Experimental Pathology* **63:** 235–241.

Bugge M, Bengtsson F, Nobin A et al (1988) Serotonin metabolism in the rat brain following ammonia administration. In Soeters PB, Wilson JHP, Meijer AJ & Holm E (eds) *Advances in Ammonia Metabolism and Hepatic Encephalopathy*, pp 461–466. Amsterdam: Elsevier Science Publishers.

Butterworth RF (1991) Pathophysiology of hepatic encephalopathy: the ammonia hypothesis revisited. In Bengtsson F, Jeppsson B, Almdal T & Vilstrup H (eds) *Hepatic Encephalopathy and Metabolic Nitrogen Exchange*, pp 9–24. Boca Raton: CRC Press.

Butterworth RF, Lavoie J, Giguere JF et al (1987) Cerebral GABA-ergic and glutamatergic function in hepatic encephalopathy. *Neurochemical Pathology* **6:** 131–144.

Conn HO & Lieberthal MM (1978) *The Hepatic Coma Syndromes and Lactulose*. Baltimore: Williams and Wilkins.

Crossley IR, Wardle EN & Williams R (1983) Biochemical mechanisms of hepatic encephalopathy. *Clinical Science* **64:** 247–252.

Cuilleret G, Pomier Layrargues G, Pons F et al (1980) Changes in brain catecholamine levels in human cirrhotic hepatic encephalopathy. *Gut* **21:** 565–569.

Cummings MG, Soeters PB, James JH et al (1976) Regional brain indoleamine metabolism following chronic portocaval anastomosis in the rat. *Journal of Neurochemistry* **27:** 501–509.

Curzon G & Knott PJ (1977) Environmental, toxicological, and related aspects of tryptophan metabolism with particular reference to the central nervous system. *CRC Critical Reviews in Toxicology* **5:** 145–187.

Eriksson LS & Conn HO (1989) Branched chain amino acids in the management of hepatic encephalopathy: an analysis of variants. *Hepatology* **10:** 228–246.

Fan P, Lavoie J, Le NLO et al (1990) Neurochemical and electrophysiological studies on the inhibitory effect of ammonium ions on synaptic transmission in slices of rat hippocampus: evidence for a postsynaptic action. *Neuroscience* **37:** 327.

Ferenci P, Schafer DF, Kleinberger G et al (1983) Serum levels of γ-aminobutyric acid like activity in patients with acute and chronic hepatocellular disease. *Lancet* **ii:** 811–814.

Fischer JE & Baldessarini RJ (1971) False neurotransmitters and hepatic failure. *Lancet* **2**: 75–80.

Freese A, Swartz KJ, During MJ & Martin JB (1990) Kynurenine metabolites of tryptophan: implications for neurologic diseases. *Neurology* **40**: 691–695.

Gammal SH, Basile AS, Geller D et al (1990) Reversal of the behavioral and electrophysiological abnormalities of an animal model of hepatic encephalopathy by benzodiazepine receptor ligands. *Hepatology* **11**: 371–378.

Gerok W (1985) Metabolische Grundlagen der hepatischen Encephalopathie. *Internist* **26**: 377–387.

Grimm G, Ferenci P, Katzenschlager R et al (1988) Improvement of hepatic encephalopathy treated with flumazenil. *Lancet* **ii**: 1392–1394.

Grüngreiff K, Wolf G, Schmidt W et al (1991a) High-affinity uptake of transmitter glutamate (GLU) in brain tissue with reference to hepatic encephalopathy (HE). *Zeitschrift für Gastroenterologie* **29 (supplement 2)**: 95–100.

Grüngreiff K, Franke D, Lößner B et al (1991b) Zinc deficiency—a factor in the pathogenesis of hepatic encephalopathy? *Zeitschrift für Gastroenterologie* **29 (supplement 2)**: 101–106.

Hardy JA, Wester P, Backstrom I et al (1987) The regional distribution of dopamine and serotonin uptake and transmitter concentrations in the human brain. *Neurochemistry International* **10(4)**: 445–450.

Häussinger D (1983) Hepatocyte heterogeneity in glutamine and ammonia metabolism and the role of an intercellular glutamine cycle during ureogenesis in perfused rat liver. *European Journal of Biochemistry* **133**: 269–275.

Hindfelt B, Plum F & Duffy TE (1977) Effect of acute ammonia intoxication on cerebral metabolism in rats with portocaval shunts. *Journal of Clinical Investigation* **59**: 386–396.

Holmin T, Agardh CD, Alinder G et al (1983) The influence of total hepatectomy on cerebral energy state, ammonia-related amino acids of the brain and plasma amino acids in the rat. *European Journal of Clinical Investigations* **13**: 215–220.

Horst D, Grace ND, Conn HO et al (1984) Comparison of dietary protein with an oral branched-chain enriched amino acid supplement in chronic portal-systemic encephalopathy: a randomized controlled study. *Hepatology* **4**: 279–287.

Huet PM, Rocheleau B, Pomier Layrargues G & Willems B (1984) Blood–brain barrier in dogs with and without hepatic encephalopathy. In Kleinberger G, Ferenci P, Riederer P & Thaler H (eds) *Advances in Hepatic Encephalopathy and Urea Cycle Diseases*, pp 261–271. Basel: Karger.

James JH, Ziparo V, Jeppsson B & Fischer JE (1979) Hyperammonaemia, plasma amino acid imbalance, and blood–brain aminoacid transport: a unified theory of portal-systemic encephalopathy. *Lancet* **ii**: 772–775.

Knudsen GM, Poulsen HE & Paulson OB (1988) Blood–brain barrier permeability in galactosamine-induced hepatic encephalopathy. No evidence for increased GABA transport. *Journal of Hepatology* **6**: 187–192.

Lavoie J, Giguere JF, Pomier Layrargues G & Butterworth RT (1987) Amino acid changes in autopsied brain tissue from cirrhotic patients with hepatic encephalopathy. *Journal of Neurochemistry* **49**: 692–697.

Levy LJ & Losowsky MS (1989) Plasma gamma-aminobutyric acid concentrations provide evidence of different mechanisms in the pathogenesis of hepatic encephalopathy in acute and chronic liver disease. *Hepatogastroenterology* **36**: 494–498.

Leweling H, Kortsik C, Gladisch R et al (1991) Effects of ornithine aspartate on plasma ammonia and plasma amino acids in patients with liver cirrhosis. A double-blind, randomized study using a four-fold crossover design. In Bengtsson F, Jeppsson B, Almdal T & Vilstrup H (eds) *Progress in Hepatic Encephalopathy and Metabolic Nitrogen Exchange*, pp 377–389. Boca Raton: CRC Press.

Maddison JE, Dodd PR, Morrison M et al (1987) Plasma GABA, GABA-like activity and the brain GABA-benzodiazepine receptor complex in rats with chronic hepatic encephalopathy. *Hepatology* **7**: 621–628.

Maier KP (1987) Progress in the treatment of portal-systemic encephalopathy (PSE). *Journal of Hepatology* **5**: 355–361.

Maier KP & Gerok W (1985) Hyperammonemia and hepatic encephalopathy. In Kleinberger G, Ferenci P, Riederer P & Thaler H (eds) *Advances in Hepatic Encephalopathy and Urea Cycle Diseases*, pp 224–231. Basel: Karger.

Maier KP, Talke A & Gerok W (1979) Activities of urea-cycle enzymes in chronic liver disease. *Klinische Wochenschrift* **57**: 661–664.

Mans AM (1991) GABA neurotransmission and the GABA/benzodiazepine receptor in hepatic encephalopathy. In Bengtsson F, Jeppsson B, Almdal T & Vilstrup H (eds) *Progress in Hepatic Encephalopathy and Metabolic Nitrogen Exchange*, pp 115–129. Boca Raton: CRC Press.

Mans AM, Consevage MW, De Joseph MR & Hawkins RA (1987) Regional brain monoamines and their metabolites after portocaval shunting. *Metabolic Brain Diseases* **2**: 183–193.

Marchesini G, Bianchi G & Zoli M (1991) Oral branched chain amino acid treatment in chronic hepatic encephalopathy. In Bengtsson F, Jeppsson B, Almdal T & Vilstrup H (eds) *Progress in Hepatic Encephalopathy and Metabolic Nitrogen Exchange*, pp 291–301. Boca Raton: CRC Press.

Meier PJ & Bansky G (1990) Neue Möglichkeiten in der Therapie der hepatischen Enzephalopathie? *Schweizerische Medizinische Wochenschrift* **120 (15)**: 553–556.

Mendenhall CL, Rouster S, Marshall L & Weesner R (1986) A new therapy for portal systemic encephalopathy. *American Journal of Gastroenterology* **81 (7)**: 540–543.

Minuk GY, Winder A, Burgess ED & Sarjeant EJ (1985) Serum gamma-aminobutyric acid (GABA) levels in patients with hepatic encephalopathy. *Hepatogastroenterology* **32**: 171–174.

Moos Knudsen G, Scmidt J, Vilstrup H & Paulson OB (1991) Amino acids and the blood–brain barrier in hepatic encephalopathy. In Bengtsson F, Jeppsson B, Almdal T & Vilstrup H (eds) *Progress in Hepatic Encephalopathy and Metabolic Nitrogen Exchange*, pp 211–217. Boca Raton: CRC Press.

Morgan MY & Hawley KE (1987) Lactitol vs. lactulose in the treatment of acute hepatic encephalopathy in cirrhotic patients: a double-blind, randomized trial. *Hepatology* **7(6)**: 1278–1284.

Morgan MY, Alonso M & Stanger LC (1989) Lactitol and lactulose for the treatment of subclinical hepatic encephalopathy in cirrhotic patients. *Journal of Hepatology* **8**: 208–217.

Moroni F, Lombardi G, Monetti G & Cortesini C (1983) The release and neosynthesis of glutamic acid are increased in experimental models of hepatic encephalopathy. *Journal of Neurochemistry* **40**: 850–854.

Moroni F, Lombardi G, Carla V et al (1986a) Increase in the context of quinolinic acid in cerebrospinal fluid and frontal cortex of patients with hepatic failure. *Journal of Neurochemistry* **47**: 1667–1671.

Moroni F, Lombardi G, Carla V et al (1986b) Content of quinolinic acid and other tryptophan metabolites increases in brain regions of rats used as experimental models of hepatic encephalopathy. *Journal of Neurochemistry* **46**: 869–874.

Moroni F, Riggio O, Carla V et al (1987) Hepatic encephalopathy: lack of changes of γ-aminobutyric acid content in plasma and cerebrospinal fluid. *Hepatology* **7**: 816–820.

Mortensen PB, Holtug K, Bonnen H & Clausen MR (1990) The degradation of amino acids, proteins, and blood to short-chain fatty acids in colon is prevented by lactulose. *Gastroenterology* **98**: 353–360.

Mullen KD, Szauter KM & Kaminsky-Russ K (1990) 'Endogenous' benzodiazepine activity in body fluids of patients with hepatic encephalopathy. *Lancet* **i**: 81–83.

Naylor CD, O'Rourke K, Detsky AS & Baker JP (1989) Parenteral nutrition with branchedchain amino acids in hepatic encephalopathy. *Gastroenterology* **97**: 1033–1042.

Nespoli A, Bevilacqua G, Staudacher C et al (1981) Pathogenesis of hepatic encephalopathy and hyperdynamic syndrome in cirrhosis. *Archives of Surgery* **116**: 1129–1138.

Norenberg MD (1987) The role of astrocytes in hepatic encephalopathy. *Neurochemical Pathology* **6**: 13–33.

Olasmaa M, Rothstein JD, Guidotti A et al (1991) Endogenous benzodiazepine receptor ligands in human and animal hepatic encephalopathy. *Journal of Neurochemistry* **55**: 2015–2023.

Ono J, Hutson DG & Dombro RS (1978) Tryptophan and hepatic coma. *Gastroenterology* **74**: 196–200.

Peterson Ch, Giguere JF, Cotman CW & Butterworth RF (1990) Selective loss of N-methyl-D-aspartate-sensitive L-(^{3}H)-glutamate binding sites in rat brain following portocaval anastomosis. *Journal of Neurochemistry* **55**: 386–390.

Record CO, Buxton B, Chase RA et al (1976) Plasma and brain amino acids in fulminant hepatic failure and their relationship to hepatic encephalopathy. *European Journal of Clinical Investigation* **6**: 387–394.

Reding P, Duchateau J & Bataille C (1984) Oral zinc supplementation improves hepatic encephalopathy. Results of a randomised controlled trial. *Lancet* **2**: 493–495.

Riggio O, Merli M & Capocaccia L (1991) The role of zinc in the management of hepatic encephalopathy. In Bengtsson F, Jeppsson B, Almdal T & Vilstrup H (eds) *Progress in Hepatic Encephalopathy and Metabolic Nitrogen Exchange*, pp 303–312. Boca Raton: CRC Press.

Rössle M, Herz R, Klein B & Gerok W (1986) Tryptophan-Metabolismus bei Leibererkrankungen: Eine pharmakokinetische und enzymatische Untersuchung. *Klinische Wochenschrift* **64**: 590–594.

Roy S, Pomier Layrargues G, Butterworth RF & Huet PM (1988) Hepatic encephalopathy in cirrhotic and portocaval shunted dogs: lack of changes in brain GABA uptake, brain GABA levels, brain glutamic acid decarboxylase activity and brain postsynaptic GABA receptors. *Hepatology* **8**: 845–849.

Schafer DF & Jones EA (1982) Hepatic encephalopathy and the γ-aminobutyric-acid neurotransmitter system. *Lancet* **i**: 18–20.

Schwarcz R, Whetsell WO & Mangano RM (1983) Quinolinic acid: an endogenous metabolite that produces axon-sparing lesions in the rat striatum. *Science* **219**: 316–318.

Smith A, Rossi-Fanelli F, Ziparo V et al (1978) Alterations in plasma and CSF amino acids, amines, and metabolites in hepatic coma. *Annals of Surgery* **187**: 343–350.

Szerb JC & Butterworth RF (1991) Pre- and postsynaptic glutamatergic dysfunction in hepatic encephalopathy. In Bengtsson F, Jeppsson B, Almdal T & Vilstrup H (eds) *Progress in Hepatic Encephalopathy and Metabolic Nitrogen Exchange*, pp 183–195. Boca Raton: CRC Press.

Tangerman A (1991) The role of mercaptans in the pathogenesis of hepatic encephalopathy. In Bengtsson F, Jeppsson B, Almdal T & Vilstrup H (eds) *Progress in Hepatic Encephalopathy and Metabolic Nitrogen Exchange*, pp 259–270. Boca Raton: CRC Press.

van Berlo CLH, van den Bogaard AEJM, van Dongen JJ et al (1987) Comparison of blood–brain transfer of α-aminoisobutyric acid (AIB) in rabbit models of acute and chronic liver disease and acute organ ischemia. *Journal of Hepatology* **4 (supplement 1)**: S5.

van der Rijt CCD, Schalm SW, Schat H et al (1991) Overt hepatic encephalopathy precipitated by zinc deficiency. *Gastroenterology* **100**: 1114–1118.

Warbritton JD, Stewart RM & Baldessarini RJ (1978) Decreased locomotor activity and attenuation of amphetamine hyperactivity with intraventricular infusion of serotonin in the rat. *Brain Research* **143**: 373–382.

Wojcik WJ, Fornal C & Radulovacki M (1980) Effect of tryptophan on sleep in the rat. *Neuropharmacology* **19**: 163–167.

Zieve L (1984a) Ammonia: the old and the new. In Capocaccia L, Fischer JE & Rossi-Fanelli F (eds) *Hepatic Encephalopathy in Chronic Liver Failure*, pp 5–14. New York: Plenum Publishing Corporation.

Zieve L (1984b) Role of synergism in the pathogenesis of hepatic encephalopathy. In Capocaccia L, Fischer JE & Rossi-Fanelli F (eds) *Hepatic Encephalopathy in Chronic Liver Failure*, pp 15–23. New York: Plenum Publishing Corporation.

Zieve L (1991) Historical remarks and recent trends in hepatic encephalopathy. In Bengtsson F, Jeppsson B, Almdal T & Vilstrup H (eds) *Progress in Hepatic Encephalopathy and Metabolic Nitrogen Exchange*, pp 3–8. Boca Raton: CRC Press.

Zieve L & Olsen RL (1977) Can hepatic coma be caused by a reduction of brain noradrenalin or dopamine? *Gut* **18**: 688–691.

Index

Note: Page numbers of article titles are in **bold** type.

Acute variceal haemorrhage, 441–442, **451–460**
Alcoholic gastritis, 486
Aldosterone antagonists, 597–598
Amino acids in treatment of hepatic encephalopathy, 625
Ammonia, 609–613
Antidiuretic hormone (ADH), 456, 589
Ascites, **581–604**
  aldosterone antagonists, 597–598
  bed rest and low sodium diet, 596–597
  loop diuretics, 598–599
  plasma expanders and high-dose diuretics, 599–600
  refractory, 600–603
  side effects of diuretic therapy, 595–596
  treatment, 594–600
Atrial natriuretic peptide (ANP), 589–590

Backward theory of portal hypertension, 426
BCAAs, 624
Benzodiazepine receptor antagonists, 625–626
β-Blockers, 567–568, 573–576
Bicuculline, 621
Bile gastritis, 486
Brain natriuretic peptide (ANP), 590–591
Bucrylate, 467
Bumetanide, 598
Butyl cyanoacrylate, 540
n-Butyl-2-cyanoacrylate *see* histoacryl

Canrenone, 598
Captopril, 589
Chronic bile duct ligation (CBDL), 429
Cirrhosis—
  hepatic vascular resistance in, 428
  liver transplantation, 520–521
  natural history of portal hypertension, 437–441
  sodium and water retention, 581–586
  sympathetic nervous system activation, 587–588
Congestive gastropathy, 432, 563

Devascularization procedure, 549
  indications for, 550–551
  operative procedures, 551–555
Dilutional hyponatraemia, 595
Disseminated intravascular coagulopathy, 487
Distal splenorenal shunt (DSRS), 503, 504–507, 509–510
Dopamine, 614–616
Drugs in portal hypertensive gastropathy, 486

End-stage liver disease, results of liver transplantation, 520
Endoscopic banding ligation of varices, 468–469
Endoscopic therapy, local—
  banding ligation, 468–469, 473–474, 475–476
  combined with other measures, 476
  complications, 470–471
  current status, 476–477
  injection of tissue adhesive, 467–468, 473, 475
  injection sclerotherapy, 465–467, 472–473, 474–475, 487
  long-term efficacy, 474–476
  repeated, schedules, 470
  techniques, 465–470
Endothelial-derived relaxing factor (EDRF), 430
Endotoxins, 591–592
Ethacrynic acid, 598
Extrahepatic portal venous obstruction, 442–443

False neurotransmitters, 614–616
Fatty acids, 613–614
Flumazenil, 621
Forward flow theory of portal hypertension, 426
Frusemide, 596, 598, 600
Fulminant hepatic failure (FHF), 615
Functional renal failure (FRF) *see* hepatorenal syndrome

Gamma-aminobutyric acid (GABA), 619–623
Gastric angiodysplasia, 486–487
Gastric circulation, changes in portal hypertension, 432–433
Gastric microcirculatory changes, 432–433
Gastric mucosal function, 489
Gastric ulcers/erosions, 486
Gastric variceal bleeding, 532–534
  surgery for, 542–543
Gastric variceal obturation, 540
Gastric variceal sclerotherapy (GVS), 538–542
  bleeding, surgery for, 542–543
  complications, 542
  elective, 541–542
  emergency, 541
  gastric variceal obturation, 540
  liver transplantation, 543–544
  sclerosants, 539
  technique, 539–540
Gastric varices—
  classification, 527–529
  coexisting, 534
  frequency of types, 529
  induction of bleeding from, 535–536
  influence on development of portal hypertensive gastropathy, 536
  influence of oesophageal variceal sclerotherapy, 524–526
  management, **527–545**
  natural history, 532–536
  pathogenesis and origin, 530–532
  profile of bleeding, 532–534
  secondary, 535
Gastritis—
  alcoholic, 486
  bile, 486
Gastro-oesophageal varices (GOV), 528
  type 1 (GOV1), 534–535, 539
  type 2 (GOV2), 535, 539
Gastropathy, **481–492**
  clinical features, 484–485
  definition, 482
  differential diagnosis, 485–487
  drugs, 486
  histology, 483–484
  macroscopic appearances, 482–483
  mild, 482
  pathogenesis, 487–489
  severe, 483
  treatment, 490–492
Generalized portal hypertension, 530–531, 543
Glucagon, 429–430
Glutamate, 619
Gynaecomastia, 595–596

Helicobacter pylori, 485

Hepatic encephalopathy, 536, **609–626**
  ammonia levels, 609–613
  mercaptans, phenols and fatty acids, 613–614
  neurotransmitters, 614–623
  pathophysiology, 609–623
  therapy, 623–626
Hepatic haemodynamics—
  abnormalities in portal hypertension, **425–433**
  changes in, in portal hypertension, 426–428
Hepatic vascular resistance in cirrhosis, 428
Hepatopulmonary syndrome, 433
Hepatorenal syndrome—
  activation of renin angiotensin aldosterone system, 588–589
  activation of sympathetic nervous system, 587–588
  antidiuretic hormone, 589
  endotoxins, 591–592
  imbalance in intrarenal vasoactive substances, 592–594
  natriuretic factors, 589–591
  pathophysiology and treatment, **581–604**
  portal hypertension, 587
  sodium and water retention, 586–594
  treatment, 600–603
High-dose diuretics, 599–600
Histoacryl, 467, 540
HRS, 604
5-Hydroxyindoleacetic acid (5-HIAA), 617–618
5-Hydroxytryptophan (5-HTP), 617–618
Hyperkalaemia, 595
Hyperkinetic circulation, 431–432
Hypokalaemia, 596

Idiopathic portal hypertension, 443–444
Increased portal venous inflow, 427, 429
Indole metabolism, 616–618
Injection sclerotherapy, 465–467, 472–473, 474–475, 487
Intra-hepatic block, 426
Intrarenal vasoactive substances, imbalance in, 592–594
Isobutyl-2-cyanoacrylate (bucrylate), 467
Isolated gastric varices (IGV), 529, 531–532, 539
Isopropylbicyclophosphate, 621

Kallikrein-kinin, 594

Lactitol, 624
Leukotrienes, role in renal disorders, 594
LeVeen shunt, 601–602
Lipiodol, 540
Liver transplantation—
  for alcoholic cirrhosis, 520–521
  incidence of bleeding varices, thrombosis, hypertension and, 518–520

INDEX

in management of bleeding oesophageal varices, **517–524**
orthotopic, 603
portosystemic shunting, 509–510
results for patients with bleeding varices, thrombosis, hypertension and, 518–520
side effects of therapy, 595–596
treatment, 594–600
Loop diuretics, 598

Mercaptans, 613–614
Metabolic acidosis, 595, 596
Metabolic alkalosis, 596
Metoclopramide, 459
Modified Sugiura procedures, 553–555

Nadolol, 573, 575, 576
Natriuretic hormone (NH), 589–590
Neurotransmitters, 614–623
Nitroglycerin, 457
Nitroprusside, 457
Nodular regenerative hyperplasia, 444
Non-cirrhotic portal hypertension, 442–444
Non-steroidal anti-inflammatory drugs (NSAIDs), 592, 596
Noradrenaline, 614–616
NSAIDs, 592, 596

Oesophageal tamponade, 451–456
complications, 454–456
historical background, 451–452
results, 453–454
technique, 452–453
Oesophageal transection and devascularization, 549
Oesophageal variceal sclerotherapy, 534–536
Oesophageal varices—
bleeding, results of liver transplantation, 520
liver transplantation in management of bleeding, **517–524**
risk of first bleeding, 438–440
risk of recurrent bleeding, 440–441
sclerotherapy, 534–536
Oesophagogastric varices—
bleeding from, **549–560**
incidence of bleeding among liver transplant recipients, 518–520
Overflow theory, 585

Paracentesis, 601
Partial portal vein ligation (PPVL), 427
Pentagastrin, 459
Percutaneous transhepatic embolization, 538
Percutaneous transjugular portosystemic stent shunt, 524
Peripheral arterial vasodilatation, 586
Peripheral vasodilatation, 431, 585
Phenols, 613–614

Piretanide, 598
Plasma expanders, 599–600
Plasma volume, expanded, 431–432
Portal decompressive surgery, 569
Portal haemodynamics, 488–489
Portal hypertension—
among liver transplant recipients, 518–520
changes in pathophysiology, 427–428
in gastropathy, 432, 489–490, 563
in hepatorenal syndrome, 587
increased vascular resistance, 427–428
Portal hypertensive gastropathy, 432, **481–492**, 563
Portal non-decompressive surgery, 569
Portal pressure gradient, 425–427
Portal pressure, haemodynamic factors influencing, 425–427
Portal vein thrombosis among liver transplant recipients, 518–520
Portosystemic collaterals, 429
Portosystemic encephalopathy, 596
Portosystemic shunting, **497–511**
elective treatment, 503–510
emergency treatment, 500–503
and liver transplantation, 509–510
prophylactic treatment, 497–500
selective versus total shunts, 504–507
shunt surgery versus sclerotherapy, 507–509
in treatment of ascites, 603
Posthepatic block, 426
Potassium canrenoate, 597
PPVL, 429
Prazosin, 459
Prehepatic block, 426
Prerenal azotaemia, 595
Prophylactic portal decompressive surgery, 569
Prophylactic portal non-decompressive surgery, 569
Prophylactic sclerotherapy, 569–573
Propranolol, 459, 573, 575, 576
Prosthetic portocaval H-graft (PCHG), 506
Pulmonary circulation, changes in portal hypertension, 432–433

Quinolinic acid (QUIN), 618, 619

RAA system, 594
Radioactive microsphere technique, 427
Recurrent bleeding, 441–442
Renal prostaglandin system, 592
Renin angiotensin aldosterone system, 585, 588–589

Saralasin, 589
Schistosomiasis, 444
Sclerosants, 466
in management of gastric varices, 539

Sclerotherapy—
 of first variceal bleeding, 566–567, 569–573
 injection, 465–467, 472–473, 474–475, 487
 oesophageal variceal, 534–536
 prophylactic, 569–573
Segmental portal hypertension, 531, 542–543
Sequential diuretic therapy, 596
Serotonin, 617
sodium and water retention—
 in ascites, 596–600
 in cirrhosis, 581–586
 in hepatorenal syndrome, 586–594
Sodium benzoate, 625
Sodium phenylacetate, 625
Somatostatin, 457–459
Spironolactone, 432, 589, 597
Splanchnic haemodynamics, 429–430
 abnormalities in portal hypertension, **425–433**
Splanchnic vasodilatation, 429
Splenectomy in segmental portal hypertension, 542–543
Splenopancreatic disconnection (SPD), 506, 507
Sugiura procedures, 552–553
 modified, 553–555
Systemic haemodynamics, 431–432

Tamponade—
 of gastric varices, 537
 oesophageal, 451–456
Terlipressin, 459
Torasemide, 598
Transabdominal stapler (EEA) transection, 553–555
Transection and devascularization procedure—
 for bleeding from oesophagogastric varices, **549–560**
 indications for, 550–551
 operative procedures, 551–555
Transjugular intrahepatic portosystemic shunt (TIPS), 524
Transthoracoabdominal oesophageal transection, 552–553
Tryptophan metabolism, 616–618

Underfilling theory, 585

Variceal bleeding—
 acute, 441–442, **451–460**
 aims of prophylaxis and treatment, 565
 β-blockers, 567–568
 clinical, randomized, controlled trials, 568–576
 emergency and elective endoscopic therapy, **465–477**
 natural history and endoscopy, 563–564
 natural history and prognosis, **437–447**
 pitfalls in assessing prognosis, 444–445
 prognosis, 441–442
 prophylaxis of first, **563–576**
 risk factors for first bleeding, 445–447
 risk signs, 564–565
 role of liver transplantation in management, 521–524
 sclerotherapy, 566–567
 surgical procedures, 566
 treatment options, 566–568
Varices—
 development of, 437–438
 endoscopic banding ligation of, 468–469
 gastric, **527–545**
 gastro-oesophageal varices (GOV), 528, 534–535, 539
 isolated gastric varices (IGV), 529, 531–532, 539
 oesophageal, 438–441, 520, 534–536
 oesophagogastric, **517–524, 549–560**
Vasopressin, 456–457, 585

Water melon stomach, 486–487

Zinc, 624–625